The History of Medicine, As Written by Its Founders
Volume 2

From *Roger's Chirurgia* (1170) to *Venarum Ostiolis* (1603)

Edited by Luis H. Toledo-Pereyra

Western Michigan University, School of Medicine
Western Michigan University, School of Arts & Sciences
Department of History
Kalamazoo, Michigan

cognella
San Diego, CA

Cover Image:
Anatomy lesson of Dr. Willem van der Meer
Pieter can Mierevelt
1617
Oil on canvas

Bassim Hamadeh, CEO and Publisher
Michael Simpson, Vice President of Acquisitions
Jamie Giganti, Managing Editor
Jess Busch, Graphic Design Supervisor
John Remington, Acquisitions Editor
Brian Fahey, Licensing Associate

First published in the United States of America in 2014 by Cognella, Inc.

Printed in the United States of America

ISBN: 978-1-62131-035-8 (pbk)/ 978-1-62131-036-5 (br)

cognella™

www.cognella.com 800.200.3908

Contents

Dedication

To the students of the History of Medicine and Healthcare at Western Michigan University and to enthusiastic advocates everywhere of this important and interesting subject.

For their support and encouragement.

Chapter 1

Preface: Recognizing the Founders of Medicine

By Luis Horacio Toledo-Pereyra

Following the publication of *The History of Medicine, As Written by Its Founders, Volume 1: From the Hammurabi Code to the Canon of Medicine,*[1] we now concentrate on the historical evolution of the teachings of the Founders of Medicine after the writings of Avicenna (980–1037), one of the great masters of his era. Medicine advanced in uneven steps for thousands of years until its scientific foundations were more clearly defined during the Renaissance and immediately thereafter.[2,3]

In this book, *The History of Medicine, As Written by Its Founders, Volume 2: From Roger's Chirurgia (1170) to Venarum Ostiolis (1603),* we continue to present the progression of the medical discipline from the late Middle Ages to the Renaissance as represented by the masters and founders of their times. As indicated in Volume 1, "The principle behind this book is that nothing can speak better for medicine than the writings of those directly involved in the history of the discipline since they were the creators of it."[1] We allow the pen of the great masters to teach us how they saw and appreciated the medicine practiced or understood during their own periods of active professional participation. We do not interpret what they wrote but rather permit interested historical readers to see the masters' writings and consequently to form their own opinions based on facts gathered from actual historical proof.

There are several deficiencies in a book of this magnitude that I would like to point out to our students of the history of medicine. Not all founders were included—those we chose had to have been translated into English, and we had to have had direct access to their work. In addition, we needed to limit the masters' contributions because of space and legal regulatory considerations. And finally, the selections were based on their importance and their personal appeal.

We followed the same details and presentation of this book as we utilized in Volume 1 except that each chapter's historical highlights appear on the opening chapter page. Then, we indicate the specific selection and pages utilized of the work to be included on the right side page of the chapter alluded to. Finally, at the bottom of the chapter's first page, we give brief remarks as to the nature and selection of the work in question.

Our goal of Volume 2 remains the same as that stated in Volume 1: to offer to students of the history of medicine a source of enlightenment so they may advance their knowledge of this exciting field of academic pursuit. As I said before, and I believe it is still true today, "If the students of the history of medicine or healthcare can validate their knowledge by reading and evaluating the original works of the fathers of the discipline, our goals will be more than well served."[1]

Our intention in introducing the Founders of Medicine as they really were and thought when they wrote their own works is as firm in this Volume 2 as it was for Volume 1 and as it was when we had the idea of developing this series of books. If our audience continues to support this concept, Volume 3 will follow in chronological order with the idea of recognizing other Founders of Medicine responsible for the great medical period of the XVII century and years thereafter.

This is the time to offer my greatest appreciation to Martha Faketty who spent long hours in locating and securing the original works of the Founders of Medicine. It took a great deal of patience and dedication to accomplish this very difficult task. Thank you, Marti.

References

1. Toledo-Pereyra L. H. *History of Medicine as Written by Its Founders. Volume 1. From the Hammurabi Code to the Cannon of Medicine.* Cognella University Readers Inc., San Diego, CA, 2012.
2. Toledo-Pereyra L. H. *Vignettes on Surgery, History and Humanities.* Landes bioscience, Georgetown, TX, 2005.
3. Porter R. *The Greatest Benefit to Mankind.* W. W. Norton and Co., New York, NY, 1997.

Chapter 2

Founders of Medicine: From Roger's *Chirurgia* (1170) to *Venarum Ostiolis* (1603)

By Luis Horacio Toledo-Pereyra

After Avicenna of Afshana (980–1039) in his seminal work *The Canon of Medicine* (1025) made important contributions to the advancement of medicine,[1] the historical tradition moved to Salerno in Italy. Here, in this medieval region, Rogerius Salernitanus or Roger Frugard (1140–1195) concentrated on innovative principles applied to anatomical and surgical ideas.[2]

Volume 2 of *The History of Medicine, As Written by Its Founders, from Roger's Chirurgia (1170) to Venarum Ostiolis (1603)* introduces the new knowledge in the progression of the history of medicine. The *Chirurgiae Magistri Rogeri* ("*The Surgery of Master Rogerius*" [1170]), as it was called originally in Latin, was considered the most important surgical work of the times. Other prominent European university cities readily accepted its value and significance. Among them were Bologna (founded 1158) in Italy and Montpellier (founded 1220) in France where medicine and particularly surgery were being forged. After Salerno (founded 848) reached its prominence, Bologna and Montpellier became, in many ways, the carriers of the medical torch. Other European cities were preparing or were in march to continue the road of improved medical knowledge.[2]

Almost 150 years after the completion of *Roger's Chirurgia* in Parma, another great anatomist, Mondino de' Luzzi (1275–1326) finished his exceptional work, *Anatomia Mundini,* in 1316.[3–5] He was professor of anatomy at the University of Bologna for 36 years (1290–1326). According to Michael McVaugh, University of North Carolina distinguished scholar in Medieval Medicine, Mondino was "universally given credit for the reintroduction of systematic human dissection into anatomy."[3] Mondino understood anatomy to the point of being "simple, concise and systematic on arranging his book."[4] He divided his advanced anatomical work into six areas: introduction to the whole body, the natural members and abdominal cavity, the generative members, the spiritual members and thoracic cavity, the animal members of the skull and face, and the peripheral parts including the spinal column and extremities.[3–5] Mondino, during his time, was the most significant figure of anatomy. Mondino was a pupil of Thaddeus Alderotti of Bologna. In this city, Mondino cemented his knowledge and contributions to anatomy. It is not well known how many human dissections he did on his own or how many he participated in while working with others.[3–4] In any case, at some point, he was an essential part of the study of anatomy during Medieval times.

In 1320, four years following the work of Mondino, a notable French surgeon, Henri de Mondeville (1260–1316), justifiably called the "Father of French Surgery", wrote his monumental surgical work entitled *La Chirurgie de Maitre Henri de Mondeville* (2 volumes). This classical treatise, though abandoned for many years, was widely comprehensive and probably one of the most advanced during the Middle Ages.[6] Mondeville clearly approached surgery "with passion" and a firm desire to succeed on the treatments he frequently utilized.[7]

Mondeville was committed to promoting a better understanding of surgery and its art. Particularly important was his management of wounds, especially those related to surgical treatment. According to Nicaise, historical expert on Medieval surgical French studies, Mondeville attempted at all times to prevent suppuration, "a useless and avoidable phenomenon."[6] Mondeville together with Theodoric developed a method "for immediate wound closure", "warm wine-soaked pads on the wound" and "dressings to protect the wound from the atmosphere."[6] His technique, although advanced for his era, did not prove to be successful on all occasions.

Following Mondeville's professional period, France produced once more perhaps the most advanced surgical personality of the Middle Ages. Guy de Chauliac (1290–1370) received his education in Toulouse, Montpellier and Bologna. He ended his surgical training in Paris; at a time when unfortunately Lanfranc, Pitart and Mondeville had already died.[8–10] De Chauliac recognized, at any rate, the surgical principles accepted by his predecessors, in particular the ones supported by Henri de Mondeville.[8]

Guy de Chauliac was well-accepted in political circles and became the private physician to three popes, Clement VI, Innocent VI and Urban V for the 28 years they resided in Avignon. While he continued his work as the pope's health advisor, he attended all his personal medical and surgical cases in the area, besides persevering in his surgical and medical writings.

In 1363, de Chauliac completed his most important surgical treatise, *Chirurgia Magna,* where he expressed many significant concepts related to the surgical discipline. In this case, de Chauliac discussed the definition of surgery, its types, the conduct of the operation, the surgical instruments used, history of surgery, anatomy, treatment of wounds, ulcers and related injuries, control of hemorrhage, the management of calculi, the use of trephine in fracture of the cranium and many other diseases with the best surgical treatment considered at the time.[8–10]

For Guy de Chauliac, the surgeon required four qualities in someone seeking to be called a surgical professional: "First, he should be learned; second, he should be expert; third, he must be ingenious; and fourth, he should be able to adapt himself."[9] In terms of its significance, the *Chirurgia Magna* of de Chauliac "was the acknowledged surgical authority in Europe for two centuries, until it was overshadowed by the most extensive treatise of Pare."[8]

Almost two centuries ahead of Guy de Chauliac, Leonardo da Vinci (1452–1519) took his turn. He was not a physician or a surgeon, but a consummate anatomist.[11] He defined the relationship between structure and function and expanded the anatomical details not seen before. He was an innovator by nature and a born scientist when attempting to decipher various anatomical differences.

Leonardo's anatomical work carefully assembled in his "*Anatomical Drawings*" (c. 1519, the exact date is undetermined), represents a series of anatomical discoveries brought about by the famous artist. His drawings did not see the public light until 1796 when Chamberlaine published them for the first time. A century and a half later O'Malley and Saunders presented, in 1952, the most up-to-date version of Leonardo's drawings. Because of the work of O'Malley and Saunders, we expanded the interpretation and appreciation of da Vinci's contributions.[11]

In 1543, *De Humani Corporis Fabrica* appeared in print under the pen of the great anatomist, Andreas Vesalius (1514–1567) with the superb anatomical drawings of Jan Calcar, student of Titian of the School of Art in Venice. Vesalius proceeded initially from Brussels, Belgium where he attended the University of Louvain for some of his art and sciences requirements prior to his medical studies. He then transferred to the more prestigious University of Paris (1533–1536) to carry on with his medical work under distinguished personalities of the times, like Guinter, Sylvius and Ferne among others.[12] In 1537, Vesalius returned to Louvain where he obtained his Bachelor of Medicine degree. At the end of the year, he directed himself to the University of Padua where after two days of examinations he was conferred the Doctor of Medicine degree *magna cum laude.*[13]

Vesalius's interest in human anatomy, already clearly evident, blossomed while on Italian soil. He completed his *opus magna* treatise *De Humani Corporis Fabrica* while at the University of Padua. In this unique book, he based almost the totality of his findings on the direct observations of the human cadaver. He opposed many of Galen's anatomical contributions which had been supported by animal dissections. C. D. O'Malley, an advanced Vesalius scholar, gave us an excellent review of who Vesalius was and what his contributions were to anatomy in particular and medicine in general.[13]

Just about the time of Vesalius, one of his contemporaries, Ambroise Paré (1510–1590), became a master barber-surgeon in 1536 out of the ranks of Hótel-Dieu, one of the most important medical centers of the world during this period in history. Sixteen years afterwards, he was named Ordinary Surgeon to Henry II and Francois II, and few years later, Premier Surgeon to Charles IX and Henry III respectively.[14] Within these developments, Ambroise Paré enjoyed a great reputation in the French Court that allowed him to dedicate enough time to the advancement of surgery.

Paré was an accomplished military surgeon as well. He actively participated in many of the frequent wars of religion so prevalent in those times, in addition to other military battles of turf, political persuasion or otherwise. What is significant here is that Paré learned a great deal from these military events and had the opportunity of putting his discoveries into practice. Namely, using boiling oil for gunshot wounds, utilizing ligatures in amputations and applying new and modified surgical instruments were the hallmarks of Paré's main contributions.[14,15] Some of his writings, such as *On Gunshot Wounds* (1545) and *The Apologie and treatise of Ambroise Paré* … (1585), reflect in great part the magnitude of Paré's developments and surgical advances.

In 1553, still within the XVIth century, the *Christianismi Restitutio* of Miguel Serveto (1509–1619) was published. In it, this courageous Spanish polymath, theologian and physician was the first European to correctly introduce and advance the pulmonary circulation concept in medicine.[16] In this book, we emphasize the ideas considered by Servetus as part of the critical scientific thinking maturing in Renaissance European medicine.

Practically during the same period, Girolamo Hieronymus Fabricius (1533–1619) completed and published his most significant contribution, *De Venarum Ostiolis* (1603). In this work, Fabricius recognized the valves of the veins, which—according to him—he had been aware of since 1574. He illustrated them for the first time in 1585.[17] The most outstanding development was perhaps the acceptance by William Harvey of the role of the vein valves in the general theory of the circulation. At this point, Volume 2 of the *History of Medicine as Written by Its Founders From Roger's Chiruigia* (1170) to *Venarum Ostiolis* (1603) ends with Fabricius at the completion of the XVIth century and the entering of the XVIIth century.

Volume 2 is ending in the same manner as we ended Volume 1: "The list of the Founders of Medicine is clearly selective and represented by those pillars of Western Medicine that have made advances well-accepted throughout the medical literature."[1]

Ultimately, our main objective was to learn from the Founders of Medicine as represented in this volume and as they wrote their experiences during their professional careers. In short, we are learning from the written words of the Founders of Medicine.

References

1. Toledo-Pereyra LH. *The History of Medicine, As Written by Its Founders, Volume 1: From the Hammurabi Code to the Canon of Medicine.* University Readers, Inc., Cognella 2012, San Diego, CA.
2. Frugard R. *The Chirurgia of Roger Frugard.* Translated into English by L.D. Rosenman. Xlibris, 2002.
3. Grant E. *A Source Book in Medieval Science.* McVaugh M, *The Anatomy of Mundinus*, pp. 729–739, 1974. Harvard University Press, Cambridge, MA.
4. Bullough VL. Mondino de Luzzi in *Dictionary of Scientific Biography. Vol. IX.* Charles Scribner's Sons, New York, 1974, pp. 467–469.
5. Mondino de Liuzzi. Wikipedia.org accessed 8/6/12.
6. Mondeville HD. The *Surgery of Henri de Mondeville.* 2 volumes. Translated from French into English by Rosenman LD. Xlibris, 1998.
7. Clarke CC, Henri de Mondeville. *Yale J. Biol. and Med.* 3:459–481, 1931.
8. Pilcher JE, Guy de Chauliac and Henri de Mondeville. *Ann. Surg.* 21: 84–102, 1985.
9. Murphy GH. *The Surgery of Guy de Chauliac. Can. Med. Assoc J.* 65:68–71, 1951.
10. Chauliac GD. *The Major Surgery of Guy de Chauliac.* Translated from French into English by Rosenman LD, Xlibris, 2005
11. O'Malley, C.D. and J.B.C.M. Saunders. *Leonardo da Vinci on the Human Body.* Henry Schuman, New York.
12. Sherzoi H. Andreas Vesalius (1514–1567) in Toledo-Pereyra LH. *Vignettes on Surgery, History and Humanities.* Landes Bioscience, Georgetown, TX, 2005.
13. O'Malley CD. *Andreas Vesalius of Brussels 1514–1564.* Berkeley, University of California Press, 1964.
14. Hamby, W.B. Paré, Ambroise in *Dictionary of Scientific Biography, Vol. X.* Charles Scribner's Sons, New York, 1974, pp. 315–317.
15. Malgaigne JF. *Surgery and Ambroise Paré.* Translated from the French into English by W.B. Hamby, University of Oklahoma Press, Norman, 1965.
16. O'Malley CD. *Michael Servetus.* Translated by O'Malley CD. American Philosophical Society, Philadelphia. 1953.
17. Zanobio B. Fabrici Girolamo in *Dictionary of Scientific Biography, Vol. IV.* Charles Scribner's Sons, New York, 1971, pp. 507–512.

Chapter 3

Roger Frugard: Roger's *Chirurgia* (1170)

HISTORICAL HIGHLIGHTS

- Roger Frugard (1140–1195)
- Originated from Parma, Italy
- Became premier surgeon in Italy
- Wrote acclaimed surgical treatise
- Completed surgical book, *Roger's Chirurgia* (1170)
- Credited with first European surgical text
- Accepted standard text in several schools of the time
- Arranged book from Head to Foot as the accepted one
- Book compiled by Roger's pupil, Guido d'Arezzo the Younger

Many of the above statements were obtained from the English translation by L.D. Rosenman.

THE WRITINGS OF ROGER FRUGARD

On manifest fracture of the skull with small external wound

If the fracture of the skull is large but the superficial wound small so that you cannot be completely certain of the extent of the fracture, a finger is to be inserted in the wound and a diligent investigation made, because there is no better method for recognizing a fracture of the skull than digital palpation.

After you have made out the extent of the fracture in this way you should incise the small scalp wound with a razor in the form of a cross and separate the scalp from the cranium with a raspatory, and if there is not too much blood in the field of operation you should remove any fragments of bone with the small forceps. If, however, the hemorrhage is sufficient to prevent this, you may change your method until you have controlled it, after which you will be able to remove the fragments successfully. With a probe thoroughly and carefully insert a cloth between the dura mater and the cranium and proceed as we

Roger Frugard, from *Annals of Medical History*, vol. 3, no. 1, trans. George W. Corner, pp. 12-13. Roger Frugard, from *The Chirurgia of Roger Frugard*, trans. Leonard D. Rosenman, pp. 25-27, 31-35, 103-108, 126-131. Copyright © 2002 by Leonard D. Rosenman. Readings selected and historical highlights written by Luis Horacio Toledo-Pereyra.

said in the previous section. Outside the cranium the wounded scalp is pressed together and the whole wound bound up with a linen cloth previously soaked in white of egg. A pad of cloth filled with feathers is laid over it and bound on according to the region of the head involved, and changed every morning or evening. If, when you dress the wound, you find the flaps swollen, it is a good sign; if, however, they are shrunken and mortified, it is a bad sign. In the course of healing when you find that the skull is entirely healed the dressing is to be reduced in size and the skin flaps are forced back to their proper situation.

On the cure of goiter by incision

If the goiter is single, with the aid of a hot iron we put in one seton lengthwise and another from side to side and apply over them a cloth soaked in egg or in lard. Every day, morning and evening, the setons are drawn toward the outside until finally the flesh is cut through. When this is done if any part of the goiter remains, powder it with powder of asphodel and purified in this way the wound will heal like other wounds. If the tumor is not provided with too many arteries it may be removed by grasping it firmly in the hands and cutting the skin carefully lengthwise. The tumor is grasped with a hook and the skin is dissected away. A finger is then inserted through the wound and the goiter removed entirely with its capsule. The wound is lightly dressed with a linen cloth. If the hemorrhage is excessive we apply those remedies which have been described above for this purpose in the chapter on arrow wounds in the neck. These remedies are continued for three days. (Styptic drugs.) Afterward if any of the tumor remains, apply powder of asphodel, following it by egg, and then proceed as in other wounds. The greatest care should be taken to avulse the capsule of the goiter completely so that nothing is left, for if the slightest part remains the patient relapses. When the wound is entirely clean, it may be dusted with red powder and sutured as we have described elsewhere, and it will be cured. If however, the goiter is very large and the patient weak or elderly, in our judgment it is best to refrain from this treatment. These large goiters usually have several lobes which make them difficult to dissect away, and we avoid treating them with a hot iron for fear of injuring the arteries or nerves. When, however, it becomes necessary to treat these patients by surgery we tie them to a table and have them held firmly in order that we may see exactly what we are doing.

The Chirurgia of Roger Frugard

A Note About The Text

Roger's Chirurgia contained four Books and an introductory Proem. The 'head-to-foot' arrangement controls the contents without special concerns for order according to types of lesions or diseases, although trauma receives the greatest emphasis.[1] Book I deals with the head, Book II with the neck, Book III with the torso and Book IV with the arms and legs. Unlike Roger, later authors arranged their treatises with head-to-foot displays of their materials in separate Books, according to the nature of the disorders: wounds, fractures, other diseases, etc. Daremberg's essay includes a discussion and examples of that change.

Roger did not provide a separate Book devoted to Cautery or an Antidotary. Therefore, I have prepared a Compendium Pharmacopeia as an appendix. It lists and briefly identifies all the simples and a

1 Tabanelli comments (p. 20) that this should be understood to be a product of the war-filled times which occupied Europe, especially the Mediterranean countries (LDR).

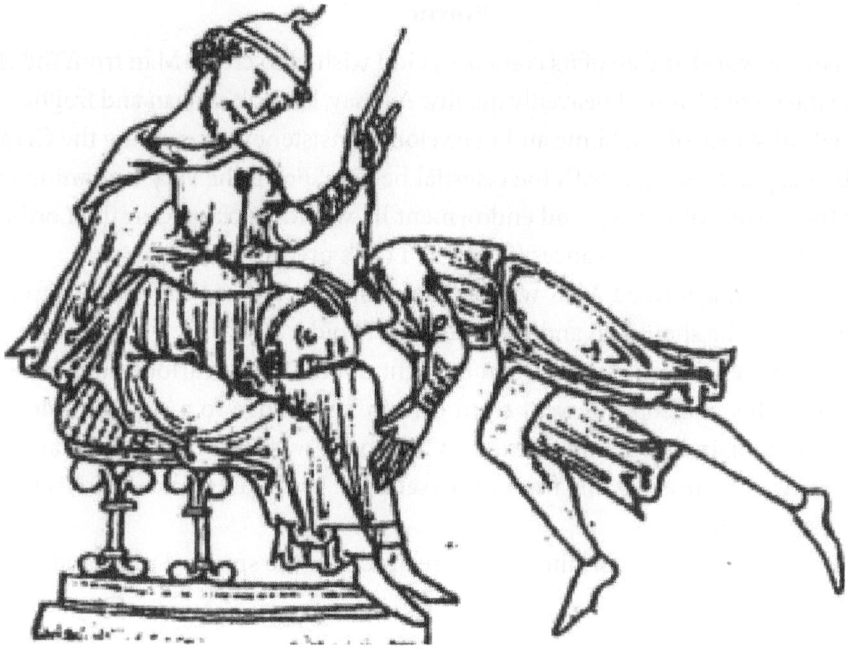

Frontispiece Surgeon Suturing A Neckwound

Reprinted with permission by Master and Fellows, Trinity College, Cambridge.

few of the compounds used by Roger and the other famous surgeons during the century and a half after him. I have culled the seven great surgical treatises written during that epoch. Roger's list is recovered in large part from Hunt's edition of the Anglo-Norman Ms, in which he provides an excellent glossary. The Roger-Roland Latin Ms and the Italian translation of Stroppiana include a rich resource of remedies in the many Addenda attributed to Roland Cappelluti. Therefore, this Compendium includes some, if not all, of the substances used by Roland other than those he found in Roger's text.

Each remedy in the Pharmacopeia and Formulary is marked with the initials of one or more authors who mentioned it. Those cited for Roger are marked **R.** In the text itself, I have used modern vernacular names for plants and metallic substances where that is feasible. Other matters identifying the medications can be found in the Pharmacopeia.

Each of the four Books in Roger's Ms was preceded by a list of the chapters by name. I have placed those lists in a Table of Contents which opens this translation.

A note on style (as presented by English translator L.D. Rosenman)

Roger's text as it appears in the Ms printed in De Renzi's Collectio and as translated by Stroppiana-Spallone will be translated in plain face type. My own parenthetical insertions in the text will be identified by (ie). Insertions taken from the other Mss and comments relevant to the text will be printed in Italic-face, and identified by H if by Hunt, by T if by Tabanelli, by D if by Daremberg and by R-R if taken from the Roger-Roland Ms in DeRenzi. The sources of footnotes will be identified in parentheses, by LDR if by me, and by the others' initials.

Proem

After the creation of the world and all of its contents[2], God wished to create Man from the clay itself and to instill in him a vital spirit of almost heavenly quality. As I say, he took a mean and fragile matter to add weight to a celestial substance of a sublime and marvelous consistency, resembling the Creator Himself, to be preserved by his grace on a par with the celestial beings.[3] From the very beginning material Man would be part of the Earth; with his second endowment he would be clasped in the Lord's embrace, so long as he continued his proper observances (ie of The Lord's precepts).

In God's wisdom he first formed Man without defects; he endowed him with a free will and he explicitly prescribed what he should do and what he must avoid.

Because he violated the Divine precepts, Man brought upon himself various punishments, assigned to the various parts of his makeup. He went from certain knowledge to a state of ignorance. From a regency over his own domain he became an exile. Where once was light now were shadows. Where he had found delight he found miser)', going from joy to sadness. In all cases, based on His fulsome justice, sadness replaced its opposite.

The Supreme Physician reserved for himself the treatment of the spiritual parts and to us physicians he relegated the treatment of the …

Wounds of the Head

The head may suffer various sorts of injuries, with or without fractures of the cranium. At times a fracture may be large and easily detected. But, large or small, the accompanying wounds (ie of the soft tissues) may be large and gaping or small simple incisions.

Whenever the cranium is broken we must ascertain if the membranes of the brain are damaged, either the pia mater or the dura mater. The signs of injury to the latter are: headache, a flushed face, wide-open eyes, blackened tongue.

The signs of injury of the pia mater are: general feebleness, loss of voice, pustules on the face, discharge of blood from the nostrils and ears, constipated bowels.

(R-R or diarrhea which is even more serious), and shaking chills three or four times a day, which foretell a fatal outcome. Furthermore, most of the above signs predict death before one hundred days. When the damage in the meninges is extensive, death will ensue at the time of the next full moon.

Although all fractures of the cranium present serious threats, we should diagnose them with care and try to intervene as best we can.

*Addenda by Roland**

1. Note that when constipation or diarrhea ensue, the risk is indeed serious that the outcome will be fatal.
2. Another bad sign: is the extremities lose their natural warmth, right to the tips to the toes.
3. The effects of the celestial bodies are noted, especially that of the moon, on the accumulation of fluid: when the moon enlarges the accumulation of fluid in the affected part increases, especially the increase of fluid in the brain, which emits froth which it cannot contain. If the brain cannot vent the fluid the patient will die.

* This likely refers to Roland of Parma, master surgeon, who succeeded Roger Frugard.

---

2 This opening phrase was used frequently rather than the simple title to identify Roger's treatise (LDR).

3 The soul had angelic properties (LDR).

Displaced Fractures With Open Wounds

When the fracture is obvious and the wound is large and open, such as made by a sword or the like, you first should remove the loose bone and other foreign matter. Remove the fragments immediately unless the hemorrhage is too brisk. Use a quill and carefully insert a piece of thin soft cloth almost all of die way between the dura mater and the fragment.[4] Then,[5] lay a linen or, even better, a silk cloth into the opening, large enough so the edges of the cloth can be tucked under the peripheral margin of the intact cranium, to prevent the discharges from the open wound from contaminating the dura mater and threatening harm to the underlying brain.

Then continue to wipe the wound dry of the accumulating pus, using a clean and dry sea sponge, as you would use blotting paper. Fill the mopped wound with pieces of linen which you have soaked in egg-whites and then squeezed almost dry. Lay a pad on top of the wound and the surrounding region and carefully wrap and tie a bandage. Change the dressing twice daily during the winter and thrice in summer time *(H: Because during the summer months wounds make more pus)*. Have the patient lie with the wounded side down *(H: to favor drainage away from the dura)* Continue this regimen faithfully until the fracture has united.

Addenda by Roland

1. Unless the depressed bone is removed promptly a syncope will occur. (*H: Sometimes the surgeon will not be called to attend a patient until days after the injury and the wound already is suppurating. In such cases the fragments of bone etc. must be removed at once.*)
2. Silk is better because its surface is less abrasive.
3. Use a quill or splinter of bone to insert the cloth.
4. The sponge must be thoroughly washed to rid it of the salts which will corrode the dura mater. All astringent substances are hot, and corrosives are hot as well as dry.

BOOK III: TORSO FROM THE SHOULDERS TO THE GROINS AND UPPER EXTREMITIES

Chapter 1. Wounds Of The Scapular Region

We treat a wound caused by a sharp weapon as follows: If fresh, we clean it and suture it, leaving an opening at one end. Then we dust on our red powder and follow with the treatments described in the chapter on suturing, in Book II.

If the wound is not recent, we first give it a good scrubbing to provoke bleeding (ie oozing) from the surfaces, and then we suture it.

In a wound caused by a penetrating projectile we introduce a strip of bacon and follow with the routine described in the chapter on projectiles.

4 A delicate maneuver to detach the loose bone fragment from the underlying dura mater (LDR).

5 Here the surgeon treats a fracture freed of loose fragments or perhaps one with a simple separation at a linear fracture (LDR).

Chapter 2. Wounds At The Sterno-Clavicular Joint

If a wound enters the joint, do this: Pack it lightly with a cloth strip or with oakum wet with egg-white. Follow that with a maturative plaster on a dry cloth to promote suppuration, varying it to suit the season (ie winter or summer).

Carefully remove any bits of bone etc. that you can find and use our black ointment. If the clavicle is fractured and if part of a bone or the joint itself is displaced, pull and lift the arm with one of your hands, and use the other to press the displaced bone into place. Then lay a pad over the reduced piece, wet with egg-white, atop which you place a bolster. Wrap it in place with a criss-cross bandage. Over that wrap a long bandage to elevate and hold the forearm (ie wrist) at the neck, taking care to take turns around a cushion under the arm at the axilla to keep the arm from slipping down. It must be kept in place until the recovery is complete.

If the wound is a compound fracture, leave an aperture in your wrappings through which you can replace drains and medications, to be used as in other wounds. An over-all bandage may cover the long bandage (ie with its opening).[6]

Chapter 3. Dislocation Of The Neck[7]

When the wound causes a displacement of the shoulder from beneath the cervical tissues, do this:

First clean the wound and scrape it to ooze blood if it is not fresh (ie when you first encounter it), and remove loose bits of matter; then suture it so: approximate the matching edges and take a deep bite (ie through-and-through) the lower edge and come out through the upper, and leave the needle in place. Then (ie to anchor the needle in place) wrap the protruding ends of the needle with the attached thread. Leave in the needle. Or, (ie instead of a single deep, suture-en-masse) you may use a row of needles taking smaller bites, each wrapped with its own thread, to obtain a neater closure. Then dust on the red powder and dress the wound, leaving open a gap at one end of the defect, as we do for other sutured wounds.

When we see that the edges of the wound are solidly joined, we remove the needles and threads. Progressively shorten the medicated drain in the wound, as in other cases. Remove the sutures and drains as you determine that the shoulder will not separate from the flap above it (ie not all at one time).

Chapter 4. Lacerations Of The Arm, Involving Nerves

When a wound transects a nerve or the bone in the arm, first lightly pack the wound with a tent soaked with egg-white, then replace it with a dry cloth and lay on a pack medicated according to the season. As usual, remove bits of loose bone, etc. Treat the nerve as we have instructed and apply the brown ointment and the others.

---

6 This outer wrap is removed whenever the surgeon changes the dressings. The inner wrap, with its aperture is not disturbed. (LDR).

7 The title is misleading. This is not a cervico-thoracic verterbral dislocation. Rather, it describes a 'saber-cut' wound which raises a flap over the shoulder and, as the flap retracts, it appears as if the shoulder is sliding away from the neck. The repair, using needles to transfix and hold the flap was not new with Roger. Some of the details in this translation are taken from H (LDR).

Addenda by Roland

1. If the bony fragments are not loose enough for easy and painless removal, leave them in place Make this paste which will loosen the bone or pieces of the arrow shaft: Grind polypodium with a little aged lard and bandage the plaster over the affected region. Or you may use the apostolicon because it contains attractive powders.

Another way to remove an arrow without pain: apply roots of saxifrage and marsh reeds with some honey ground to make a plaster. Be aware of the wound that oozes oily blood. That means that the marrow cavity (ie of the humerus) has been entered and that the wound will be fatal.

Chapter 5. Swellings,Tumors And Hardness Of Nerves[8]

When nerves are painlessly swollen or are hard and contracted you have only to use a medicine of althea. Take two pounds of the gum of the roots of althea, one pound of greek-fennel seeds, five pounds of squills, three pounds of oil, one pound of wax. Take one ounce each of turpentine, galbanum, and gum of clematis. Take five pounds each of colophony and tar. Chop the roots and grind them; do the same with the linseeds (ie not mentioned in the foregoing), fennel seeds and squills. Soak the mash in six pounds of water for three days. On the fourth boil the lot until the liquid is thick. Filter it through a cloth sack; you may add some hot water to facilitate the filtration of the viscous juice. Take two pounds of it with four pounds of oil and boil it until the water is gone. You will know that when the oil no longer floats. Now add the wax; when it melts add the turpentine, then the gum of the chopped clematis and galbanum, and, last of all, add the colophony and tar. Let it cool a while after taking it from the fire. It will be ready when a droplet placed on a marble tile spreads. Filter it again and save it. Rewarm it for use.

It is good for treating pleurisy and chest-pains due to cold. Re-warm about an egg-shell full, enough to anoint a healing chest. It warms the cold and moistens and softens the dry.

Chapter 6. To Clean A Suppurating Wound

If a foul wound begins to suppurate you may treat it with this ointment: Take one pound of oil, five pounds of ram's fat, two ounces of white wax, three ounces of greek tar, a large handful each of salvia, horse-mint, St. Mary's herb, soapwort, dill and rue. Mix the oil, lard and wax and strain them. Mix in the others which have been mashed and set it aside for use.

Another paste for the same purpose: Take a handful each of wild and domestic salvias, daphne, centinervia, saxifrage, artemisia and bugloss. Grind them in a mortar with one pound of ram's fat and make soft balls. Later on, drop a ball in a pound of oil and boil until the herbs precipitate. Remove from the fire and filter off the liquid. Boil it again before adding three ounces of wax in the summer, two ounces in the winter. When the wax melts add one ounce each of powdered mastic, olibanum, and colophony, while stirring assiduously with a spatula. Remove from the fire and stir in a little turpentine. Now you may set it aside for use. This ointment is very effective for cleaning away pus and for regenerating and nourishing healthy tissues.

8 "Nerves" included tendons, aponeuroses, ligaments as well as nerves (LDR).

Chapter 7. Superfluous Granulation Tissue In Wounds

When proud flesh overgrows in a wound use a powder of hermodactyl dusted on a fluff of cotton soaked with saliva, which you stuff into the wound.

Another remedy: Take four ounces of quick-lime, one ounce of yellow arsenic and some warm water. Mix it well until everything is dissolved. Set it over a flame until it is completely dry. Grind the residue to make the powder, which you can save.

Another: Take equal amounts of hermodactyl, round clematis and verdigris. Grind them together to make a powder which will eat away the proud flesh without a violent action.

Another powder for use to corrode cancers: Take lime moistened with a little honey to make a paste which you shape into loaf and place on a tile. Grind it into a powder.

Chapter 8. Erysipelas In A Wound

Wounds may be complicated by several things, only one being erysipelas. The differential diagnosis and treatment for erysipelas follow here. Pustules may appear; the white ones are amenable to treatment, and they are a good sign. The black ones, usually hard, represent invasive erysipelas and carry an evil prognosis.

We should intervene with cool remedies. First lay on a pad wet with juices of house-leeks, henbane, stone-crop, umbellicus venus and hyoscyamus. Mix them with egg-white, oil of roses and white and red sandalwood oil. If you cannot obtain any of these ingredients, use what you have in the amounts available and do not go to something else. If the wound is excavated, fill it with the following: Take one pound of filtered lard, six ounces of colophony, four ounces of wax, two ampoules of oil and three ounces each of mastic, olibanum and myrrh. Mix the melted wax, lard and oil and filter them. Add the powders while grinding. When a paste is formed, use it.

Addendum by Roland

1. The excavation in the wound has three causes. 1. The original wound. 2. Failure to treat in the deeper region of the wound, thereby promoting the collection of pus. 3. The lack of skill on the part of the surgeon who treated only the upper part of the wound.

Chapter 42. Displacing A Stone From The Bladder-Neck

When you seek to relieve the obstruction at the bladder-neck by displacing a stone, first use fomentations and inunctions, and insert some oil via a syringe. After a brief wait, insert the syringe all the way to the bladder-neck. Then, very gently and carefully push the stone back into the bladder.

Ours is the most reliable and the least distressing technique. First we foment and anoint. Then we examine (ie as above) and make certain the diagnosis with the bimanual method, and we gently displace the impacted stone, carefully pushing it down and back. You will provide lasting relief.

Chapter 43. Special Precautions For Removing Bladder-Stones

Always limit the diet in preparation, and have the patient eat almost nothing for two days before the operation. On the third day, having established the diagnosis as we described, you push and hold the stone in the bladder neck with the intrarectal fingers while you cut down on it through a vertical incision in the perineum, and you extract it.

Dress the wound for nine clays with twice-daily fomentations of acanthus, pellitory and malva, and use topicals of egg-yolk on oakum pads in the winter. In the summer use whole eggs.

Addenda by Roland

1. Do not enforce the dietary restrictions if the patient cannot fast or is feeble or is a child.
2. Take care not to cut the central perineal ligament. Always incise on one side or other.

Chapter 44. Superfluous Proud Flesh At The Bladder-Neck Incision

The accumulation (ie after lithotomy) is removed with a sharp knife, and the defect is closed with sutures. Then medicate.

Take special care: If the stone is so large that you cannot extract it, treat it only by displacing it, as we have instructed.

Chapter 45. Wounds Of The Back Which Involve The Spinal Cord And Nerves

We will not repeat the material dealing with the dorsal regions (including the bladder) except to mention that vertical wounds deep into the back which may involve a nerve can be treated. But you treat in vain a wound which transects the spinal cord.

Chapter 46. Wounds Of The Rectum

When a sword or other sharp weapon cuts into the rectum in its long axis, treat it as an ordinary laceration. But if there is a transection with complete or partial retraction of the cut ends, tie off the open end of the rectum with a sturdy cord to block the feces. Keep the sturdy ligature in place until the tissues beyond it slough away. Then treat that wound with our medications.[9]

When the rectal wound does not penetrate, an ill-advised medication (ie probably a corrosive) will make matters worse.

If the weapon is a projectile, treat the wound as a laceration.

Addendum by Roland

1. The longano is the end section of the rectum, between the sacrum and the coccyx, including the ampulla (LDR).

Chapter 47. Wounds Of The Kidney

These are rarely encountered. Such cases are best trusted to divine interventions rather than to the surgeon. However, if he is conscientious he may be able to be of some help, taxing his ingenuity according to the magnitude of the injury. If a fistula ensues, he may treat it in the ways he now knows.

9 The consequences of this treatment are beyond fantasy (LDR).

Chapter 48. Perianal Abscess, Carbuncle, Cancer And Fistula

An abscess may appear near the anus and present itself as a hard ball, a carbuncle, which may drain spontaneously and then re-form and become a fistula. In your initial assessment ask the patient if flatus escapes via the fistula; that will indicate an opening within the rectum. Treat it so:

Insert your greased long finger and explore within the rectum especially to feel if a probe can easily be passed from outside through the inner opening of the fistula.

If so, thread a seton, using the probe as the needle, and tie it in place. On a later day cut down on the probe. If you wish to avoid cutting, introduce a good amount of corrosive ointment along the tract, as you tighten up on the seton. When it is laid bare, treat the defect as an open wound.

Chapter 49. Hemorrhoids

There are three types: 1. The Internal, causing bleeding and pain. 2. External, with or without pus. 3. Enlarging clusters, resembling figs, which are very constrictive (ie sphincter-spasm) and painful.

When hemorrhoids are internal, you should make them empty their blood, first fumigating the region to relieve the pain. Use mullein, marrubium and horsemint, and take chestnut shells, pumpkin rind and old shoe-leather. Set all on hot coals to create fumes over which you seat the patient on a perforated bench. Repeat the treatments until the bleeding stops and the pain subsides. Then apply leeches to complete the treatment.

In treating the external clusters use an instrument as for a clyster. Inject the juice of wild watermelon to be retained for one or two hours. Repeat until the burning discomfort subsides. Then anoint with white ointment made without vinegar. Then fumigate as above.

When external hemorrhoids enlarge and no pus appears, take the leaves of artemisia and absinthe and grind them and boil them in linseed oil. Apply that as hot as the patient will accept, for three or four days. This usually is a good remedy. But if you do not observe any shrinkage, place some honeysuckle fruit in an earthenware pot and incinerate it and make a powder of the ashes. Apply it after you anoint the piles with honey. Then rub on raw sheep's wool with your hands (or feet!). Apply the powder immediately. Continue the measures until the hemorrhoids no longer shrink.

If later on you want a complete cure, ligate each 'grape' with a silk thread. When the region is not sensitive you may cut off the pile. If not numb, let the ligated tissue slough away without cutting. Apply a bit of corrosive ointment to each site or apply a hot iron.

On occasion the hemorrhoid will not bleed but will drain pus. In such a case look to determine the direction in which to drain, either down toward the buttocks or into the anus. In the latter case you need do nothing. In the former, either insert a hot cautery (ie a stab) or use a corrosive ointment. Follow with the routine wound-care.

Addenda by Roland

1. Another remedy: Sorrel roots boiled in a fine white wine. Use it to fumigate the seated patient. This treatment dries and destroys the hemorrhoids. The smoke should be directed through a funnel.
2. The juice of pellitory, egg-yolk and oil of roses will decrease the swelling.

Chapter 50. Strangury After Wounds

A suprapubic or perineal wound may cause strangury. We can offer some relief.

Make a plaster of the ashes of the leaves and the roots of elder trees boiled at length. Put some it in a sac and lay it over the pubis, as hot as tolerated. It will not delay urination.

Chapter 51. The Application Points Of The Cautery From The Shoulders To The Groins

Knowing die great benefits of the cautery everywhere in the body, I must comment here on the special therapeutic applications in the trunk, from the shoulders to the genitalia. We use them against swollen and inflamed joints in the hands and the arms and we use the arm to treat painful hands, and we apply it three finger-breadths away from a specific painful joint.

To treat inflammation and pain in a hand, burn in the dorsal hollow between the thumb and hand and in a web between two fingers on the other hand. To treat the upper arm, shoulders and eyes, burn the hollow at the elbow, both the inner and the outer surfaces. For asthma burn in the suprasternal notch. For liver disease burn directly over the organ.

Chapter 52. Setons

For splenic disorders, place a seton over the spleen. You may use two, placed well apart.. For pain in the umbilicus, place one three fingerbreadths below.

For pain in the flank, place one in the lumbar hollow, and another three fingerbreadths below. For pain in the back, place two: one three fingerbreadths above, the other the same distance below.[10]

For pain in the testicles place a seton behind the scrotum, over the ischium.

For hemorrhoids place a seton above the anus.

10 The Seton Cautery was inserted through a fold of skin. When the track was charred, the seton was withdrawn and a probe with an 'eye' was inserted. The eye was threaded and the probe was withdrawn, leaving the thread in the channel (LDR).

Chapter 4

Mondino de Luzzi: *Anathomia Corporis Humani* (1316)

HISTORICAL HIGHLIGHTS

- Mondino de Luzzi (1215–1326)
- Originated from Bologna, Italy
- Studied at Bologna at the College of Medicine, graduated 1290
- Was a disciple of Thaddeus of Florence (Taddeo Alderotti)
- Became the first to integrate anatomical studies and dissection with medical school teachings
- Performed first public human dissection in Bologna (1315)
- Published *Anathomia Mundini* (1316) with some inaccurate information and following Galen's principles and findings
- No evidence of accepted use of this text by other universities

THE WRITINGS OF MONDINO DE LUZZI

Of Diseases Of The Mirach [Abdominal Wall] And Siphac [Peritoneum] And Of Their Cure

In the cure of ascitic hydropsy proceed thus, following the authorities. This method, which greatly hangeth on anatomy, is the extraction of the watery matter by incision. The manner is to bring back over the guts the part of the *mirach* [abdominal wall] which thou hast not incised, that it standeth as before. After having placed the patient on his back draw the skin upward. Then take a knife and pierce as far as siphac [peritoneum] so as to make an incision in siphac also. Have to hand a canula and place it in the puncture and draw away as much of the watery matter as the patient may endure. But bear ever in mind that it were better to take too little than to wholly, for the loss of strength that cometh thereby.

Then release the skin for it will return to its own place and cover the wound that no more water escape. When thou wouldst draw more, pull back the skin as at first. Do not make this incision save at the sides; first for that a wound made in the middle doth not unite speedily since there siphac is thicker and more solid; second for that, owing to the cords, the wound is apt to induce convulsions; and third for that water, being heavy, ever cometh forth more freely an [if] it hath a downward leading.

Mondino de Luzzi, "Of Diseases of the Mirach [Abdominal Wall] and Siphac [Peritoneum] and of Their Cure," *Fasciculo di Medicina*, trans. Charles Singer, pp. 63-64. Readings selected and historical highlights written by Luis Horacio Toledo-Pereyra.

If the venter [abdomen] doth suffer interruption of continuity, then this interruption either goeth deeply or no. If it be not deep the cure is by no means hard. But if it go deep then some of the contents may come forth from the wound. If they do so, that which doth come forth is either *zirbus* [omentum] or some other part of the contents. If zirbus, sew with silk or tie as near the skin as may be, then cut off, since all that the air doth touch is infect, and, if put back, raiseth corruption of the other parts. After cutting off it must be returned and the thread brought outward. The lip of the wound is to be left open, for Nature will unite the zirbus and expel the thread. Afterward heal the wound.

If, however, what hath come forth be bowel, then it is either hurt or no. An [if] it be not hurt nor no other substance be involved, put back as speedily as may be. Yet should any substance such as dust or even blood cleave thereto, wash in warm water ere thou return it. If owing to lapse of time there be wind therein and it be distended that it may not be returned, lay thereon a solvent cataplasm or a sponge moistened in a solvent decoction. The swelling will thereby decrease that it may be returned. The wound of the mirach can be enlarged at need for the gut to be put back.

But it may be that the gut itself hath been cut. Then if it be one of the larger bowels the edges must be sewed with silk as are the edges of the other organs. But if one of the small bowels it will not bear sewing save the stitches be deep, and that would hinder his action. Therefore 'tis better to join together the edges of the wound in the bowel with heads of large ants. Unite the edges of the intestine and have large ants ready and cause them to bite the joined edges of the wound. Then cut off the head at once. Do this until the edges be united. Then return the gut as before.

I now return to the cure of wounds of the wall of the venter. Such wound must be cured by the union of the edges. These, when brought together by the fingers, must be held by silk stitches as thus followeth. In the first stitch take the whole of the mirach with the siphac on one side and on the opposite only the mirach. In the second stitch, on the side on which the siphac was omitted take both siphac and mirach, and on the side on which the siphac and mirach were first taken, take of mirach and omit siphac. Continue thus till the edge of the siphac be joined and brought again to the edge of the fleshy member that the junction of the wound may be made firm and sure. The same method is followed with the wound if nothing hath come forth.

Editor's Note: It is important to mention that we would have preferred to feature a larger selection by de Luzzi. However, we were limited on the use of Mondino's writings due to rights holder restrictions on republication. We direct the interested reader to consult **The Anatomy of Mundinus.** ***Translated and annotated by Charles Singer, with additional notes by Michael McVaugh, from*** **A Source Book in Medical Science,** ***ed. Edward Grant, Harvard University Press, 1974.***

Chapter 5

Henri de Mondeville: *La Chirurgie de Maitre Henri de Mondeville*, 2 volumes (1320)

Contributions:
- Surgical ethics
- Causes of ulcers / how to cure
- Dividing ulcers into 3 categories
- 3 things that distinguish cancerous ulcers
- Believed that stimulating the spirit also stimulates the mind for better cure
- 2 types of cauteries; actual, potential. Actual is more reliable / easier to use
- Blood letting / what veins to use

HISTORICAL HIGHLIGHTS

- Henri de Mondeville (1260–1316)
- From Normandy, France
- Studied medicine as a clerk at Paris and Montpellier
- Studied surgery in Bologna under Theodoric
- Supported "pus abolitionists" such as Hugh of Lucca and Theodoric
- Became surgeon to French King Philip the Fair
- Admired Galen and Aristotle
- Padua remained center of Greek medical studies in Europe
- His book, *La Chirurgie de Maitre Henri de Mondeville,* enjoyed preference in the Middle Ages until de Chauliac's work became available

THE WRITINGS OF HENRI DE MONDEVILLE

The Surgery of Henri De Mondeville, Volume II: Treatise II, Doctrine II

Introduction

Nicaise's (earlier translator into modern French) Note: After completing Doctrine I of Treatise II, Mondeville stopped work on his "Surgery," which he had begun in 1306. He added Doctrine II which follows here in 1312 and he altered, his original plan for the chapters, as he restated, it in the Introduction below.

Here begins the Particular Introduction to Doctrine II of Treatise II of the Chirurgia of Master Henri de Mondeville, Surgeon to our Illustrious Leader, The King Of France.

Having completed Treatise I of this *Surgery*, which contains the Anatomy limited to what is useful for a surgeon, and having completed Doctrine I of Treatise II on the treatment of wounds, I now undertake with the support of God to write Doctrine II to be followed directly by Treatise III. My plan is to devote an entire chapter to an ailment, to describe it, to offer treatments for it, and to follow with explanations to clarify the more obscure items.

I shall deal with each ailment in four ways: 1. Define it and describe it. 2. Describe in detail only those varieties which come within the purview of a surgeon, and the various sources of certain difficulties that he may encounter. 3. The causes of the ailments themselves. 4. The symptoms (ie signs) in common for all the varieties, and those which distinguish each particular case.

Then I shall provide up to three methods for treating each ailment, but only if they have rational bases. First will come preventive measures, followed by curative treatments and then by palliation.

I. Preventive Treatments are the medical and surgical measures that will deter the progress of an illness. Here I quote Galen *(Commentaries on the Aphorisms,* 22), "If an impending cause is aborted, that is an anticipation, not a cure." He said the same in *Techni, Tr. of Causes,* Ch. 27. Haly agreed (*Commentaries),* "This treatment (ie prevention) can be used in some but not all surgical conditions. For example, a person may suffer from chilblains in his feet all winter long, whereas he could have avoided the suffering with proper treatment." The same is true for many conditions; many persons can be spared illness with preventive measures. However, such are not applicable in cases of wounds, contusions, fractured bones, etc., conditions which are not predictable. As Aristotle wrote *(On Harmony,* Bk. I and *Physics,* Bk. II), "There is no science that can foretell and prevent all chance events; one cannot tell in advance, but once they begin, one may get some inkling of what will happen."

I. The preventive treatments are vised by some medical practitioners in certain cases when they are indicated, as one may read in Galen's *De Ingenio,* Bk. XII. Ch. 3, where he tells us to treat syncope in anticipation of it happening. "You who are wise physicians will be put to shame if you allow your patient to faint."[1]

II. Second, I will describe Curative Treatments and include references to the recommendations of the medical and surgical authorities, especially to Galen, the citations where he describes his own treatments. I shall deal with the treatments first by giving the General Precepts that I have garnered both from the older authorities and from the moderns. Those are the principles and canons from which one may abstract and infer nearly all the procedures designed for particular cases and for the special operations.

I shall refer to authorities for their treatments in all except three types of cases in which surgeons, simply to earn fees, will perform operations really designed for palliation. 1. When the patient is absolutely incurable by surgery, as in internal cancers, when fistulas communicate with the urinary system or with the marrow-cavities of bones and in other similarly evil conditions that you cannot cure with surgical procedures unless you can radically extirpate the entire lesion, roots and all; when it is clear that the patient's vital forces cannot withstand such procedures which are depleting or lethal. 2. Some curable illnesses do not warrant surgical procedures. Avicenna (Bk. IV. Fol. 4, Tr. Ill, Ch. on unhealed fistulas) wrote this about the treatment of chronic fistulas, "The treatment consists of a total ablation with the knife or the cautery or with caustic medications, procedures that cause such profound suffering that a patient will choose to live with his disorder rather than submit to the treatment." 3. When a disorder is curable by a surgical procedure that both the surgeon and the patient agree to undertake, but the treatment will produce another disorder that is worse than the original one. In that category

1 I cannot trace this reference. I assume that Galen rebukes the physician who bleeds his patient until he faints (LDR).

are operations for a fistula in ano that is a complication of chronic hemorrhoids, and when the internal opening of the fistula is above the anal muscles.[2] Another example is a case of extensive malmort.[3] The surgical procedures in such cases lead to disorders and to suffering that are worse than the original. Hippocrates (*Aphorisms*, Part 6) said the same. Later on in this Treatise if you are attentive, you will read how common sense will demonstrate the truth of the foregoing.

III. Palliative Surgical Treatments aim to ease and to diminish the effects of a disease, but do not attempt to cure the patient. The surgeon can blunt the severity of the illness and render it more tolerable to the patient. All the medical authors palliate with dietary regimens for incurable patients and for cases when there is no advantage to treat for cure when a condition is incurable. Hippocrates), in many places (*Aphorisms*, Part 6) and Galen and Haly (*Techni, Treatise on Causes*, Ch. 33) all advised that we fall back on palliative treatment when curative measures avail little or cannot be used, saying, "a curative treatment should get rid of a disease. If you cannot accomplish that, palliate it by changing it to a less serious form." These treatments are not the same as in the three cases where curative treatment are not at all suitable. There the patient is absolutely incurable, or if he is curable, the patient will be unable to withstand the radical treatment, or when the treatment causes a more serious disorder. In all three kinds of cases, curative treatments are contraindicated.

However, when the patient wishes to obtain relief and he can afford to pay for his services, which may include palliative treatments,[4] the surgeon will provide a suitable diet and will take care of all the patient's needs, and will fulfill all the orders which are the concerns of a supervising physician, all of it to the extent of the patient's generosity in payments already received and those to be anticipated. The palliative treatments in the last two cases often come when the patient has refused to accept the recommendations to undergo curative treatments. In my own experience in Paris, I have seen that happen many times when my colleagues have disagreed with my judgment.[5]

Treatise II: Chapter 1: The Treatment of Ulcers Three General Comments

A. Description of Ulcer

Definition: An ulcer is a wound that has suppurated or has been caused to suppurate (ie by medications), or it discharges other impure matter for a long time or in great quantity, or simply one which has not begun to heal within the expected usual time. According to the Salernitans that was about two days.[6] However, Galen (*De Ingenio*, Bk. IV, Ch.4) fixed die time at seven days, stating "one may blame our All-Powerful God and cast blame for prolonging the time for healing up to a year, when it should take place within a week."

The Varieties: One type of ulcer is called apparent, it can be flat or concave. There are five types of the latter: the virulent, dirty (ie sordid), corrosive, putrid and simply slow-to-heal. We shall discuss the treatments of each variety later on in this chapter. Now we shall go on to describe their similarities and differences.

2 An incision through the sphincters may lead to permanent incontinence of feces (LDR).
3 A chronic ulcer with necrotic slough; often a deep stasis ulcer 011 the leg or a necrotizing ulcer anywhere (LDR).
4 The patient is wealthy enough to maintain a personal resident-surgeon to attend him (LDR).
5 When he accepted the patients for palliation (LDR).
6 The expected time for a properly treated wound to show signs of healing (LDR).

Other than the principal varieties there are ulcers that develop after certain complications or dispositions, and they do not fall into the categories that are listed in surgical handbooks (ie Practicas). The medical authors, especially Avicenna (Bk. IV, Fol. 4, Tr. 3, Ch. 1) said "one ulcer derives from an internal source, another from an external; one is painful, another is not; some are complicated by an abscess or tumor, others not; some are accompanied by heat, others by cold; some with fever, others not; some are caused by humors that cause burning pain, in others the humors do not burn; some are venomous or cause poisoning, others do not; some have indurated margins or beds; some are livid or black or green; some are granular and shed hair, and others do not. Some provoke spasms, some develop in fleshy tissues, others in nerve-bearing regions. Some produce superfluous granulation tissues, whereas none appears in others. In some the ulcer-bed is a gangrenous bone. Some appear in persons or in parts of their bodies endowed with healthy complexions, others are to the contrary. Some merely are damp, some are very wet, others are moderately so. Some are recent, others very old and others are in between. Some are round, some are irregular. Some have lost much tissue, some none, some only a small amount, some a moderate amount. Some bleed. Some bulge with superfluous humors (ie edema), others have none."

In addition to the apparent and the deep ulcers, other types exhibit more differences than we have already listed. Some of those differences include cancers, esthiomene, fistulas, mal-mort etc., as we will see in the chapters that define them. All these varieties, differences, conditions of ulcers and other matters should be known by a surgeon who wants his treatments to succeed. Indeed, one must treat according to what he encounters in any ulcer. These generalities will apply in all subsequent chapters.

The Causes And The Varieties Of Causes'. Some are proximate (ie material) and others are predispositions. That is what Avicenna wrote (Bk. I, Fol. 2, Ch. 27 "Causes of Ulcers"). The materials which cause ulcers are blood, bile, phlegm, melancholy, wind and water.

The predisposing causes are the innate tendency of a part of the body to impel the bad humors to the ulcer and the weakness of the ulcerated part which receives them; the two cooperate in forming the ulcer. Another predisposition is the looseness of the tissue, its sponginess or its thinness, such as found in glands or emunctories. Another predisposition derives from the diameters and the lengths of the blood vessels and other channels that are directed toward the ulcer. Another cause is the location of the parts that are ulcerated. For example, the legs and the feet are lower than the rest of the body.[7]Another cause is an excess of nutritive matter delivered to a sick region which cannot convert it, and another is superfluous heat attracted to the part.[8] Other causes are venomous bites and stings and the lack of resistance to them. Excessive exercise of a limb may attract humors, as well as a contusion, a fracture, a dislocation and a tight constriction. Another cause is pain that attracts heat and the vital spirits.

Furthermore, we see certain ulcers come from external causes and others from internal ones. The ignorant mob speaks of and believes in chance or of Divine intervention as the internal cause of these disorders, sent to us by our glorious and sublime God. The common folk, say that it is He who sends them, and we should not interfere and use our man-made treatments. The outcome of the treatment is as it pleases the Lord. They support their opinions by insisting that God alone cures us of our chronic debility; he wounds and he provides the remedies. What he has given he can take away. Others think differently and they defend God by saying that diseases with internal causes do not come from him but from the bad luck of the patient.

The surgeon must understand all of this; the causes and their effects as listed here, and others, too.

The Symptoms: There are two kinds, those which are common to all ulcers and those that belong to each variety. The symptoms in common are described in all the surgical handbooks and by the medical

7 To explain why the legs are common sites for what we today call stasis ulcers (LDR).
8 To explain dependent edema and the frequent company of low-grade cellulitis (LDR).

writers. You can infer others from the name of the ulcers in our list. Every good surgeon knows them. The particular symptoms will be described when we get to their treatments.

B. The Treatment of Ulcers

We divide them into Preventive, Curative and Palliative.

I. Preventive Measures consist of defending against and eliminating all the causes which we have described, which favor the development of these maladies, especially those which are proximate or impending. Indeed, even if we do intervene, an ulcer may be inevitable, yet often we are effective and no ulcer will form. That is what we mean by the preventive (ie preservative) treatment of wounds. The prevention of inflammation (aposthems) keeps wounds from forming pus and from bursting open (ie to become ulcers). By prevention we avoid ulcers.

II. Treatments For Cure: 39 General Guides:

1. When a specific dyscrasia complicates an ulcer, such as inflammation or swelling (ie edema), treat it for cure before you attack the ulcer. That is Avicenna's rule (Bk. I, Fol. 4, Ch. 21; and Bk. IV, Fol. 4, Tr. 3, Ch. 1). The medications for ulcers have drying actions, and they interfere with the wet medicines needed to dissolve and cleanse the complicating dyscrasia, which must be treated first.
2. Whenever the ulcer is extremely painful, you try to relieve it before acting on the preceding Rule. So said Avicenna (ibid., Ch. "On Relief of Pain"). And Galen said it, too, *(Acute Regimens,* Bk. Ill).
3. Your medication for healing (ie closing) the ulcer will fail until you get rid of the dry crusts and the filthy matter. (Galen, *Megatechni,* Ch. 3, and Avicenna, Ch. on Ulcers).
4. When the ulcer or the rest of the body suffers a dyscrasia, treat that with evacuants, proper diets and topicals directed against the dyscrasia. Then treat the ulcer. (Avicenna, ibid.)
5. If the liver, the spleen or the stomach suffers dyscrasias, restore their health first. Those organs are necessary for the health of the entire body; they make healthy blood. When they are sick, the blood from them is not strong enough to heal ulcers.
6. When the humors of the entire body or of the ulcerated member alone or of an organ that usually provides normal humors for the body show signs of deterioration or diminution or both, you should get rid of them with evacuations, or temper them with phlebotomies or laxatives or both and with a healthy dietary regimen that acts contrary to the impaired humors. Those humors are not suitable for replacing ulcerated tissue or for keeping the region healthy.
7. Inasmuch as the humors which cause ulcers come from other parts of the body, we try to intercept or deflect (ie repercuss) them (Avicenna, ibid.)
8. All ulcers are treated by foods, by internal medicines and by suitable topicals which are desiccative and by a regimen that is proper in its six non-natural elements and is contrary to the causes of the ulcer, (Avicenna, ibid.).
9. When you treat ulcers, avoid using suppuratives (Avicenna, ibid.), both internally and in your topicals.
10. Avoid using naturally humid medicines, because, as Avicenna explained, we should emphasize desiccatives.
11. When ulcers are exposed during the mid-day to warm moist air, the cure is retarded, nor can we find any favorable air that does not cause ulcers to suppurate and thereby to interfere with the healing.
12. Do not use active cold medicines. Hippocrates (*Aphorisms,* Part 5) said that cold irritates ulcers.

13. You may apply cool medicines on ulcers that tend to be warm, and use the warm topicals when the ulcers tend to be cool. Galen (*Commentaries on the Aphorisms,* Part 2) said we should always treat with contraries, and Hippocrates agreed *(Aphorisms,* at the end of Part 2).
14. Do not apply corrosive topicals on internal ulcers and on those that penetrate, such as those that enter the chest cavity, because the medicaments then cannot be extracted (ie before they damage vital organs).
15. On deeper and more moist ulcers use drier topicals. As it works its way into the depths of the ulcer the medicine loses its strength. Therefore, when the distance is great you must resort to the most potent compounds.
16. In some cases you must take care not to allow cohesion of adjacent thin layers of tissue, for example the eyelid must not adhere to the eye, and fingers should not be allowed to adhere to each other. This principle really is self-evident.
17. Ulcers which come after other illnesses are difficult to treat because in curing the illness Nature traps the residues of the corrupt superfluidities in the ulcer.
18. The skin surrounding some ulcers may lose its hair. That is a sign that the bad humors have corrupted the region. That ulcer is difficult to cure. So said Galen (*Commentaries on the Aphorisms,* Part 6).
19. Ulcers at the coccyx are not easy to cure (Avicenna, Bk. I, ibid.) for four reasons, a. Many nerves end there, and they separate the parts.[9] b. It is near the immodest openings, c. It is a low part. d. When the patient strains to expel feces he distends the region and prevents the ulcer from closing. Galen *(Megalechni,* Bk. V, Ch. 3, in the part where he discusses wounds of the lung) said that immobility is necessary (ie for healing) in a wounded or an ulcerated part.
20. Ulcers at the knee and at the tip of the elbow lie over joints which move and stretch or contract the edges of the lesion. The same is true for the lips, the eyelids, the penis et al. Treatments are difficult (Avicenna, ibid.). Again, the reason is that the regions cannot be put at rest.
21. Ulcers in nerve-bearing regions are difficult to cure because they are very painful. Galen (*Commentaries on the Aphorisms,* Part 5) said that pain impairs the flow of humors, and, since nerves are spermatic structures, their tissues are not easily repaired.
22. Round ulcers are difficult to cure. a. They have lost more tissues and need more time to regenerate them. b. Nature cannot decide where to begin the repair; a circle has no sides, no beginning and no ending, c. The margins are equally separated, whereas in oblong ulcers the opposing sides can be brought together by traction at the ends.
23. Round ulcers can be very painful and babies may suffer unto death from pain. That must be relieved. Avicenna (Bk. IV, ibid.) said that the vital force is depleted and overcome by strong pain.
24. Ulcers over or near the dorsal spine, and those in the front of the lower leg are difficult to treat and because they are near large nerve-bearing muscles they are disposed to spasm and they cause much trouble (Avicenna, ibid.)
25. If the ulcer is the only ailment, apply the topicals as the only treatment. (Theodoric, Bk. I, Ch. 8.)
26. Laxatives and emetics help in the treatment of old and painful ulcers, (ibid).
27. Round and excavated ulcers will persist until you can elongate them by incising opposite margins to convert them to ovals, (ibid.)

9 Nerve-tendon-ligament: here is another example of the confusion. The 'nerves' were contractile structures. They form clusters and plexuses which separate the fleshy tissues. By definition, a wound is a separation! (LDR).

28. When the surfaces of the ulcer are indurated, cut them away with a knife or a cautery, to allow the granulation tissue to adhere.[10]
29. Purge away and obstruct the return of humors that have accumulated in an ulcer. Use good purges to deflect them. If the influx has ceased but the stench of the ulcer remains, evacuate the region by cupping and bleeding, and use desiccatives in the ulcer. If once is not enough, purge again.
30. A resistant chronic ulcer may be treated by making a fresh wound alongside it, and keeping it open while the primary ulcer heals. That will intercept and deflect the humors which caused the first ulcer. When that heals, the second ulcer will be easy to cure. (ibid. Ch. 10).
31. Whoever treats ulcers should have available plasters and other medications that attract bony fragments and any other abnormal stuff that may be lodged in ulcers. (Avicenna, Bk. I, ibid.).
32. When you first encounter an ulcer do not bathe it or the patient with hot water. However, when it is well along and is healing, and when it drains healthy pus, you may bathe it or irrigate it as we have instructed. When the ulcer is new and you have to bathe the patient, cover the ulcer with a sparadrap [11] or wrap it. Galen taught us how to wash an ulcer *(Megatechni,* Ch. 1). But, if you wash it at the outset you attract more humors and bring on inflammation (Avicenna, Bk. I, ibid.).
33. A deep or an obscure ulcer needs stronger medications than does the exposed kind. The deeper and the less exposed they are the more potent the medications must be, because as they work into the depths they lose some of their power, (Avicenna, ibid.)
34. Whenever some of the bad humor is attracted (ie from nearby) to an ulcer you have to deflect it before reaches the ulcer, but you should not be too aggressive (ie with potent medicines) and make matters worse by attracting even more (ie by injuring the member).
35. Also, when the humors come from elsewhere in the body, you should use evacuants in a distant part. On the other hand, if the all the inflow is from nearby, evacuate from nearby. The first method requires more potent measures because of its distance, but the same is not true for the nearby source. If we are too violent there we will bring in more of the humors than we pull out. If there are no distant sources, we need only to evacuate locally.
36. If the ulcer is complicated by another ailment or an abscess or by severe pain, use a topical that will treat the ulcer as well as the complication. A complicated lesion requires a complicated compound (ie not just a Simple).
37. The topicals must take into account the delicacy of the site and the sensitivity of the region and of the noble and principal organs nearby. Consider the needs of the whole region and all the other things. Therefore, we should apply topicals which are suitable in strength: weak, medium-strong or very energetic.
38. If worms[12] appear in an ulcer, kill them with the juice of river-calamint, persicaria, leaves of parsley, absinthe, centaury and wild mint and the like. (Avicenna, Bk. IV, ibid.).[13]
39. Ulcers that have internal causes or are due to repletion of the body (ie dropsy) or others that occur in doddering old folks, and ulcers that provoke much pain in muscles, or cause fevers, Or those that derive from burned tissues or from poisonous matter, or those which are indurated, dark, livid or sickly green, or are accompanied by spasm, or which form excessive amounts of proud flesh, or those that hide a patch of gangrenous bone or a foreign body, or are very wet or very old (ie chronic), or have lost substance, especially if the loss is extensive, and occurred with hemorrhage, and those

10 Mondeville means that healthy blood will adhere to the surfaces and be the source of the granulation tissue (LDR)
11 A section of cloth made sticky with egg-white. It will seal the ulcer during the immersion (LDR).
12 Maggots (LDR).
13 All of the medications are described in the pharmacopeia of the Antidotary, Treatise V (LDR).

which received their offensive matter from other sites, all of them are more difficult to treat, all other things being equal, than are ulcers that occur in conditions opposite to the foregoing. I have already given a partial explanation for that. A curious student should pay attention to the following sections where we will deal with what already has not been specifically discussed.

A practicing surgeon should be well-prepared to offer prognoses as to which ulcers are curable, and which of those are easier to cure if he has learned our definitions and the explanations, the causes, clinical signs, and the guiding principles for treatments as we have disclosed them. And he can infer what nearly all the treatments will consist of, both in general and in what will apply in specific types of ulcers. All the principles given above are the bases for the particular treatments which follow.

Treatise II: Chapter 4: The Treatment Of Cancerous Ulcers

I. The Diagnosis of Cancerous Ulcers: Six Items

A. The two words of the term, 'Cancerous Ulcer' have different meanings. To know what we deal with here we shall clearly indicate either a non-ulcerating cancer or a cancerous ulcer, to avoid ambiguity.

B. The Definition of a non-ulcerating cancer:[14] It is an abnormal mass or an inflammation formed from corrupted or putrefied melancholic humors. It contains no exterior openings or wounds. We shall not concern ourselves with them here; the inflamed (ie abscessed) cancers will be an item in the chapter on aposthems.

C. The cancerous ulcer, however, has an opening, an obvious, rounded, fetid ulcer with rolled raised edges and an excavated interior. The substance is hard and uneven, livid or black in color.

D. The Varieties of Cancerous Ulcers: One type has an internal cause; a burned[15] and putrefied melancholic (ie black bile) humor collects somewhere in the body. Another type has external causes, such as a badly treated wound or ulcer. Occasionally a cancerous ulcer is the effect of both internal and external causes, such as a contusion that becomes a cancer, or when we incise to drain a cancerous aposthem.

Some cancerous ulcers are curable, if they are small, are entirely in soft tissues and are of recent origin. Others are incurable, such as one that arises in nervous regions, or one that grows deep during a long existence, or grows in or near principal or noble organs.

E. Causes: The curable one derives from a burnt and putrefied melancholy which comes from the combustion of a natural melancholy, the incurable one derives from a burnt and putrefied melancholy which is a product of other burned humors, which by their combustion became a non-natural melancholy. After they have undergone a second combustion, they putrefy and become more malignant.

---

14 The word 'cancer' was applied to many tumors, ranging from true neoplasms to other lesions, both the ulcerated and those with intact overlying skin. The 14thC French term was 'chancre' (EN). In this chapter Mondeville takes great pains to define neoplasms in various grades of malignancy, invasiveness, rates of growth, etc. He is equally 'painful' in assigning to each variety its own causative humors, and is disdainful in his condemnation of the erroneous identification of cancers with other ulcers. However, his own terms confuse cancers, gangrene, etc. as was the common confusion in ancient and medieval times. Bear it in mind that all these lesions are visible, palpable and smeilable on or just beneath the surface of the body. The medieval surgeon did not deal with neoplasms of the viscera. Furthermore, we must view Nicaise's translation as the work of man who was newborn in the era when the cellular nature of cancers was first elucidated. Few pathologists in the last half of the 19'" C had a solid grasp of the concepts introduced by Virchow. Nicaise's circumlocutions reflect his own attitudes about what he read in Mondeville's pages (LDR).

15 'Burned' does not mean incinerated. One's natural heat may be overactive, not necessarily a fever. The natural heat may 'burn' the bile etc. Unnatural heat is defined later in the chapter (LDR).

One kind of cancerous ulcer involves the upper parts of the body. Most often it comes from burnt and putrefied (ie non-natural) melancholy, from burnt bile. It is a very corrosive humor because it comes from a thin fluid that has been heated twice.

The other kind involves the lower parts of the body. It derives from a burnt and putrefied melancholy which was produced by the combustion of true natural black bile. This cancer is more curable and benign and has less corrosive features than the other kind.

One type involves soft flesh, another involves nerves, a third is in bone.

One kind grows deep, another is on the surface. One involves only external structures, another the internal.

Their ages vary from recent to old. Some appear in robust and strong people, others affect the debilitated and the delicate. Not all patients are willing to be cured and they refuse to give themselves to the surgeons and undergo operations.

A drainage incision or a spontaneous eruption of a putative non-ulcerating cancer that really is an abscess is a wound that becomes an ulcer because the treatment was wrong; that ulcer, if treated badly, may become a cancerous ulcer when it attracts more putrefied melancholic humors. At times, the attracted humors have not yet putrefied and do not undergo putrefaction until they arrive at the corrupted site.

Other causes can be inferred from those described above.

F. The Symptoms (ie signs) are described in the section on Definitions. We shall add here the three things that distinguish cancerous ulcers from the sordid ulcers which they resemble. 1. When you irrigate the cancer with lye it becomes even more unsightly than before; its color fades to that of ashes. After the wash has dried, a viscous, sticky stuff remains as an adherent film or membrane. But, when you wash the sordid ulcer with lye, you clean it, and its color improves (ie pink).

2. The stench of a cancer is horrible beyond description. Anyone exposed to it will know the diagnosis before he sees the patient. The odor of the ulcer is bad enough, but not intolerable, and it is very different from that of the cancer, which has the stench of a cadaver.

3. After you apply corrosives on the cancerous ulcer you can see that you have made it worse. After the eschar separates, the malignancy has increased in size. The reaction of the ulcer is different.

II: The Treatments: Three Kinds

A Preventive Measures

1. If a cancerous ulcer is the result of the faulty treatment of a wound or ulcer, intervene with the measures that we use for the prevention, the cure and the palliation of wounds and ulcers. If you do it properly, you will never see a cancer develop. 2. To prevent a non-ulcerating cancer from becoming a cancerous ulcer, observe the caveat of the preceding paragraph. I shall add more detail in Doctrine II of Treatise III in the chapter on non-ulcerating cancers.

B. Curative Treatments: General Measures:

In addition to all the items in our Precepts (ie rules) for treating ulcers and fistulas which an operating surgeon must know, I shall add fifteen Precepts for cancers.

1. In all cases of both kinds of cancers, for prevention and cure and palliation, always use the general purges as well as those designed for local evacuations, which eliminate the faulty humors.
2. After the evacuations, take pains to identify the type of the cancer that may be curable.
3. If you cannot prevent the accretion of cancerous matter, at least try to fortify the affected region to resist the influx of humors and to reject some of it.
4. For cancers of internal origin, cancers in nervous regions, cancers in the upper part of the body, for old and established cancers that penetrate deeply[16], for those that derive from the twice-burned melancholic humors, for those that arise in feeble and delicate patients and for those in patients who may refuse treatments, and when a cancer obviously is incurable, in all and any similarly daunting situations, you should know that the treatment for cure, if at all feasible, will be difficult.
5. Both kinds of cancers may be curable: if they have external causes, if they are small, recent and superficial, if they lie in fleshy regions and are not near nerves or important structures, if they appear alone without complicating factors and if they occur in robust persons who are eager to be cured.
6. Both kinds of cancers are incurable: if they are long-established and complicated, when they grow deeply or are situated in nervous or bony regions, if they are near important or vital organs, if they derive from twice-burned melancholic humors and if the victim is debilitated and feeble.
7. When you treat any kind of cancer, the patient must agree to abide by the dietary regimen that is the same for all persons: it contains the six non-natural things. However, the topicals will differ from case to case.
8. You can cure a cancer only by radically extirpating all of it, leaving none of it behind. The malignancy is greater in the roots, as both Serapion (Tr. V, Ch. 25) and Rhazes (*The Divisions)* claimed.
9. It follows from what I have said that you must not undertake a radical operation to cure a cancer unless it is situated in a region where nothing stands in the way of a total extirpation. As Serapion aptly remarked (ibid.), the treatment itself is violent and, if it fails, it will destroy the patient by exacerbating the cancer.
10. It follows, also, that you cannot assume that you can cure a hidden internal cancer [17] when it cannot be encompassed by your surgical operation. Again I cite Serapion (ibid.) and Hippocrates (*Aphorisms*, 38, Part 6) who add that those who are treated with the knife, cautery or with caustic medicines die sooner than the untreated. The untreated live longer because they have not been burned or incised or injured by painfully caustic medicines; rather, they have received proper palliative treatment.
11. We conclude from the preceding that we should not try to destroy a cancer piecemeal with corrosives, as is commonly done. In fact, while you can burn away one part, the roots become even more malignant. You must eliminate it all at one time (ie for cure), and not in parts.
12. When you try to cure a cancer by radical measures, apply defensives on the surrounding area.
13. The best way to accomplish a cure is to cut it all out with its roots. Then wipe out the blood and cauterize the surfaces (Galen, *Megatechni.*, Bk. XIV, Ch. 4).
14. After cauterizing or applying corrosives, follow the practices stated in Precept 9 in Chapter 3 on fistulas.
15. Deal with the eschar after using the cautery or corrosives as in Precept 10 in that chapter, and in 8, 9, and 10, above.

---

16 'Deeply': the term meant the extension beyond the subcutaneous tissues and rarely into a viscus. The cancerous breast was an exception (LDR).

17 'Internal' denotes the inward extension of a cancer on the surface, not a visceral neoplasm (LDR).

Operative Techniques

In the preceding sections we have emphasized the incurable types of cancer, in which the surgeon should avoid attempts at radical cures, because palliative measures alone will help the patient. Furthermore, you should understand that curative efforts are very difficult, whereas at times a palliative treatment may cure, if the surgeon prudently conducts it with great care. The surgeon should not undertake a cure until he has been entreated to go ahead with it, and has been assured a larger-than-usual fee.

The three elements of a curative treatment are:

1. The Diet: The diet for both types of cancers should continue without change from the beginning to the conclusion of the course of treatments, until the patient recovers or dies. As Galen wrote (*Megatechni*, Bk. XIV, ibid.), the diet should consist only of cool foods: well leavened bread; fresh meats of lambs, kids, calves, capons, hens, partridges, small birds of the meadow with narrow beaks; soups made with borage and spinach and broths made with the listed meats to which you may add eggs, which also may be eaten raw. The beverages should include barley water, aged white or red wines which are clarified and diluted with water. The patient should abstain from other beverages and from the flesh of goats, cows and bulls, hares, of aquatic birds and from all garden vegetables except for chickpeas, and from all salted, acidic, roasted and broiled foods, as well as from cheeses and cabbages.
2. The Evacuations: a. The General Purges evacuate and distract the humors from the cancers. The evacuation is by phlebotomy and laxatives. The distraction is by emetics for cancers below the umbilicus.[18] For lesions above that level use laxatives to empty the bowels and phlebotomies from saphenous veins, and massage of and applications of cords around the legs. b. For evacuating a particular region, the head for example, when the cancer is in the face, after the General Evacuations, use massage, scarifications, cups, and leeches applied near the site. Those maneuvers consume the residue of humors that have infiltrated the surrounding tissues.
3. Operative Techniques: Two Parts:

A. The Artificial[19]

Having followed the proper sequence outlined above, you incise and excise the cancer with all its roots. Then you get rid of the contaminated blood that floods the defect. Then you repeatedly apply a hot cautery to all the surfaces.

If, in the second maneuver the patient cannot tolerate the hot iron, apply a defensive around the defect and lay on a large amount of corrosives on all the surfaces within the wound. Do that once only (ie unlike the repeated applications of the hot cautery). An eschar remains after the terrible suffering has abated, much like that after the actual cautery,

The treatment continues: 1. Apply defensives. 2. Use coolants on the surface of the eschar. 3. Then apply suppuratives to cause the eschar to come away. 4. Then use detergents and, 5. desiccatives, and 6. regeneratives, and 7. cicatrizers.

The medications themselves, how to use them and the special virtues of each are described in Chapter 10 of Doctrine I of Treatise II. The techniques for making incisions and for using defensives and mondificatives are described in Chapter 1 of this Doctrine, on Ulcers. The way to get rid of the blood is not very 'surgical' (ie a mop-up). The techniques for the use of the

18 The opposite part of the body is used for the evacuation, that is, for distracting the bad humors from a distance (LDR).
19 'Artificial': The surgeon's artifice (LDR).

cautery are in the chapter on cauteries. The repercussives and mitigatives used to relieve the pains after burning, and the suppuratives and the corrosives are to be found in the Antidotary.

B. The Empirical Techniques[20]: Two Methods

1. Medications that act only when carried by the patient (in a sack): the small liver-wort; piloselle, which is gathered in the meadows while reciting the Pater Noster; St. John's herb and agrimony. Use all together or separately. Ceterach works well and some say that it prevents cancers.
2. Medications that act when applied to the outer surface of a cancer: powdered Herb Robert; powdered myrtle-leaves; crushed lesser consolida, alone or with the fat of a castrated male animal; scabious; incinerated dill; crushed clover in honey; juice of honeysuckle or leaves of sorrel and potentilla. The latter is like tormentilla but it lacks nodes on its roots.

Palliative Measures

These are similar to what we described for fistulas in the preceding chapter. Here, too, are three categories.

A. The Diet is the same as when we are treating for cure.

B. The purgatives are the same, with the following restrictions: Here we use purges only during the spring and the autumn, and only when recommended by a wise physician.[21] They are repeated about twice a week, at dawn, during those seasons. Use a small amount of goat's milk in which you infuse 5 dr. of a good quality epithyme.

C. The topicals: 1. The defensives are those we use for all wounds. 2. Ointments: Equal parts of ceruse and tuthie—well washed to remove irritants—and oil of roses or the like in which is a quarter-part of the juice of morel or of a similar plant in an amount deemed suitable at the time. Grind all with a lead pestle in a lead mortar bowl which you rub vigorously to obtain some lead in the mixture. This ointment inhibits the influx of humors, it restricts the infiltrative corrosion of the cancer and it reduces its malignancy. It allows the sufferer to have comfortable sleep at night.

You can compound many similar useful ointments, some cool, some warm; each kind will work better in the cases for which it is specially designed. They are listed by many authors and we need not repeat them here.

D. The Humectants are made with decoctions and juices of morel, purslane, etc. You may use them at every dressing instead of the ointments, or, if you see any benefit, you may use them together by placing a cloth or some oakum saturated with one of the humectants on top of the wound in which you have put the ointment. The warmer the topicals the more comforting they will be all. Renew them frequently.

You may temper all the topicals to suit the case. When the disease eats into the nearby tissues and causes more suffering, more pricking and burning pain, and if the patient is a feeble sort, increase the coolness by adding ceruse and other cool substances. You can increase the warming actions by adding tuthie and oil of roses and some white wax.

Never increase the coolness of the topicals unless constrained to do so by the need to relieve the pain. In so doing you will make them thick and fatty, and make the pain worse later on. Similarly, do not add to the warming effects unless you must, lest you increase the invasive tendency of cancers in warmed patients. You should be most circumspect and use only a few well-tested topicals, and you should completely abandon those with which you have had little experience. An error on your part will

---

20 'Empirical': In common use and not Artificial, but not necessarily in disfavor by the professionals (LDR).

21 The Physician gave the orders and the surgeon carried them out: the clysters, cups, phlebotomies, etc.(LDR).

cause irremediable and permanent damage. The surgeon must use his own common sense in treating these patients; he should not rely on hearsay or on what some author has recommended.

The better to understand this subject, I suggest that you review what I wrote in the General Precepts, and in the chapter on the treatment of ulcers and fistulas in this Doctrine. You should know all of it, and I shall not repeat it here. Besides, an experienced operating surgeon should know where to find what he needs in those pages.

Seventen Explanations

I. All the famous authorities have written about the treatment of cancerous ulcers. Many of them combine that with the treatment of non-ulcerating cancers. Hippocrates (*Aphorisms*, 38, Part 6), Avicenna (Bk. IV, Fol. 3, Doct. 3), Galen (*Megatechni*, Bk. XIV, Ch. 4) and Rhazes *(Divisions,* at the end; and *Almansor,* Bk. VII) and Serapion (*Practica,* Doct. 5, Ch. 15) all deal at length with this subject, as did Theodoric *(Grand Chirurgia,* Bk. IV, Ch.6) and many others. Yet, none of them has given a complete definition of an ulcerating cancer.

II. A cancerous ulcer is an ulcer. Here the generic term is 'ulcer', and it excludes all other lesions. Other definitions also are exclusive: the word 'apparent' excludes deep ulcers and fistulas; 'round' excludes oval ulcers; 'fetid' is limited to the horrible stench of cancers. When we say, "which have thick, heaped up and folded and raised margins which are separated from the base (ie undermined), or are excavated (ie cavernous), that is, they have cavities beneath the smaller opening atop, or that they are hard and nodular, livid or black", we exclude all the other apparent ulcers.

III. We have four reasons for calling these lesions 'cancers': a. The external ulcer often is round, an unusual shape for other ulcers. Here the shape is like the carapace of the marine animal we call cancer, which in France is called crab. b. It clings to where it lies. c. It is surrounded by many long and tortuous veins that suggest the appendages of a crab. d. It eats in any or all directions, a movement that suggest the sidling of a crab that can move forward or backwards or to a side.

IV. Avicenna (Bk. IV., Fol. 3. Doct. 3, Ch. on Treatment of Non-ulcerating Cancers) claims that it derives from a melancholic inflammation. He said that he encountered this astonishing anecdote in the works of another famous authority. "A woman's cancerous breast was totally extirpated and she seemed to be cured. Almost immediately, the other breast was attacked by cancer." Avicenna reasoned that the second breast had been attacked by the cancer before the first breast was removed, and the humors which had been deflected from it had flowed to the second side. I think that is a good explanation.

V. Avicenna (ibid.) and nearly all the authorities agree that the best treatment for an ulcerated cancer is to keep continuously in place a linen cloth saturated with the juice of morel and never to let it go dry and become warm; re-wet it as often as needed. Hippocrates seems to have had a contrary opinion (*Aphorisms,* Part 1). Avicenna later gave a another opinion (Bk. I, Fol. 4, Ch. 29, and Bk. IV Fol. 3). I believe that those two authorities meant that cold is not good when you are treating the ulcer itself, but it is good when you are trying to relieve pain.

When the pain is really severe, you should use narcotics.

VI. Here I give evidence for my claims that there are two kinds of melancholic humors. One derives from natural[22] black bile; it is called sclerotic, which means hard. We should not call it cancerous. The second derives from non-natural black bile. It is a melancholy which is no longer in its original state. It has been corrupted and burned. That is cancer, and the term itself connotes two types. One derives from

22 'Natural': Black bile from its first beginnings, not the product of the changed or burned humors which were not black bile at their beginnings (LDR).

the burnt black bile that has not undergone putrefaction during a long existence. That cancer remains unchanged; it does not ulcerate on its own, and it causes little harm. If by chance the overlying skin erodes, and it ulcerates, it does not enlarge because its substance does not putrefy.[23]

The second type derives from a more intensely burned and putrefied melancholy, which causes a cancer that usually does not ulcerate. In the course of time it may ulcerate, indicating different kinds of matter and different locations in the body and different lifestyles of the patients. This cancer exists in two forms. One derives from a natural melancholy that is the residue, the lees of the other humors.[24] It becomes the non-natural melancholy when it is burned. The other cancer derives from a non-natural melancholy which is made by burning other natural humors or their ashes, not their lees.

Now let us return to the first category, those formed from melancholy, that is, from putrefied and burnt lees. There are two types. One is formed from a more solid matter, the other from the more liquid (ie subtle). The first, coming from a feebler and unusual substance, is less malignant. It causes less damage and erodes less. The second type is more malignant because it derives from more invasive (ie biting) matter.

A cancer that derives from melancholic humors themselves (ie not the lees) which have been burned and then undergo a second combustion, and therefore are twice-burnt—they acquire evil properties for some reason and they become corrupt and putrefy—the cancer of such an origin is more damaging, more erosive and it does more harm to the patient. It is very hard to cure.

The medical authors describe all the ways that combustion and putrefaction happen, in the parts of their books where they discuss putrid and quartan fevers.

VII. Galen (*Techni*, Ch. 5) and Haly (ibid.) explain that there are two kinds of melancholic humors. One is the lees of other humors, the other is result of the combustion or the ashes of others, of salt-phlegm, blood, yellow bile. When they are burned they become melancholy. You can see it in a child who has a hot liver and large veins; when he becomes an adolescent, he burns his bile to form melancholy.[25]

VIII. Non-natural melancholy has two forms, putrefied and not putrefied.

The putrefied type has three varieties, a. One fills the great veins near the principal organs and accounts for the continuous quartan fever, b. Another is found in varying amounts in medium-size or small-caliber veins anywhere in the body. It provokes a quartan or a double fever.[26] c. The third is found in capillary veins or at their tips. They cause a cancerous aposthem.

There are two types of non-putrefied melancholy, a. One occurs only in soft tissues and causes leprosy, b. The other appears only in the skin. This variety has two classes. 1. One appears in all the body's skin and is called black jaundice. 2. The other is local. It causes black morphia, other dark spots and sometimes cancers, pustules, et al.

IX. Excoriations, inflammations (ie supercalefactions), small ulcers on the gums and on the penis,[27] all of which are shallow and recent, are not true cancers, in spite of what many authors, practitioners and common folk say. Instead, we call them corrosions (ie erosions). They do not fit any of our definitions

---

23 Mondeville struggles to explain benign neoplasia (LDR).

24 See Tr. III, Doct. I, Ch. 3 on Phlebotomy, on the examination of the layered blood-clot (LDR).

25 I can find no suitable interpretation of this statement. Perhaps Mondeville was explaining the behavior of the rebellious teenager in his own century (LDR).

26 This curious apposition of terms, 'quartan' and 'double', may confuse the modern reader. John Halle, a surgeon of the Elizabethan era (fl 1550), explained it nicely in his edition of Lanfranchi's *Chirurgia*. "Quarta febris is used either for an intermittent or, for an exquisite continuous fever called quartan continua. … It is rarely seen, and sometimes is known as daily fever." (abstracted from pp 92–93 of his Interpretive Table (ie Glossary), see our bibliography for Treatise V, The Antidotary (LDR).

27 Possibly herpes of the lips and the genitals (LDR).

of cancers, and they should not be treated as cancers in ways we have described in this chapter. Gentle treatments will suffice, as you will find them in the chapters devoted to the them.

X. The persons who believe that cancers simply are ulcers risk serious consequences First, when they cannot extirpate a cancer, they apply strong corrosives, such as used for ulcers, and they exacerbate the cancer. Second, when they really have an opportunity to extirpate a cancer, they use weak corrosives, too feeble to get into the cancer, and they just stimulate the growth of its roots. On the other hand, they who wrongly believe that an ulcer is a cancer make three grave errors. First they apply corrosives that are stronger than necessary, in too large amounts, as if they were treating cancers, and they cause needless suffering. Second, they destroy more tissue than is necessary. Third, they attract humors which make the ulcer itself erosive and cancerous.

XI. I am amazed at Avicenna's statement (ibid.) that a cancerous ulcer is no longer an ulcer after it has been cauterized with the hot iron, because that makes its surfaces thicker and tougher. That statement is contrary to our General Precepts that a cancer cannot be cured except by a radical extirpation. You should not make it worse with the use of the cautery. Therefore, when a cancerous ulcer has not been totally removed it continues to grow and the ulcer persists. Furthermore, I added this Precept: you cannot cure a cancer piecemeal. Rhazes *(Almansor,* Bk. VII) wrote, "When someone is unsuccessful in an attempt to cure a non-ulcerating cancer, he does nothing more than to convert what previously was curable into an incurable cancerous ulcer. He hastens the patient's death. And when he cannot completely remove a cancerous ulcer he leaves an ulcer which is not just a simple ulcer." My view is that Avicenna did not mean that a cancerous ulcer could stop being ulcerated, a statement contrary to his own teaching and that of the authorities who have dealt with cancer. Rather, he meant that after a cancer has been treated, a non-ulcerated cancer can grow at the same site, because the humors that formerly produced the ulcerated cancer continue to work.

XII. Avicenna (Bk. IV, Fol. 3, Ch. "on Leprosy") said that a cancer in a single place can be dealt with as if it was leprosy simply because it also is beyond cure. When you treat lepers with potent medications you do so to sustain the patient's spirits but you do not affect the lesions. That is not the case for cancers.[28]

XIII. Rhazes (*Almansor*, Bk. VII) wrote, "When you treat a cancer early in its course knowing that it is a cancer that has not ulcerated, perhaps it grows very little at first, and then over time it increases and ulcerates, that is a bad affair. If it impinges the respiratory passages it will lead to a day of anguish and terror and death." etc. And he added that such is a well known sign of incurability. And, further, when a cancer has grown larger, you should avoid heating it and causing it to spread inward as well as on the surface. In his book *(On Divisions)* he advises against the patient lying on his cancer when he is in bed.

XIV. All the authorities and all the books and all the practitioners agree that the sublimate of arsenic is the corrosive of choice for treating a curable cancer; it is very potent and can be precisely placed to corrode more at one time than other corrosives do in two. If need be, it can be attenuated for use in a less aggressive cancer, or for use in a nerve-bearing or sensitive region, or near noble organs, or in debilitated or delicate patients, in hot seasons and in hot countries. Grind it and mix it with guimauve, juice of plantain, et al. (ie to attenuate it).[29]

XV. More about the established methods (the Artificial): Consider here certain empirical facts, as we often do. Many items are thought to be empirical by some people simply because they have no ready explanations for them, and the same items are said to be part of a surgeon's (artificial) armamentarium by those professionals who can offer rationales. The *Aphorisms* of Urso[30] give rational explanations for

28 Where you direct your attention at the lesion (LDR).

29 This seems to contradict Mondeville's statements that one can cure a cancer only by a radical extirpation (LDR).

30 Urso of Calabria, fl. @1150, A physician and philosopher at Salerno (LDR).

things that commonly are accepted as unproved, such as why a magnet attracts iron and why a red shield placed over a deeply submerged cadaver in a stream will resist the flow and remain motionless, and reveal the location of the body which could not be found in other ways. In his *Aphorisms* we can find explanations for many things that seem even more astonishing, where the common folk have beliefs and fears, and the savants can identify specific causes.

XVI. In our chapter on empirics we mentioned the medications in the small sacks hung about the necks, etc. We questioned the usefulness of some of them, as testified by Constantine in his book *(Incantations, Magic, Sorcerers, Evil-doers, Remedies Suspended From Necks and Other Parts of the Body).* He offers proofs from authorities, citing Aristotle, and Medical authors. Avicenna (Bk. II, Ch. on Coral), said that Galen hung coral over the outlet of the stomach (ie epigastrium) to treat severe pain, and the pain subsided at once, only to return when he removed the coral, and to ease again when the coral was replaced. He tells of many marvelous experiences with coral and he describes other empirics used successfully in certain desperate cases in which all the standard prescriptions had failed. Therefore, Constantine supported the proposition held by the ancient philosophers, that the vital force (ie virtue) of the spirit controls (modifies) the body. The statements of The Savants prove it. Plato wrote, "When the human spirit believes that something will avail it, a thing that itself offers no benefits, it becomes useful; simply by its effects on the imagination it will help the body. In the same way, something felt to be harmful will do harm, because the complexion of the body befits the virtue of the spirit. That is why, when a physician stirs the spirit of his patient with incantations and the like, and he offers great assurances while he treats the patient's body with suitable medicines, he hastens the cure." Do the incantations etc. have any direct therapeutic effects? We seek answers from Constantine (ibid.) and Ovid *(Ars Amatopia).* The latter wrote, "Whoever asks for help from our Art, extends his faith to include magical beverages and incantations."

The fact that stimulating the spirit also stirs the body is illustrated in the following. Anyone who tries to walk on a narrow rail will fall if he thinks that it will happen, but when that is not on his mind, he will succeed. Similarly, after a bad fall, some will escape while others will die, even without obvious injuries, as I once saw happen at Paris. A man and his friends met someone on the Marmoset Street, and he said to his friends, "Do you see at that fellow? He thinks that I detest him enough to kill him, although I really don't dislike him at all, but I am going to cast some fear into him without touching him." He drew his sword and made a powerful thrust at the fellow, but did not touch him, and the man immediately fell dead.

Treatise III: Chapter 2: On Cauteries

Their Necessary And Elective Uses Where The Skin Is Intact Including Removal Of Excrescences And Draining Aposthems Anywhere In The Body According To The Arts Of Medicine And Surgery

As indicated in the title of this chapter, we will exclude the applications of cauteries which are not surgical. Our concern is with the metallic instruments and substances such as cantharides (ie vesicants) and eruptors. We shall exclude the treatment of plethoric persons who have not had preliminary purgation and healthy persons who have nothing special to prevent and no diseased matter to evacuate, who simply want a cauterization as a passing fancy. We exclude cauterization as follow-up (ie touch up) measures for healed wounds, ulcers, cancers, fistulas etc in whom some skin had been lost. And, finally, we exclude cases where superficial growths have been extirpated or aposthems have subsided without need for open drainage. We will deal with those topics elsewhere in special sections. Here we shall limit ourselves to the use of metallic cauteries, cantharides and other caustics when they have definite artificial indications.[31]

Five General Items

A. The Description: Four Points

1. Definitions: A Cautery is an instrument for special surgical procedures, which is beneficial for preventing certain maladies in predisposed persons, for palliating and for curing maladies already in effect. We will name them as we come to them. To cauterize, to burn, to cook and to 'filet' as the peasants say, are four terms with the same meaning. To cauterize is to burn or to cook and to filet. The last suggests (ie as a pun) the need for prolonged diligent surgical care, as if he treated his own daughter, 'fille'.
2. The Two Varieties: The Actual Cauteries are metallic, iron or other, instruments that are hot enough to burn tissues. The Potential Cauteries are medicaments: A simple such as cantharides or a Compound such as various emptors. They are not intrinsically hot nor are they heated for use, but they have an innate burning quality.
3. Similarities and Differences: They are alike in that both are destructive, and both burn, evacuate and consume. There are other minor similarities. They differ in that an actual cautery causes less damage; heat is a simple element and its effects are manifest only when its virtue is transmitted directly to a material substance. It works more rapidly and its injurious quality disappears more quickly. Its action is at the place of contact and does not extend beyond the member in which it is used. Because it has no distant effects, it does not attract humors from other parts of the body.[32] It can be applied in all kinds of weather and at any season, especially when the patient has acute pain, and in all sorts of ailments with all kinds of complexions, and the surgeon weighs all the factors and excludes some cases such as certain hot illnesses in which there is nothing to drain.

As I say, it can be used in any weather and at any time of the day in all maladies caused by humors that have not yielded to other measures. The cautery may be applied as a last resource, as stated by Rhazes (*Albucasis*, Bk, I, Ch. 1). We apply the iron after all other medicines have failed. Rhazes continued, saying that the 'any time, anywhere' tenet held if other circumstances permitted it. That is, the benefits of the cautery are greatest when the chosen time is correct, especially when you use it to relieve intolerable pain.

The Potential Cautery produces a large lesion because its effects are not immediate; some time is needed for it to do its work. The natural heat of a region has been activated and it waits for the burning potential of the medication to take effect. Thus there is a prolonged conflict between the body's spirit and the burning power of the medicine applied on it. That combat weakens the forces of Nature. As Galen said (*de Ingenio,* Bk. Ill, Ch. 1, and *Aphorisms,* Part 5) suffering attracts humors from the entire body toward the source. In that way the distant parts suffer by depletion and the cauterized region becomes an inflamed mass (ie an aposthem). Furthermore, the lesion caused by the caustic endures; the painful

31 'artificial' means 'according to the art of surgery', that is, according to the Rules (EN).
32 Mondeville contradicts this statement later, when he describes diverting cauterizations (LDR).

local inflammation cannot just be waved away. All caustics have some venomous qualities, and the evil residues linger in the body.

4. Comparing the Two Types: three items:
   a. Actual versus Potential Cauteries: From what I have stated above and from what follows you will conclude that the actual cautery is favored as more reliable and easier to use. I offer ten reasons: 1. It is less destructive. 2. The burn heals more rapidly. 3. It is less attractive of humors. 4. It does not harm structures at a distance from the primary lesion. 5. It is useful in more kinds of disorders. 6. It leaves behind no venomous residue. 7. We can terminate the burning simply by removing the cautery which we control with our hands. We are more precise in directing the instrument. 8. Thanks to the forego-ing we can also control the intensity of the application. That is not possible with the potential cautery; after it has been applied, it is on its own. 9. When we cauterize to stop bleeding from large veins we must be aware that the eschar will come away sometime later and the hemorrhage may resume. In such a case we can reapply the hot cautery, but we dare not reapply the caustics. 10. According to Rhazes (ibid.) the potential cautery often creates an incurable lesion, such as a lethal cancerous ulcer, whereas that never happens when we use the actual cautery.
   b. Comparing the various kinds of cauteries: We take counsel from the authorities: Rhazes (idem. Ch. 2), Avicenna (Bk. II, Fol. 4, Ch. 29) and other illustrious writers all agree that the finest instruments are made of Gold. Then come the silver and then the iron and the steel. All other things being equal, the gold is chosen because it has the most temperate complexion and is more pure than silver. Silver is better than iron for the same reasons. That which is more temperate and more pure causes less damage. However, we cannot assess the degree of heat in the gold and silver instruments because their colors do not change when they are heated. On the other hand, iron changes from black to white. All cauteries function only when they are hot enough, but when gold and silver are too hot they bend and they melt. Furthermore, they cool rapidly when they are removed from the fire. On the other hand, the iron cautery retains its heat and retains its shape. For all these reasons and with concerns for the inconveniences, I generally prefer the iron cautery. However, if, by chance an expert with gold and silver can provide the properly heated cauteries we can avoid some of the defects and use them. But, all in all, the iron cautery is the most trustworthy,
   c. Comparing the potential cauteries. In some cases the emptors are better than vesicants (cantharides), in other cases the opposite is true.[33] The eruptors are preferred when we wish to attract humors from distant regions and attract bad humors to the surface, with a long-acting effect. After the eschar comes loose and the abscess is evacuated, the drainage wound can be kept open for a long time. Eventually a firm, dry, thick and dark scar forms.

Cantharides is better when we want only to attract from beneath the skin, not from deeper tissues. It has a more rapid action and it does not form a crust; an excoriation remains after the blister breaks. Those lesions drain suddenly and release watery matter and they do not have to be kept open. They usually heal within six days.

33 Eruptors and cantharides: Some intensely caustic substances eat their way through the skin and cause the underlying collections of pus to burst through, hence 'eruptor'. Cantharides, or the Spanish Fly was an irritating vesicant, blistering the surface of the skin. More detail is given in the Antidotary. (LDR).

How To Use Cauteries

The Actual Cautery: Nine General Principles

1. Before using the cautery, especially if the patient is plethoric, evacuate the patient with purges, bleeds, etc., and apply all the proper topicals, ointments, etc.[34]
2. The operator must know the anatomy, the numbers, the location, the complexions and the functions of the site he will cauterize, as well as know the causes, the complications and the duration of the illness of the entire region in which he will cauterize. In some cases he will recognize that the cautery rarely will be of value.
3. In cases where persisting pain has not yielded to treatment with properly used evacuations and topicals, the actual cautery usually will work well after the necessary preliminaries are carried out.
4. Never use a cautery on a patient who is well filled with healthy humors before carrying out a proper phlebotomy, and until he has abstained from wine, and you have not observed improvement. The good humors usually are sanguinous and the phlebotomy and the abstinence are useful. Unless you follow those precepts, your cautery may do harm (see William of Saliceto, Bk. V, Ch. l).[35]
5. In fleshy tissues the cautery easily can penetrate too deeply. In nervous tissues and in places rich in arteries and veins, as at the elbow and in the popliteal region, you should press no deeper than the skin. If a cautery touches a nerve it will cause a contraction, and if it touches a large artery or vein it will provoke a hemorrhage.
6. If some of the old harmful matter persists in the body after an evacuation, apply the cautery on the knob in the hollow just below the knee (ie head of the fibula). If the malady persists in only one part of the body, apply the cautery in the hollow below but near the affected organ.
7. Even when properly used, the result of the cauterization may be less than satisfactory. When it is successful you need not repeat an applicadon. However, if the application and the purges and the topicals all had been used correctly and the patient is no better off than he was before the treatments, repeat the cauterization. Hippocrates (*Aphorisms*, Part 2) wrote, "Do everything reasonable". After the second applications always prescribe a rich diet with good wine until the depleted vital forces have recovered. Then repeat the purge once or twice and repeat the cauterization and prescribe a diet containing foods that are contrary to the cause of the ailment. Repeat this routine several times if necessary, until the patient is completely cured. Remember, a persistent drip of water can erode a rock!

   When the initial treatment is partially effective, you can be confident that the malady is curable if you persist and follow the established rules. Reapply the cautery in the fontanelle (ie the hollow) where you had the initial success, or in another favorable place.
8. Comparing the actual and the potential cauteries: Never use a caustic if you can find another way to do what is necessary and is tolerable for the patient. If he is not cowardly nor unwilling to accept the hot instrument, and he has a very cool and moist complexion, use it. A caustic, which by its very nature has a poisonous complexion, will inflame and corrupt the complexion of the region where it is applied, especially when it meets up with a potent contrary which is very cool and very moist, and when it is applied during the winter. The place for the application of a caustic should not be near a principal organ in the torso, or near the heart.

34 See footnote 299, Tr. II, Doct. I, Ch. 2 (LDR).

35 Chapters 1, 2 and 9 of William's Book V are devoted to Cauteries. Most of that material, in turn, came from Albucasis' book on Surgical Instruments. William. was a teacher of Lanfi-anchi, who taught Mondeville. (LDR).

9. In consequence if the foregoing, we conclude that the actual cautery is better suited for treating ailments caused by hot dry humors, and we never should use the potential cautery in patients with those complexions with those ailments. After it has destroyed the bad substances its actions continue and its lingering effects are harmful in a body with a warm and dry complexion.

B. The Techniques For Using Actual Cauteries: Two Items

1. The Instruments in Common Use: Rhazes (*Albucasis*)[36] described the many shapes and varieties; William of Saliceto listed six; Lanfranchi gave ten. They and others described what each had found useful in his day-to-day practices, but they did not describe the cauteries for special cases. That is not surprising, because every day we encounter new cases that call for novel instruments and new ways to use them. The types which they recommend for surgeons are those we should have ready-made and at hand keeping one or more suitable to the case, adding or eliminating some of them, or exchanging all of them for the special kinds we will need as we antipate it. You cannot put all of that in a book. Really, one can ridicule the idea that everything good already has been invented and that there is no room for anything new. Damascenus (*Aphorisms*, II, Part 3) said, "Native genius enhances our Art, and vice versa."

The surgeon can and should vary his instruments to suit his intentions, and to befit the anatomy of the parts he will treat.

Seven types of cautery have been in common use from ancient times until the present:

a. The Nut (ie node), used by the barbers and the untrained rustic operators. Usually, they put a perforated cold metal plaque on the place they will treat—sometimes they will substitute a piece of thick shoe-leather with a perforation—and they introduce the hot 'nut;' through the hole. That serves three purposes: a. It keeps the hot nut from slipping away from the desired spot. b. It avoids burning the nearby tissues, c. A pin or cuff near the tip will be stopped by the plaque and prevent the tip from burning too deeply into the subcutaneous tissues, (see No. 17, p. 524).

b. The Seton Cautery (Nos 19–23). You pinch a fold of skin and subcutaneous tissues with the special perforated tenaculum, with holes set over the place you will cauterize. Push the red hot needle through the holes, and quickly pull it out and insert a cold threaded needle. The thread will remain as a seton after you knot the ends, and it will keep open the cautery tract as long as you wish it.

c. The Round-Tip makes a slightly deeper burn. In other words, it cauterizes through the skin when you treat a lesion near a nerve. It burns at either end, with a large or a small tip.

d. A Pointed or Needle Tip makes very small burns, as after the extraction of hairs to prevent regrowth. You bend it to the angle you need.

e. Some make oblong burns, often large and deep. They are the Cutters, the Olivaries and the Tongue-like instruments, all with at least one cutting edge (Nos. 14, 15, 16).

f. Some cauteries have a Rod or a flat Blade at the end. You heat it and insert it through a cold tube to avoid burning the surrounding tissues when you insert it to burn only with the tips, as in treating within the nose or mouth. (Nos. 18, 18a, 18b).

36 Rhazes and Albucasis: see fn 234, Notable XIII, in Tr. II, Doct. I, and the Bibliography in the Engl. Translator's Introduction Vol. I (LDR).

g. One is called the Circular or Dactylary cautery, because it is a flat disc to which are attached several prongs (ie like bent fingers)[37], one in the center and several attached to the circumference. The projections are heated and applied through the perforations in a cold metal plate which is made to fit the dactyls (No. 24), allowing the surgeon to apply them easily and accurately. The cold plate protects the surrounding skin. This instrument is most often used in treating pain in the hips and buttocks.

2. How To Cauterize With These Instruments

First gently palpate with the balls of your finger-tips and mark the spot for the application with red ink. If you use a perforated plate set the opening over the red spot. Hold the plate firmly in place and tell the patient to look away while your assistant hands you the red-hot cautery. Insert it for as long as necessary. The cautery may be used without the plate.

3. When, Where And What To Do After The Burn

Immediately apply a mitigative ointment, such as lard or butter or some medication that will ease the pain and comfort the patient. After it has subsided, apply suppuratives such as rancid lard or bitter porridges such as contain liver-wort and the like, until the eschar sloughs. Then put a small green pea in the defect and press it in. Later, after removing the pea, fill the defect with a pill of ivy-wood or similar, a bit larger than the pea. Leave it in until pus appears at the edge of the defect. Then begin a twice-daily change of dressings, gently wiping the area dry with a linen cloth before covering it with a folded (about twelve plies) cloth pad, atop which you lay on some leaves of ivy, oxalis or grape-vine. Place over all a disc of gold or silver or copper metal, or, even better, of sole-leather which you can lace in place with a strip of raw-hide. This will protect the cauterized site from further injury.

The burn wound should drain pus for exactly three months, unless there is a good reason to change the rule. If it drains beyond that time, one of two disturbances, or both, may occur. First, after the essence of the burn has evaporated, the open wound will attract all sorts of humors, good as well as bad, mostly watery liquids. That will revive the pain of the cauterization.[38] Second, there will be a chronic discharge from the wound which the patient cannot bear, and the surgeon cannot stop. He will not be able to discontinue his care of the patient as soon as he may wish, and, even if he is allowed to do so, he would not dare to. As Master Arnold of Villanova said, a very old wound should not be allowed to close lest a serious complication appear. That is, the chronic drainage of humors will no longer find a means of escape unless there is another wound nearby. That is why one should not prolong the procedure beyond the time when the cauterization loses its burning and consumptive quality and its virtue, unless there is a strong reason. Then no longer is it a cauterization, it has become an ulcer.

Rather than useful, it is harmful, except in two instances. First, when the overload of bad humors is too great for the cauterization to eliminate during the usual limited term, and the patient is too cowardly to permit you to make another burn nearby. In such a case, I prefer to keep open the draining ulcer rather than dam back the superfluidities. Second, the draining ulcer may be kept open in a person who had practiced hygienic phlebotomies.[39] In such a case, a chronic ulcer as well as an over-due cauterization may be useful in treating a chronic fistula which had not been cured with other measures.

When the cauterization has been concluded, we must let the wound close by itself, using no surgical measures other than pruning away excessive granulation tissues to allow a scar to form.

---

37 No. 17 is labeled 'pointed' but corresponds to Mondeville's 'Nut'. with its stop-pin The instrument and its perforated plate is labeled 'clactylaiy'. What is called 'round' in the text corresponds to Appendix I, Item D in Wm. of Saliceto's Plate 1. The names in Mondeville's text should be used as translated here, whereas the Figures which are taken from Guy de Chauliac's text as written fifty years later see Vol. I. Appendix I (LDR).

38 Edema and cellulitis (LDR).

39 Who is familiar with the procedure (LDR).

Therefore, when it is conducted properly, whether or not it has been partly or entirely successful, and when the hoped for cure has not yet been attained, you may repeat the procedure if there has been some sign of improvement, as we stated in the seventh rule. If the goals of the treatment have been attained, there is no need to repeat. If a good result is not complete, you will do well to repeat the cauterization.

When the initial site was not a good one and the patient had suffered excessively, go to a nearby spot, in the same fontanelle or in another close to it, where you should have burned in the first place.

Sometimes, you may go to an altogether different region when a repeated cauterization is deemed necessary.

Treatise III: Chapter 3: Phlebotomy

The Therapeutic Diminution Of Blood, Useful and Necessary For The Body, As It Should Be Practiced In Individual Cases, According To The Art Of Medicine and Surgery[40]

Phlebotomy is a medical measure that uses a surgical operation. A physician determines the need and the surgeon carries it out; both of them have the same goal, the health of the patient. Long ago the physicians ceased doing it themselves as beneath their dignity, so they say, and ceded it to the surgeons. More recently, the surgeons have ceded the operation to barbers, with two excuses. 1. It does not pay well. 2. It requires little skill. For these two reasons and others: 3. Today, few people other than those with surgical ailments seek a surgeon's recommendations about when to bleed. Most of those are well-to-do, or part of the nobility or are prelates in the care of physicians. The common folk put themselves in the hands of the barbers. Since all the medical and surgical hand-books deal with phlebotomy in great detail, I simply will briefly review the subject in this chapter, and I will include a summary of the indications given by other authors. If you seek more complete information go to the authors whom I will cite below and to the chapters noted there.

I will consider thirteen issues here: 1. The definition. 2. The uses and its effects. 3. For whom it is suitable, and for whom it is not. 4. Certain General Principles. 5. Which veins to use, and for what ailments. 6. The qualifications required of a good phlebotomist. 7. The proper timing. 8. Preparing the patient. 9. How to phlebotomize. 10. The care after the bleed. 11. Examining the shed blood. 12. Precautions. 13. Explanations of obscure points.

I. Definitions

A bleed is the therapeutic removal of a small amount of blood from veins and arteries. It really serves the purpose of a General Evacuation to rid the patient of a multitude of humors. The definitions, all and parts, are well known and need no explanation and amplification beyond what is found in the hand-books.

II. The Uses And The Benefits

We bleed for three purposes: l. To preserve health. 2. To prevent illness. 3. To treat maladies already in effect. The first two have elective bleeds, the third is a necessity.

40 See Ch. 1 of this Doct., Part I On Incisions, and Fig. 16 (LDR).

The time for the elective as well as the necessary, and other related matters are taken up in Chapter 1 of this Doctrine I. As stated there we have six uses for phlebotomies: l. To evacuate blood and humors that are offensive in quantity and quality or both. 2. To induce distraction or a separation of humors such as when you treat an abscess you bleed from the opposite side to divert the bad humors from the aposthem by attracting them to he site of the bleed. 3. Simply to attract the bad matter, as when you bleed from a saphenous vein to attract blood to the womb and induce menstruation. 4. To modify some humors, as when you bleed because we sense that the blood in the veins is too hot. 5. To prevent certain disorders that are suspect or threatening. 6. To lighten Nature's burden and improve its curative powers.

III. Indications and Contraindications; Two Parts

A. When Bleeding Is Not Indicated, 6 causes: 1. Factors relevant to the Causative Humors: Too dense, too thin, too viscous, too adherent, too cool, too lumpy, too watery. For example, if the matter is too dense, the bleed will attract only the liquid parts and will leave behind an even thicker residue. The other features will reveal the objections and you will draw your own conclusions. 2. When the patient's vital force is feeble, a bleed will deplete it even more. 3. Certain aspects of the disease itself: here are three negative reasons: a. When the causative humor is poisonous or violent, as in anthrax. b. When the pus already is too abundant, as in quinsy. c. When the lesion is very serious, as an injured or inflamed eye. 4. When complications take effect, and the bad humors suddenly are disturbed. When Nature already is fully occupied in defeating the illness and has enough to do to digest the pus and evacuate it. A phlebotomy at that time will distract Nature and the illness may prevail. 5. Certain elements in the Complexion: the air, the lifestyle the geographic region, the weather, the customary use and disposition of the body (ie vigor, robustness, etc.). All the foregoing deter you from bleeding lest you further enfeeble the vital force. For example, a melancholic complexion is a sign of anemia, and the same holds for phlegmatic humors. One easily can review the other features and find more information in the works of other authors. 6. Certain conditions affecting the stomach and other internal organs. If the patient has overeaten or is anoretic, or if he is constipated or has diarrhea, you need no help to understand why you should not bleed, or why it is not necessary (ie to bleed an already 'evacuated' patient).

Children younger than nine years should not be bled excepting in some urgent circumstances such as when they are suffocating due to an excess of blood as in quinsy. Even then, the physician must not be rigid; he must leave the final decision to the parents and friends. Old folks who are slipping into the decline of their dotage, after age seventy, especially if they are not robust; convalescents who have passed the critical phases of their illnesses; pregnant women, especially during the first and thirds trimesters; young but washed-out people with small and hard-to-see veins and scanty beards; those with clumped humors and scanty blood. All those persons should not be bled; let them treasure their limited supply.

The same policy will exclude persons who have been poisoned—internally or externally; those who have early cataracts and dropsy, excepting those with amenorrhea or hemorrhoids. Exclude women during their menses and persons who are obese (ie difficult veins) and who have recovered from colic or from vomiting, lest you attract bile into their stomachs. Exclude those who have recovered after another evacuation, or after long spells of insomnia and after a spell of hard labor. Exclude those with delicate stomachs and livers who often fall prey to cool maladies. There are many more conditions that you will encounter.

B. When Phlebotomies Are Indicated:.We bleed patients who suffer from recurring abscesses and boils, from anthrax, fevers and overindulgence with meats and cheeses and wine and sweets, and those who are idle and foppish, and those who eat too much broiled food and then generate too much blood and those who drink too much heavy wine, and those who have too much melancholic blood, that is, the red humors which accompany blood as it flows through the body, and those in whom you suspect there may be an internal overheating (ie combustion) of humors and the like, or who may have an inflammation on the surface of the body accompanied by a fever, and in those who may have had a prolonged course of treatment of a malady during the warm seasons, and those with strong vital spirits and a sanguinous complexion and who grow bushy hair. We include those who suffer gout and other kinds of inflamed joints, and those with paroxysms that occur with sanguinous disorders, who have continuous fevers and large inflamed internal or external masses or pleurisy or buboes, and those who suffer spasms of repletion and various similar maladies.

IV. Precepts Taken From Older Treatises

A. We bleed for one of three reasons: to preserve health, to forestall an illness and to treat it.

B. All therapeutic (ie 'artificial') bleeds aim to reduce an excess of sanguinous humors or remove it if is defective, or both.[41]

C. When you bleed during the springtime months, take special care to avoid collapse of the patient.

D. Victims of torture, flagellation, rackings with body blows should be bled immediately, using standard methods, to prevent aposthems from appearing (ie hematomas becoming abcesses).

E. You will have more success if you bleed a person to prevent a suspected illness than if you wait for it to develop fully. That is, bleed at the very onset when the humors are in flux toward the site of the malady and are well mixed with healthy blood, before the malady is fully under way. Later, when the signs indicate that the sick humors are already being digested, after the stage of evolution has passed, you may bleed even then, using our standard techniques.

F. When the sick humors already are agitated (ie but not yet digested) and on the move, withhold the bleed lest you make matters worse by impeding the Natural process of digestion of the bad humors.

G. When the malady is past the stable state, discontinue your phlebotomies. However, when you think it is worthwhile, you may use small bleeds which do not deplete the patient. For the same reason, you should not bleed during the cool months of fall and winter.

H. Diversive bleeds, that is from the opposite side, will most often succeed in arresting the flow of the humors to the site of the disease.

I. Avoid bleeding when it is very cold or very hot, and soon after coitus.

J. Repeated small bleeds are better than a single large one. When the arm you have used for those bleeds is inflamed, use the other arm and apply naturally cool topicals, which you have warmed, to the inflamed arm.

K. When you bleed from a cephalic vein do not repeat too often at the same site lest you cause an inflammation.

L. Bleeding from the index finger-thumb web is good for illnesses of the liver and the diaphragm, Galen advises it.

M. When you bleed for ailments in which sanguinous humors predominate do it as you would for other humoral maladies. Bleeding evacuates all humors, and if the cause is only sanguinous, bleeding alone is a sufficient treatment. When other humors also are involved, bleed as appropriate for the affected part as well as to evacuate the body as a whole.

N. Scrawny persons are more liable to faint during a phlebotomy because they have less blood.

---

41 Normal venous blood consists mostly of sanguinous humor, carrying with it various amounts of each of the other three (LDR).

O. You should not bleed when there are signs of repletion (ie spasms) or when raw humors are in excess (ie an undrained abscess affecting nerves).

P. When you have to bleed in those cases, they should bathe beforehand or take exercise or take some relaxant.

Q. In weak patients, use several small bleeds rather than a single large one.

R. A bleed through a small incision removes more of the thin part of the blood and leaves behind the thicker. That is better for the summer months. A larger incision is favored for the winter when it is serves better to sap the vitality. A major bleed from a large opening is suitable only when the vitality is energetic, when the blood is thicker as during the cold months. Smaller incisions are suited when the opposite conditions prevail.[42]

S. Even when it may seem unnecessary, you may bleed to treat certain fevers, to enhance the patient's vital forces in their action to get rid of the residues of the bad humors and cure the ailment.

T. Always obey the 'two diameter rule' as Avicenna insisted (Bk. I, Fol. 4, Ch. 3.)[43]

U. Bleed only after you know the correct diagnosis.

V. Bleed when the veins are distended with blood, before the blood becomes corrupted, against established medical principles as stated above.

W. You may bleed at any time in an acute situation, even when you may impair the patient's own natural forces which are digesting the bad matter.

X. Do not bleed when the patient is constipated or when the air is windless and heavy (humid).

Y. Use the cephalic vein for conditions of repletion in the head and neck. Use the basilic vein for repletions below the neck. For ordinary repletions use the median vein. The exceptions are cases when another vein is selected by the referring physician.

Z. It is unwise or harmful to bleed for cool and dry ailments and further deplete the patient's blood.

AA. Galen said *(Megatechni,* Bk. XIV, Ch. 3) that after the bleed have the patient sleep for two hours.

BB. If the veins are full, the blood may putrefy if you do not evacuate it.

CC. Bleed when an overabundance of humors causes putrefaction.

DD. Bleed a febrile patient on the first day, at the latest on the fifth clay. If you wait until the seventh you will create a crisis.

EE. Bleed a patient who harbors an aposthem. Nature then can combust and digest and get rid of the residue after the bleed.

FF. A disorder with several humors at fault should be treated by bleeding. When only one humor is at fault, purges alone will be sufficient.

GG. A phlebotomy is better than a purge when treating pleurisy, and it cannot do harm.

HH. Phlebotomy is the best treatment for ailments caused by blood-born humors.

JJ. Even when the humors are in the large veins, a phlebotomy (ie which uses small veins) can get rid of some of them.

V. The Selection of Veins and Arteries for Bleeding

Before proceeding, let us review these facts. Veins of all sizes derive from the kylous (the many-branched) vein as the trunk of a tree which comes up from the roots gives off many branches, as we described it in our Anatomy. Among the many veins are the few that we commonly use for phlebotomies (see Chapters 6 and 12 and Fig. 5 in Treatise I).

---

42 The temperature and other elements are more fully discussed in Section VII of this chapter (LDR).

43 Bleed from an opposite side or the opposite half (upper or lower) but do not cross both diameters (LDR).

In each arm there are three veins used for most phlebotomies: 1. The Cephalic Vein is opened in two places: at the elbow and in the web between the thumb and the index finger, near the base. Bleeds from that vein treat warm affections of the head and the neck. Bleeds from the web are preferred and are more effective (by weakening the patient) for disorders of the head, yet they are not dangerous or subject to error (ie missed by the phlebotome). 2. The Basilic Vein (hepatic) is opened on the inner side of the elbow-crease and between the small finger and the auricular finger[44] on the dorsum of the hand, and in between, in the forearm. The bleeds are for treating all cool maladies of the body below the clavicles. It is useful in preventing disorders of the head. Use the right hand for disorders of the liver and the left for the spleen. 3. The Median Vein derives from branches from the other two. It also is called the Cardiac, the Purple, the Brown and the Black Vein. It lies centered in the elbow fold. One bleeds here to treat maladies anywhere in the body, but especially those of the heart and the chest.

Bleed from a vein on the forehead for illnesses of the rear of the head to divert the bad humors and as curative measures for illnesses in the front of the head. Sometimes we use it to treat delirium, and for chronic disorders of the head it is better than the other three evacuative measures.[45] A bleed from this vein near the vertex of the scalp is good for treating ulcers of the scalp, saffati and tinea. Use the blood to rub on the tineas while it still is warm.

Bleed from the arteries as well as the veins on the temples to treat migraine and ocular disorders. It adds support to other treatments in preventing recurrences. Sometimes, after a bleed you may apply a hot cautery or a corrosive topical to keep open the wound.

The veins beneath the cars (ie external jugulars) are useful against pustules on the scalp and for migraine. Veins just between or beneath the nostrils are useful against delirium and other maladies of the head. The sublingual veins up front near the teeth are used for treating quinsy, tonsillitis, throat disorders, acute and hot inflammations of the eyes, itching, pustules of the nose, scotomas and vertigo. In such cases first bleed from a cephalic vein.

Bleed from veins on the inner surface of the lips to treat small ulcers and pustules in the mouth (ie aphthous), gingivitis and the defects after dental extractions. Use a vein between the chin and the lower lip to treat halitosis.

The guide veins (ie external jugulars) are useful against leprosy and suffication due to congestion of neck veins.

Bleed from the large vein on the inner surface of the thigh about one foot above the knee, which feeds the entire leg and fills the varices and causes stasis ulcers (ie mal-mort). It will treat all those maladies. To stop bleeding from that site insert a small pill of sublimated arsenic or similar into the phlebotomy. It will corrode the vein and form a kind of flesh in the opening, but will not shut off the vein itself.

Bleed from a vein in the popliteal hollow to treat disorders of the uterus or to induce menstruation.

The Saphenous Vein between the ankle and the heel is bled for uterine problems in women and for ailments of the testicles, groins and penis in men. Corresponding to this vein on the lateral surface of the foot is the Sciatic Vein which is very good for treating pain in the upper thighs and sciatica which extends from the hip to the toenails. Also, it is useful for internal disorders of the kidneys and nearby organs within the body and on the surface. Bleeds from both the saphenous and the sciatic veins have been used for delirium.

Bleed from a vein between the fourth and fifth toes to treat salt phlegm, stasis ulcer (mal-mort), cancer, esthiomene and all kinds of melancholic disorders of the legs.

---

44 This conflicts with the classical terminology: the little finger is auricularis (for cleaning the ear!); the fourth is the ring finger, annularis; the middle finger, impudicus, is the signal of contempt; the first finger is index; the thumb is pollex. (LDR).

45 Laxatives, clysters, cauterizations (LDR).

I know a Parisian physician who is unusual only with his experiences using certain difficult treatments with which he has claimed miraculous cures. He bleeds from the same single vein in patients whom he personally knows, and always had bled (ie hygienic) when they were in good health. He believes that, whenever they are sick, Nature will send the faulty humors to the same spot where the customary bleeds had been made, and nowhere else.

VI. The Necessary Qualifications For A Phlebotomist[46]

He should be of middle-age, have sturdy limbs and steady hands. His eyesight should be good so he can identify the veins commonly used for phlebotomy and recognize arteries and the nerves that lie beneath them so he can avoid them. He must not bleed a sick person unless that has been requested by a physician or a credited surgeon. Nor should he bleed a child or a domestic or other kind of servant, nor the mistress of the house without her husband's permission, especially if he is a rich or famous or noble person. He should own a good supply of sharp, clean and polished lancets with narrow blades set at angles of various degrees. He must be able to use all of them skillfully, as suited for each case. He should profess himself to be as skillful in the procedure as any other, or at least state that one cannot find another phlebotomist as capable as himself because he then will be trusted above others. He should make that claim before performing the phlebotomy and other simple and commonly performed operations. In that way the patient's imagination and confidence will help, and will assure success without doing any harm.

VII. The Timing

A bleed may be scheduled (ie elective) or be required on short notice (ie necessary). I explained those terms in Chapter 1 On Incisions.

The elective bleed aims to preserve and conserve health. It is performed at the wish of the patient during the spring and autums because the weather is more temperated in those seasons. That is what Hippocrates prescribed (*Aphorisms*, Part 6.) The precise time is determined by several factors. For example, when you are concerned that the humors will putrefy more than showing a few bubbles[47], then bleed early in the spring. When the opposite is the case do it later in the season. Many other things are involved in that decision, subjects for the surgeon to judge. If the temperature is rising, wait for a north wind, preferably during the morning. But if the day is cool, bleed while there is a southerly breeze, toward noontime. At what epoch or age or during what phase of the moon? The four phases of lunation are known to all: The first quarter belongs to springtime and adolescence. The second phase is warm and dry and is associated with summertime. The third is cool and dry and associates with autumn and age. The fourth is cool and moist and is tied with winter and senility. Therefore, since Nature rules and the physician is only the servant, so it is that young girls want normal menstruation during the moon's first quarter, young women want it during the second, mature women during the third and older women during the fourth, just so do we decide in prescribing phlebotomies, taking into account the patient's age and the quarter of the moon. That is what the Poet (ie Ovid) meant when he said, "The old moon needs old people, the new moon needs youths, and the middle-aged moon wants middle-aged people. That is how women purge themselves."

46 Here it is clear that Mondeville is instructing lay practitioners and barbers (LDR).

47 The appearance of the blood spilled into the collecting dish (LDR).

As to the time of day, Avicenna (Bk. I, Fol. 4, Ch. 'On Phlebotomy') said that when we bleed to evacuate blood (ie sanguinous humors) do so from early in the third hour (9 A.M.) to the end of the fifth. Others have said to wait until a meal has been digested and the bowels have been emptied and the weather is most temperate. Therefore, we should bleed when we are near the time when the blood is moving, that is, between sunrise until the third hour, because a humor in motion is more easily evacuated.

If we wish to evacuate blood that is bilious, we should bleed between the first and the ninth hours. For melancholic blood, do it between the ninth hour and evening, and the same for phlegm.

As to the day itself, some recommend that we follow the Egyptian calendar (see Guy de Chauliac, p. 566), where some clays are excluded.[48] I have five good reasons why that choice is unwise, a. The plagues and the persecutions that befall us today come at different times (ie than in ancient Egypt) and unlike the influences of astrology and of Nature on earth, theirs were caused by miracles. b. The effects then were limited to the Jews and the Pharaoh. c. They affected only the Jews in Egypt, not others. d. The calendaric effects did not exist before or after other such(ie historical) plagues. e. The Egyptian calendaric pattern has no effects on any other medical or surgical procedures that are just as serious as phlebotomy. Therefore, there should be no prohibited days for bleeding. Whenever the patient or somebody else says something about suspected days before you begin your procedure, defer the act on the advice of the referring physician. If you go ahead with it and something bad ensues, even when no fault can be found in any part of the treatment and the complication was fortuitous, people will blame only the physician for negligence in knowingly permitting a surgical phlebotomy on a banned day.

Some persons claim to have documents or writings that determine when a bleed on such and such a day and month will lead to a specific person's death, and when the event can happen without a complicating illness or death. Don't believe any of that drivel, because even the Heavens (ie astrologic) lack such general influences, so fixed and determined. Indeed, the influence changes continuously as the Earth moves. So it is that on the first day of May or of September its influence will change from year to year, and the same is true for every day and every month. The reasons are clear.

In summary, when the Moon is embarrassed in any way, as when it is in opposition or conjunction with the Sun, or is in the sign of Gemini, and when any of all the other ways that we must know will prevail, then we should abstain from phlebotomy. We discussed them in greater detail in the chapter on Incisions. You will find there the protocol for necessary (ie emergency) phlebotomies.

VIII. The General Regimen For Patients Who Want Phlebotomy

When a patient needs a phlebotomy to relieve a thickening of humors, he should bathe during the preceding evening to cause his blood to be thin and to flow more readily. If his stomach is weak, let him eat a mouthful of bread soaked in the juice of oxalis leaves or similar until the belly tightens a bit and is comforted and repels bile. For those who fear phlebotomy or who have had no experience with it and may be cowardly, offer bread soaked in wine or syrup or sugar of roses (rosat), etc. Let those who can do so chose the day when they can be free of such emotions and bodily disturbances. They should fast during the preceding evening, including dinner, If they insist on eating something, let them simply nibble. They should not be constipated on the day of the bleed, but if they had a considerable (ie debilitating) evacuation during the night before or in the morning, such as a major sweat or other, you may delay or cancel the operation, then and there.

48 The days of the Ten Plagues that preceded the Exodus, as described in the Pentateuch (LDR).

IX. How To Perform A Phlebotomy

When he is at work, the phlebotomist should exhibit a smiling and agreeable face and he should please the patient. Preparations are made near a source of water and should include a hand-towel, a strip if cotton and a wood rod (ie to twist the torniquet), some oakum pads and some hemostatic topicals. He should eschew many assistants for five reasons. 1. They will get in the way. 2. The patient may be alarmed by a hovering crowd. 3. One of them may faint and present an unwanted added patient. 4. They are not accustomed to the fearful reactions of the patient, which are not uncommon. 5. Some people believe that if more than one incision fails to strike a bleeding vein, a serious or lethal outcome will occur in their presence.

When everything is ready, search for and find the site for the incision and insert a blade in the usual way, observing all the precautions already described and others to follow. When the patient is a poor man, let the patient himself hold the twisting rod in his other hand. A physician should stand by and instruct the operator, perhaps to tell him to make a larger incision during the winter, and to inform him when the humors are cold and thick, and to tell him how much to bleed, because they are more readily expelled through such an incision. In warm weather and when the humors are thin and are flowing briskly and the patient's vitality is already feeble, the smaller incision will allow less vital spirit and heat escape. When the patient is weak, let him lie supine during the bleed, supported by his back, the strongest part of the body. As Avicenna (*Canon*, Bk. I) and others have asserted, the body is built up from the spine, as a ship is built from its keel. To pursue the analogy we call the vein that courses along the spine 'the keel vein' (ie inf. Vena cava).

X. The Postoperative Care

The patient should rest in place where the air is fresh, mild and dry, in a room that also is dry and not rheumatic, where it has been warmed by a fire if it is too cool. If it is too warm let it: be cooled with cold water and clumps of green plants. Keep all the doors and windows closed to keep out the heat.

For two or three days he should eat small amounts of easily digested foods that are known to generate good blood, such as hen's eggs, small chickens, roasted or cooked without water. In spite of the admonitions of Isaac[49] urging abstinence from wine and offering a profusion of food, I say that you should diminish both when the patient's vitality is low (ie due to the bleed), but restrict the food rather than the wine.

The patient should rest in bed on his back or on the side opposite the bleed for an hour or longer. Then he may begin to eat a little, but he must remain in-house for three days, abstaining from other evacuations (ie purgation, sweats, etc.) and from tub baths. All of this is for two purposes: 1. To prevent the humors that were attracted by the bleed from returning to the diseased site. 2. Lest the heated and the thinned humors which are caused by bathing will break open the sealed vein.

To prevent complications caused by disturbed emotions, the patient should keep himself happy and satisfied by enjoying the company of his companions, playing at dice and bones to gamble for food and wine.[50] He should not be irritated or be bored. He may hire a musician who can play several instruments, but who is of his own sex to avoid suspicions and nasty gossip.

As to sleep, etc.: Galen said (*de Ingernio*, Bk. IX, Ch.2) that he should sleep for two hours after the bleed, giving two reasons. 1. The patient should be nursed during the weakness caused by the bleed. 2. Sleep will come easily for those who frequently nap during the day. 3. For a healthy and robust person with no organs susceptible to disease, whose nerves are not too cold, the post-bleed nap may

49 Isaac Judaeus, the Elder. Tunis, fl. 10thC (LDR).

50 Here we see that games with dice so common in today's bars and clubs are indeed very ancient (LDR).

be unnecessary. However, Avicenna seems to have had a different view *(Canon*, Bk. I, Fol. 4, Ch. On Phlebotomy), claiming that sleep is not at all necessary. But I agree with Galen. Avicenna gave three reasons for his opinion: a. Sleep immediately after a bleed will induce contractions of the nerves in persons who have cold and weak nerves; it produces deep within them—the common folk say, "in the very marrow of their bones"—a painful heaviness not unlike that at the onset of a quartan fever. That heaviness causes the heat and the natural spirit and humors to withdraw deep within the body. Thus, the already debilitated nerves experience a new coldness, and from that comes the painful contractions. b. Anyone with a debilitated member is at risk for aposthems. The humors which are withdrawn from the body by the bleed or are driven inward by the sleep, become more liquid and are attracted to the ailing member and engender an aposthem. c. All persons who have been bled fear that in their sleep they will roll over on the incised arm (ie and reopen the incised vein).

When the illness requires a copious bleed, as in a case of quinsy or a continuous fever or some other very intense affair, or when it is caused by an excess of blood, such as in inflammations of the shoulder, take measure of the vital force at the time and if the vitality is strong, at one session remove as much blood as is necessary. But if the patient is feeble, use repeated smaller bleeds at fairly long intervals (days). The latter method is used with more care and is called secondation. The phlebotomist can use his fingernail to reopen the vein in the depths and release a thin liquid blood (ie the serum) and leave behind the thicker elements (ie the coagulum). If he uses a knife he will release the corrupted clot. A second sharp incision should always be used if the patient can tolerate it rather than the fingernail method.[51] When the bleeding makes bilious humors flow to the patient's tongue and cause thirst, slake it with barley water.

51 The tradition was carried until recent times. Even in this century, many surgeons kept one of their index fingernails long to assist in their dissections, notwithstanding their use of rubber gloves (LDR).

Chapter 6

Guy de Chauliac: *Chirurgia Magna* (1363)

HISTORICAL HIGHLIGHTS

- Guy de Chauliac (1290–1368)
- Born in Chauliac, Auvergne, France
- Studied medicine at Tolouse, Montpellier and Bologna
- Became a pupil of Nicholas Bertrucius in Bologna
- Earned Master of Medicine degree from Montpellier
- Became physician to the Popes: Clement VI, Innocent VI and Urban V while in Avignon
- Completed outstanding surgery book: *Chirurgia Magna* (1363)
- His book came to be acknowledged surgical text 'par excellence' in Europe for two centuries
- Ambroise Paré surgical works later dethroned Guy de Chauliac treatise
- Chauliac anatomy was as good as Mondeville but not as precise as post-Vesalians
- Accused of believing that "pus was part of the healing process"

THE WRITINGS OF GUY DE CHAULIAC

The History of Surgery

The workers in this art, from whom I have had knowledge and theory, and from whom you will find observations and maxims in this work, in order that you may know which has spoken better than the other, should be arranged in a certain order.

The first of all was Hippocrates [5th century B.C.] who (as one reads in the *Introduction to Medicine)* surpassed all the others, and first among the Greeks led medicine to perfect enlightenment. For according to Macrobius and Isidore, in the fourth book of the *Etymologies* ... medicine had been silent for the space of five hundred years before Hippocrates, since the time of Apollo and Aesculapius, who were its first discoverers. He lived ninety-five years, and wrote many books on surgery, as it appears from the fourth of the *Therapeutics* and many other passages of Galen. But I believe that on account of the good arrangement of the books of Galen the books of Hippocrates and of many others have been neglected.

Galen [2nd century A.D.] followed him, and what Hippocrates sowed, as a good labourer he cultivated and increased. He wrote many books, indeed, in which he included much about surgery, and especially the *Book on Tumors Contrary to Nature,* written in summary; and the six first *Books on Therapeutics,* containing wounds and ulcers, and the last two concerning boils and many other maladies which require manual operation. In addition, seven books which he arranged, *Catageni* (that is, about the composition of medicaments according to kinds), of which we have only a summary. Now he was a master in demonstrative science in the time of the Emperor Antoninus [Marcus Aurelius], after Jesus Christ about one hundred and fifty years. He lived eighty years, as is told in *The Book of the Life and Customs of the Philosophers.* Between Hippocrates and Galen there was a very long time, as Avicenna says in the fourth of the *Fractures,* three hundred and twenty-five years, as they gloss it there, but in truth there were five hundred and eighty-six years.

After Galen we find Paul [of Aegina, 7th century] who ... did many things in surgery; however, I have found only the sixth book of his *Surgery.*

Going on we find Rhazes [d. c. 923], Albucasis [d. c. 1013], and Alcaran [?], who (whether they were all one and the same, or several) did very well, especially in the *Books for Almansor* [by Rhazes] and in the *Divisions,* and in the *Surgery* called Albucasis. In these as Haly Abbas [late 10th century] says, he put all his particulars, and in all the *Continens* (which is called *Helham* in Arabic) he repeated the same things, and he collected all the sayings of the ancients, his predecessors; but because he did not select and is long and without conclusion, he has been less prized.

Haly Abbas was a great master, and besides what he sowed in the books on *The Royal Disposition,* he arranged on surgery the ninth part of his *Second Sermon.*

Avicenna [980–1037], illustrious prince, followed him, and in very good order (as in other things) treated surgery in his fourth book.

And we find that up to him all were both physicians and surgeons, but since then, either through refinement or because of too great occupation with cures, surgery was separated and left in the hands of *mechanics.* Of these the first were Roger [of Salerno, fl. c. 1170], Roland [of Parma, fl. c. 1200], and the Four Masters [anonymous], who wrote separate books on surgery, and put in them much that was empirical. Then we find Jamerius [fl. c. 1230–1252] who did some rude surgery in which he included a lot of nonsense; however, in many things he followed Roger. Later, we find Bruno [of Longoburgo, fl. c. 1252], who, prudently enough, made a summary of the findings of Galen and Avicenna, and of the operations of Albucasis; however, he did not have all the translation of the books of Galen and entirely omitted anatomy. Immediately after him came Theodoric [Borgognoni, 1205–1298], who gathering up all that Bruno said, with some fables of Hugh of Lucca [d. c. 1252–1258], his master, made a book out of them.

William of Saliceto [c. 1210–c. 1280] was a man of worth who composed two compendia, one on medicine and the other on surgery; and in my opinion, what he treated he did very well. Lanfranc [d. before 1306] also wrote a book in which he put scarcely anything but what he took from William; however, he changed the arrangement.

At that time Master Arnald of Villanova [d. 1311] was flourishing in both skills, and wrote many fine works. Henry of Mondeville [d. c. 1325] began in Paris a very notable treatise in which he tried to make a marriage between Theodoric and Lanfranc, but being prevented by death he did not finish the treatise.

In this present time, in Calabria, Master Nicholas of Reggio [d. 1350], very expert in Greek and Latin, has translated at the order of King Robert many books of Galen and has sent them to us at court; they seem to be of finer and more perfect style than those which have been translated from the Arabic. Finally there appeared a faded English rose [*Rosa Anglica* of John of Gaddesden, d. 1361] which was sent to me, and I have seen it. I had thought to find in it sweetness of odour, but I have found only the fables of the Spaniard, of Gilbert, and of Theodoric.

In my time there have been operating surgeons, at Toulouse, Master Nicholas Catalan; at Montpellier, Master Bonet, son of Lanfranc; at Bologna, Masters Peregrin and Mercadant; at Paris, Master Peter of Argentière; at Lyons (where I have practised for a long time), Peter of Bonant; at Avignon, Master Peter of Aries and my companion, Jean of Parma.

And I, Guy of Chauliac, surgeon and master in medicine, from the borders of Auvergne, diocese of Mende, doctor and personal chaplain to our lord the pope, I have seen many operations and many of the writings of the masters mentioned, principally of Galen; for as many books of his as are found in the two translations, I have seen and studied with as much diligence as possible, and for a long time I have operated in many places. And at present I am in Avignon, in the year of our Lord 1363, the first year of the pontificate of Urban V. In which year, from the teachings of the above named, and from my experiences, with the aid of my companions, I have compiled this work, as God has willed.

The sects which were current in my time among the workers in this art, besides the two general ones, which are still in vigour, namely, that of the Logicians or rationalists, and that of the Empiricists (condemned by Galen in the *Book of Sects* and throughout the *Therapeutics),* were five.

The first was of Roger, Roland, and the Four Masters who, indiscriminately for all wounds and boils, produced healing or suppuration with their poultices and cataplasms; relying for this on the fifth of the *Aphorisms,* "The loose are good, the hard are bad."

The second was of Bruno and Theodoric who indiscriminately dried up all wounds with wine alone, relying for this on the fourth of the *Therapeutics,* "The dry comes closer to the healthy, and the wet to the unhealthy."

The third sect was of Wiliam of Saliceto and of Lanfranc, who wishing to hold the middle ground between the above, cared for or dressed all wounds with unguents and sweet salves, relying for this on the fourth of the *Therapeutics,* that there is only one way to healing, namely, that it be done safely and painlessly.

The fourth sect is composed of all the men at arms or Teutonic Knights and others following war; who treat all wounds with conjurations and liquors, oil, wool, and cabbage leaves, relying on this, that God has put his efficacy in words, in herbs, and in stones.

The fifth sect is composed of women and many ignorant ones who entrust those sick with all maladies only to the saints, relying on this: the Lord has given it to me as it has pleased Him; the Lord will take it from me when it shall please Him; blessed be the name of the Lord, Amen.

And because such sects will be refuted in the course of this book, let them be put aside for the present. But I am amazed at one thing, that they follow each other like cranes. For one says only what the other has said. I do not know whether it is from fear or love that they scorn to hear anything except what is traditional or proved by authority. They have read Aristotle badly in the second of the *Metaphysics* where he shows that these two things most of all prevent the sight and knowledge of the truth. Let us abandon such friendships and fears, for Socrates or Plato is our friend, but truth is still more a friend. It is a holy and worthy thing to honour truth in the first place. Let them follow the dogmatic doctrine of Galen approved in the *Book of Sects* and throughout the *Therapeutics,* which is entirely composed of experience and reason, in which one seeks things and scorns words. And he himself has taught the means of seeking truth, in the book on *The Constitution of the Dogmatic Art,* chapter seven, which under a certain epilogue he put in the third book of the *Natural Faculties,* chapter ten, in this way: he who would know something better than the others must suddenly be very different from the others (that is, at the beginning and by nature, and by first knowledge). And when he is a boy, or at the age of puberty, he must be seized with a certain amorous rage for the truth; he must not cease to study day and night, to learn all that has been said by the most famous of the ancients. And when he shall reach the flower of his age and learning, then he must judge what he has learned by examining it very well for a long time and perceive all that agrees with the things which are clearly apparent, and all that disagrees with them, and thus choose the one, and reject the other. To such a one, I hope my observations will be very useful; but to the others, these writings will be as superfluous as a fable told to an ass.

I do not say, however, that it is not a very good thing to cite witnesses in ones discourse, for Galen in many places, besides reason and experience, which are for all men the two instruments of judging (as he says in the first of the *Therapeutics*, chapter three), brings in the third, by witnesses. Of which in the first of the *Miamin* or *Compositions according to Plans*, he says that the belief in things which one writes increases with the agreement of those who repeat them; and therefore he says that he will write down all the medicaments which have been made up by expert doctors. And thus I shall do (as I have said) in my procedure, with the aid of the glorious God.

Let us return to our theme, and put down the conditions which are requisite to every surgeon, who wishes by art to exercise on the human body the aforesaid manner and form of operating, which conditions Hippocrates, who guides us well in everything, concludes with a certain subtle implication, in the first of the *Aphorisms:* life is short, and art prolix, time and chance sharp or sudden, experience fallacious and dangerous, judgment difficult. But not only the doctor must busy himself in doing his duty but also the sick person and the attendants, and he must also put in order external things.

There are then four conditions which are valued here, according to Arnald, a very eloquent Latinist. Some are required of the surgeon, others of the sick, others of those present, others in those things which come in from outside.

The conditions required of a surgeon are four: the first is that he be educated; the second, that he be skilled; the third, that he be ingenious; the fourth, that he be well behaved. It is then required in the first place that the surgeon be educated, not only in the principles of surgery, but also of medicine, both in theory and practice.

In theory he must know things natural, non-natural and unnatural. And first, he must understand natural things, principally anatomy, for without it nothing can be done in surgery, as will appear below. He must also understand temperament, for according to the diversity of the nature of bodies it is necessary to diversify the medicament (Galen against Thessales, in all the *Therapeutics*). This is shown by the virtue and strength of the patient. He must also know the things which are not natural, such as air, meat, drink, etc., for these are the causes of all sickness and health. He must also know the things which are contrary to nature, that is sickness, for from this rightly comes the curative purpose. Let him not be ignorant in any way of the cause; for if he cures without the knowledge of that, the cure will not be by his abilities but by chance. Let him not forget or scorn accidents; for sometimes they override their cause, and deceive or divert, and pervert the whole cure, as is said in the first to Glauconius.

In practice, he must know how to put in order the way of living and the medicaments; for without this surgery, which is the third instrument of medicine, is not perfect. Of which Galen speaks in the *Introduction:* as pharmacy has need of regimen and of surgery, so surgery has need of regimen and pharmacy.

Thus it appears that the surgeon working in his art should know the principles of medicine. And with this, it is very fitting that he know something of the other arts. That is what Galen says in the first of his *Therapeutics* against Thessales, that if the doctors have nothing to do with geometry, or astronomy, or dialectics, or any other good discipline, soon the leather workers, carpenters, smiths, and others, leaving their own occupations, will run to medicine and make themselves into doctors.

In the second place, I have said he must be skilled and have seen others operate; I add the maxim of the sage Avenzoar [12th century], that every doctor must have knowledge first of all, and after that he must have practice and experience. To the same testify Rhazes, in the fourth *Book for Almansor,* and Haly Abbas on the testimony of Hippocrates, in the first of his *Theory.*

Thirdly, he must be ingenious, and of good judgment and good memory. That is what Haly Rodan [11th century] says in the third of his *Techni;* the doctor must have good memory, good judgment, good motives, good presence, and sound understanding, and that he be well formed, for example, that he have slender fingers, hands steady and not trembling, clear eyes, etc.

Fourth, I have said, he should be well mannered. Let him be bold in safe things, fearful in dangers, let him flee false cures or practices. Let him be gracious to the sick, benevolent to his companions, wise in his predictions. Let him be chaste, sober, compassionate, and merciful; not covetous, or extortionate, so that he may reasonably receive a salary in proportion to his work, the ability of his patient to pay, the nature of the outcome, and his own dignity.

The conditions required of the sick man are three: that he be obedient to the doctor, as the servant is to the master, in the first of the *Therapeutics;* that he have faith in the doctor, in the first of the *Prognostics;* that he be patient, for patience conquers malice, as it is said in other writing.

The conditions for the attendants are four, that they be peaceable, polite or agreeable, faithful, and discreet.

The conditions for things coming from outside are many, all of which ought to be arranged for the advantage of the sick, as Galen says, at the end of the commentary of the *Aphorisms* mentioned above.

Treatise 3: On Wounds

Doctrine 2: Wounds in Compound Organs. Chapter 6: Concerning Wounds in the Belly and Its Parts

As there are two parts in the belly, namely that which is contained and that which contains (as was explained in the Anatomy [in the first Treatise of the *Inventarium]),* so also wounds sometimes occur in the containing part and sometimes in the contents. Thus, wounds of the belly are sometimes external and do not penetrate to the inner parts, and sometimes they do penetrate to the inner parts. Of those that penetrate to the inner parts, some are of such a nature that nothing of the interior members protrudes; but sometimes the omentum protrudes, or the intestines, or something else. Wounds in the contained parts are sometimes in the omentum, sometimes in the intestines, sometimes in the stomach, and so forth. These are the distinctions on which indications and treatments are based.

The **causes** of these wounds are the same as those of other [wounds]: sword, lance, arrow, and anything capable of cutting and perforating.

Signs and indications. A sign that a wound in the belly does not penetrate is obtained by visual inspection, by [exploration with] a probe, and by the fact that nothing comes out of it. But a sign that it does penetrate is obtained when the probe enters deeply and when the omentum, intestine, or some other member comes out of it. A sign that the omentum has protruded and has been altered is when its substance, fatty and full of veins, is visible, and when it appears livid and dark. A sign that the intestines are wounded is the issue of feces from [the wound]. The sign indicating whether it is the large or small intestine is deduced from the location, for the small intestine is above the navel and the large intestine below. A sign that the stomach is wounded is that chyle issues from it and that [the wound] is located in the front. A sign that the liver is wounded is the issue of blood and [the wound] is located on the right side. A sign that it is the spleen is the issue Of feculent matter and [the wound] is located on the left side. A sign that it is the kidneys is the issue of watery blood, and also the site. In *Therapeutic Method* book 6, Galen expresses the view that wounds and sutures are more dangerous and difficult when they are in the middle of the belly than when they are on the flanks, because the [middle] parts contract more due to their muscles and the intestines can more easily protrude. It is also judged that unless one comes quickly to their aid and reintroduces them, the intestines will swell up and inflate because of the coldness of the air, and then it will be difficult to reintroduce them. Hippocrates in the sixth part of the *Aphorisms* also concludes that unless one counteracts the protrusion of the epiploon or omentum or *zirbus* quickly, it will very rapidly be altered and corrupted. For this reason, physicians cut off what is exposed and altered. According to Galen's commentary [on the *Aphorisms*], while this is not always the case, it is ! for the most part the case. In *Therapeutic Method* book 6, Galen also expresses the view that the large intestine can readily heal, but the small intestine heals with difficulty, and the jejunum not at all, because of the multitude and magnitude of the vessels and the thinness and sinewy character of the tunic. Also, this intestine receives bile in its undiluted form and is closer to the liver than the other [organs]. Moreover, one may venture to treat the lower parts of the stomach because they are fleshy and also because medications can remain in that location; but in the orifice of the stomach, [medication] touches the afflicted parts only in passing, and its sensitive nature repels treatment. …

Treatment. There is nothing distinctive about the treatment of wounds of the belly which do not penetrate, apart from the ligature. … Their treatment is the same as that of flesh wounds: with a suture if they need it, and with other things that help the production of flesh. Penetrating wounds where no internal part protrudes or is wounded are treated in the same way, except that they have their own particular suture.

Suture of the belly. This suture takes different forms according to different circumstances. Some, such as Galen, prescribe that [the belly] be sutured so that the peritoneum is joined to the abdominal wall, because being in itself without flesh (since it is bloodless and sinewy), it cannot readily be consolidated, and because of the laxity of the abdominal wall a rupture may follow. The first stitch is made by inserting the point of the needle through one lip [of the wound] so that it does not touch the peritoneum; then by piercing the other lip from the inside, it penetrates all [layers] including the peritoneum, and it is knotted on the outside. In the next stitch, the needle, entering through the lip, pierces everything, including peritoneum and abdominal wall; re-entering through the other lip, it avoids the peritoneum and only pierces the abdominal wall, and it is knotted on the outside. Let the other stitches be made in this way until the whole [wound] is adequately sutured.

Galen relates another method, which Albucasis [*Abû al-Qâsim al-Zahrâwî* fl. ca 1000] adopts. It is the general method, and it is easier, but not safer, and it is to suture all four margins of the two lips together with a single stitch and a knot. As many stitches are made as are necessary.

Albucasis describes a third method. One pierces [the lips] with needles, as he says, and then leaving the needles in place, one winds a thread over their tops as women do in [lacing up] sleeves. …

The fourth method is Lanfranc's and Henri [of Mondeville] adopts it. A threaded needle is stuck in on the outside of one lip and pierces the whole peritoneum and abdominal wall; then coming out through the other lip from; the inside, it again pierces the peritoneum and abdominal wall. Then, at a distance of one's little finger from the first stitch, make a second stitch with the same needle and thread, without cutting or knotting it, in this way: insert the needle in the lip that was last perforated from the outside towards the inside, then insert it in the other lip from the inside towards the outside, always including both the peritoneum and the abdominal wall. Near the needle, you will find the end of the thread, which you initially left outside. Tie the two ends of the thread together, making a single knot on the side for every two stitches, because in this way the thread will never pass on top of the lips of the wound, but will only appear on the sides. When the suture is finished, apply other remedies, and bandage up. …

In a penetrating wound of the belly in which the inner organs are wounded and do not protrude, if the belly wound is large enough (and if it is not large enough, it can be enlarged with an appropriate instrument, to be described below), let [the internal parts] be carefully pulled out. If they need to be sutured and if this can be done successfully—as for example the fundus of the stomach or the large intestine let them be sutured with a furrier's stitch and not with ants' heads, as some practitioners say (for so Albucasis testifies), because it is both disagreeable and ineffective, as the facts show. Some, such as Roger [of Parma], Jamerius, and Teodorico, insert a tube made of elder wood into the intestine so that the feces do not corrupt the suture; but others, as Gugliemo [of Saliceto] relates, put in a section of the intestine of some animal, or according to the Four Masters, a piece of a trachea. This does not seem reasonable to me, because nature, bent on expelling foreign bodies, expels and removes it from the suture, and so the purpose for which these things were applied is frustrated. In my view, it is better, after the intestine has been sutured as stated above and cleaned of all filth, to apply externally a powder which will preserve the suture, and that [the organs] be reinserted into the belly according to the method which will be described.

If the omentum has protruded and is blackened and corrupted, let the blackened parts be tied up with a loop, and let the part outside the loop in the lower end of the sewing of the belly be cut away, leaving the heads of the loop and of the thread which sutures the said intestines outside, so that suppurating matter may drain out of the wound. When the omentum has been sutured or ligatured, it should be reinserted into the belly as stated, and let the wound in the belly be immediately sutured as stated. Under no circumstances should it be opened until the internal organs are healed, as Jamerius and Roger prescribe, and Lanfranc follows them on this point. This is be cause nothing is more harmful to internal members and to natural heat than contact with air which has not been altered by [the body's] nature. Because of this [patients] fall victim to that pernicious occurrence, pain and griping of the intestines, and this causes them to fall into spasms and consequently die.

And along with this, the open wound, which was of necessity large because of the operation, continually predisposes the guts to extrude, which is harmful and dangerous in the extreme.

Things of this nature are provided from the outside; but on the inside, let there be administered what Avicenna says—centaury and terra sigillata—and the things that are mentioned in connection with wounds of internal organs of the chest, because they will also be suitable for these [wounds]; and in Galen's *On Simple Drugs* 6, horse-tail is highly recommended by some for wounds of the intestines and bladder. And Galen in *Therapeutic Method* 6 prescribes clysters of sharp, black, tepid wine, especially in a case where the perforation is right down to the inner cavity.

At least for the first seven days, let the diet be light and such that it does not produce stool or superfluities that cause putrefaction, but rather, those that consolidate. … If [the patient's] strength is weak, one can give chicken broth [simmered] to the point where the cooked parts dissolve; and if some tragacanth and gum arabic can be added in, which will not make it taste sharper, this would be best. And Guglielmo praises effusively water from the decoction of incense and mastic.

In a penetrating belly wound in which the intestines or some other part protrude, wounded or not, sutured or bandaged, Galen and Avicenna identify four tasks: the first is to restore what is protruding to its proper place; the second, to suture the wound; the third, to apply drugs; and consequently the fourth is to ensure that no internal part suffers swelling or pain.

The first [task] is accomplished if the wound is large enough that [the protruding part] can be introduced with the hands, using a gentle pressure; or [the patient] can be shaken by elevating the hands and feet, and in this way [the organs] are re-introduced, according to Roger. If they cannot be replaced in this way, because they are swollen or because the wound is small, is it not then necessary (says Galen) to do one of two things: either evacuate the windiness, or make the wound larger? But I think that the first [option] is better, if it can be carried out successfully. How will it be carried out successfully? By removing the cause of the windiness. And what is this? The coldness of the surrounding air; and so healing is carried out by heating. One must therefore steep a soft sponge in hot water and warm the guts with it. In the meantime, let some sharp warm wine be prepared, because this warms much more than water does, and strengthens the guts. Some, indeed, like Roger and Teodorico, split suckling pigs or other animals down the middle and apply them to the guts as warm as they can, and they repeat this until the guts are warmed and deflated and go back to their place. Haly Abbas prescribes that the patient be suspended by his extremities over a bath and shaken, or that the guts be anointed with oil of violets (or with warm pig grease, as Jamerius says), and in this way the guts will go back to their place.

But if, after you have done all this, the guts remain swollen, Galen and the others prescribe that one cut open the belly wound enough to allow what is protruding to be replaced. Suitable (according to [Galen]) for such incisions are what are called double-headed syringotomes, namely those which are curved and rounded back and at the end—not pointed—the shape of which Albucasis describes thus:

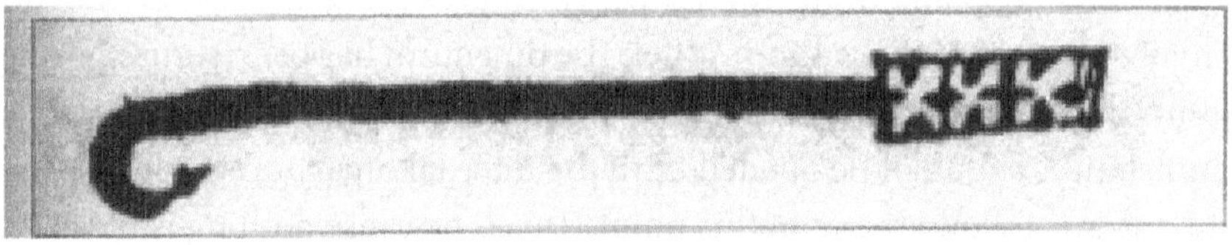

A suitable position for the patient is on his back, but with the wounded part elevated; the point of both is to avoid any harm to the protruding part from the other internal organs.

The second task is accomplished when a competent assistant brings the whole gash together by pressing from outside with his hands, and then opens it little by little while the entire wound is sutured by the physician in an assured manner. How the suture of the belly is made has been described above.

The third task is accomplished, according to Galen, with the drugs called sanguinolentive [*promoting the flow of blood*] and which, as we have shown in previous [sections of this book], consolidate wounds in other parts. These are, namely, the powder that conserves sutures, and stupes with wine, and plasters, and other remedies that generate flesh. A bandage on the outside is in this case more necessary than the bandage which we said ought to be worn in the case of the chest.

The fourth part of the treatment does not differ greatly from that used in other cases. However, one ought to measure out soft wool in proportion to warm oil, to infuse everything in the vicinity, and to cover the area between the swelling and the armpits. But it is better to introduce something into the intestines with a clyster for such a purpose. Concerning the treatment of abdominal dropsy by incision, Avicenna in *Canon* book 3 says that it may transpire that pain and perforation follow the incision, and then it is necessary to administer an effusion of oil of dill and camomile to the perforation, and to place upon the spot where the incision was made a plaster made from fenugreek and linseed and the seed of marsh mallow and the like. But some, such as Henri [of Mondeville], in order to eliminate such unbearable perforative griping, boil salt with wine, and add bran until it thickens, and place it in a sack which they apply to all the painful parts, as hot as possible, and a bandage is put over it. And when it has cooled down, it is changed for another of the same kind, and this is repeated until the pain and griping subside. There is no need to attend much to any matter which might remain in the cavity of the belly, because it cannot be of any great quantity, since these parts are not heavily supplied with blood. And as Guglielmo says, nature resolves it or else dispatches it to the inguinal region, and there let it be treated as is customary for other swellings in this area. …

English Translator's Preface (L.D. Rosenman)

Edward Nicaise (the French translator), the indefatigable surgeon-historian-editor, provided wonderful editions in French of three giants in the history of French Surgery: Guy de Chauliac in 1890, Henri de Mondeville in 1893, and Pierre Franco in 1895. In that remarkable series he completed what Malgaigne did for Ambroise Paré in 1840–42, and together they opened the eyes of curious readers during the latter half of the 19th C, to see the accomplishments of the Medieval and Renaissance surgeons who were the torch- bearers of our Art until the 18th C. Yet, as Ulysses spoke for Shakespeare,

"*Time hath, my lord, a wallet at his back wherein he puts alms for oblivion.*"[1] Even the brightest lights grow dim if they are not attended and the great torch-bearers and their works need refreshment. After Nicaise all the Europeans, except the English speaking people, had new editions and translations of the three, and recent English editions of Henri and Pierre are available. Yet, when we seek modern English editions of Guy de Chauliac we find only one, a translation of a small part of Guy's *Major Surgery* by W. A. Brennan, published in 1923. And here now is a complete new English Edition.[2]

Let me explain the title. Guy's Latin Manuscript was named the *Chirurgia Magna,* and a small probably spurious French work was titled the *Chirurgie Petite.* My terms refer to the sizes of the books: the *Major Surgery* and the *Minor Surgery,* and in no way indicate the extent, or the difficulties, or the perils of certain manual procedures performed by surgeons, as we today call them major or minor operations. Certainly, in Guy's era there were few operations, perhaps excepting amputations, repairs of hernias, and removal of bladder stones that we would call major.

Little need be said to supplement the ample and appropriate comments provided by Nicaise and Joubert in their long discursive Introductions and footnotes, and I have inserted only a few footnotes and explanatory interjections. Indeed, as Nicaise wrote in the historical Introduction to his edition of Pierre Franco, if we were to combine the introductions in his editions of Henri de Mondeville, Pierre Franco, and Guy de Chauliac with Malgaigne's Introduction to his Ambroise Paré, we will have a complete history of European Surgery before the modern era.

Nicaise took pains to explain his difficulties with 14th C Latin and 16th C French. I will add a note of apology for my own misconceptions of what Nicaise called obscurities. The Reader should know that this book is a translation of a work that was transformed from what had been written in 1353 in the strange Latin of southern France (see Fn. 135 and page 127). It was submitted to scribes and copyists through several centuries, and no two manuscripts were alike in all details, in the Latin, old French or other languages. Many printed editions appeared after the 15th C, and the many variances were retained, based on the various manuscripts, which were their sources. And they were printed in many languages. Joubert reviewed several of them and published several editions. In 1659 he edited the book used by

1 Troilus and Cressida, Act III, Scene 3 (LDR).

2 This Edition abbreviates some of Nicaise's repetitions, and eliminates most of his section of Supporting Documents (ie Pieces Justificatives), and all of his Glossary of Old French Terms. They are redefined in English as they appear in the text (LDR).

Nicaise, who based his own selection after a careful research among all the mss and printed editions available to him. He chose Joubert's printed edition for his own of 1890. Joubert's edition used the French language that was spoken during his own epoch, and Nicaise repeated what he found there with few emendations. Joubert had encountered many passages and terms which he translated with apologies, and Nicaise did the same; both of them submitted many footnotes that provided the reader with variants from which to choose. I accept and follow their paths.

Many passages seem obscure, clumsy, and difficult to translate, even to transliterate. The Reader must blame. The Author must explain.

Guy hoped to produce a treatise that summarized the best of what he could find in the surgical lore of the ancient and more recent treatises to which he had access, and he would indicate what he thought were the better methods, as they were recommended by the Masters whom he revered, or which he himself had tested. He is prolix and repetitive. His conservative, almost reluctant acceptance of manual surgical procedures, and his explicit details of treatments with diets and medications, repeated often ad nauseam, reflects his situation among the church-educated physicians who dominated Academic Medicines in his epoch. That position was strong in the Schools, and it explains why Guy's treatise was the bible for surgeons during the ensuing two centuries, and why it was referred to with respect until the late 18th C.

Guy's era was that of the Great Plague, and his book was written afterwards. Its respectful attitude toward his colleagues and his suave gentility secured him as an officer of the Church, and as a Surgeon for The Popes at Avignon. However, he lacked the vigor, the wit, and the critical outlook of Henri de Mondeville whose bitter reflections on the churchmen, the surgeons who were less critical than himself, and all the other qualities of a burdened surgeon who wrote—but did not live to complete—his remarkable *Surgery.* If only one great medieval surgical text was available to a curious Reader, I would name Henri de Mondeville's.

Format

Nicaise's (the French translator) text is in a standard type face.

All titles of Books and Manuscripts are in Italics.

THE MAJOR SURGERY

In The Name Of The Lord
HERE BEGINS THE ENTIRE TREATISE
OF THE SURGICAL AND MEDICAL TOPICS
COMPILED AND COMPLETED IN THE YEAR OF THE LORD MCCCLXIII
By **GUY DE CHAULIAC,** SURGEON, MASTER IN MEDICINE IN THE VERY ILLUSTRIOUS
STUDIA OF MONTPELLIER

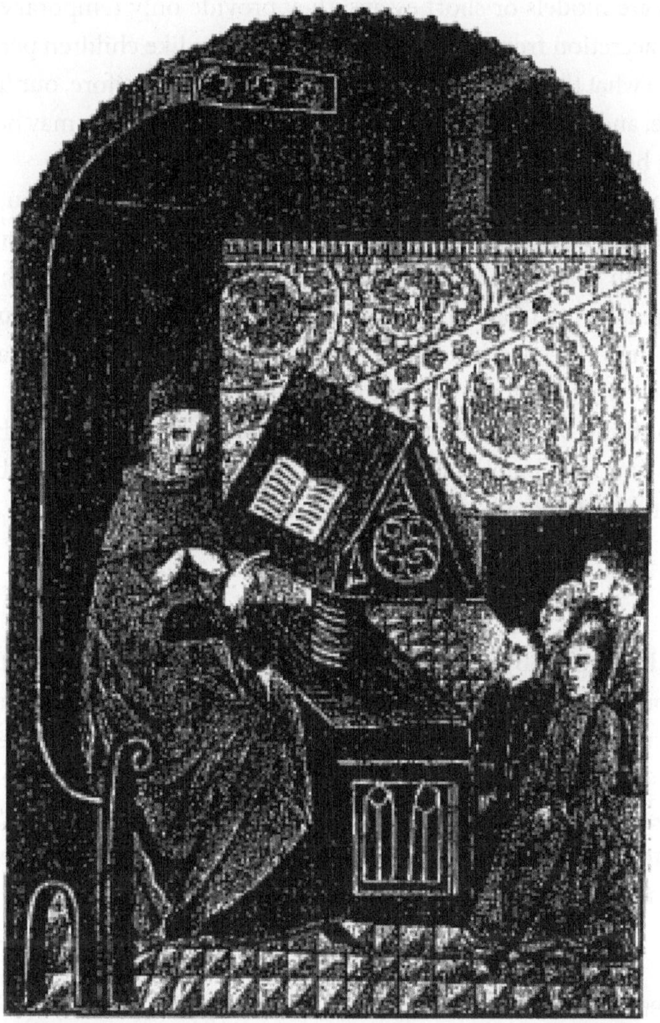

Figure 2. A Lecture in the 15th C A Miniature As A Frontispiece For A French Ms of Guy de Chauliac Ms 396 Bibliotheque Nationale of Paris Fol. 1. Copyright in the Public Domain.

GUY DE CHAULIAC'S PREFACE TO *CHIRURGIA MAGNA*

Having first thanked the Lord who has given me a long life and has spared my body and granted me peace and has kept me active, who has given me knowledge of the Art of Medicine and of the way to heal with divinely inspired efforts, now I will try hard to discuss what I have garnered. Before I comment on the collection of matters dealing with the Art of Surgery and Medicine, I must thank the living and true Lord for giving me all the materials without which this kind of introduction would be impossible. I will give him my heartfelt devotion here and throughout this work, and elsewhere, and plead for His continued assistance and for the protection of his Son. They gave me a happy start and provided the milieu in which to accomplish something useful, and by his command I will bring it to a good ending.

What led me to this collection was not the lack of books, but the need to unify and find a useful concordance. None of us has at hand all of the books, and none of us has been able to read them all cover-to-cover and to remember everything he has read. A lecture may serve a good purpose, but it has limited value, as are models or short essays; they provide only temporary benefits. Knowledge (ie science) has been an accretion from its very beginning. We are like children perched on the shoulders of giants, and we can see what they see; and yet somewhat farther. Therefore, our hypotheses and constructions may be valuable, and, as noble Plato wrote, even brief written notes may be less obscure than a long lecture, and they can be re-read and remembered.

And for the sake of my old age and to keep my wits alive, this book is for you, the Masters of Medicine at Montpellier, Bologna, Paris, and Avignon, and especially for those who served the Popes and have been my companions in that service, with whom I have been nourished, and have studied, read (ie lectured), and operated, trying to avoid mediocrity. Here I will try to re-state and to modify to a degree the principles set forth in the speeches and writings of the sages and savants as they have put them in their surgical treatises. That is why my book should be called an Inventory, A Surgical Collection. I have added almost nothing of my own other than a bit here and there that I think may be worthwhile. Certainly it is not perfect, and doubtlessly it will be superfluous in places and obscure in others. I ask for your emendations; and I ask that you pardon my ignorance.

Here are the Premises:

The Matters To Be Known By Anyone Who Wishes To Avail Himself Of The Art Of Surgery[3]

Dear Readers: You will see that this Chapter (ie Commentary) is arranged similar to the Inventories of civil wills, where the most common and the most valuable items of an estate are listed first. This Singular Chapter describes how I have done that here. First come the usual (ie common) and the most important matters needed by anyone who wishes to avail himself of the Art of Surgery. That is what the Philosopher (ie Aristotle) wrote in his *Physics,* "We know that the proper process of science is to go first to the more general and then to the particulars."

The Definition of Surgery

Let us begin by asking what Surgery means. Although there have been many definitions, they all take root from our father, Galen, in his *Introduction to Medicine,* where he wrote, "Surgery is part of the curative art that makes use of incisions, cauteries, and the setting of broken bones." In Book I of his *Treatment of Fevers,* He added this to his definition, "and other manual operations."

That is a good definition of what now is considered a third category of Medicine; it is broadly defined as the science of treatments of maladies that require manual procedures which are not to be used before

3 In the Venetian Editions *The Singular Chapter* is called *The Universal Chapter.* In it Guy states the Generalities applicable to the entire work; they contain material s needed by whoever wants to profit as a *surgeon, et al.* The meaning of the term Singular has been debated. I will say only that the word derives from the Latin 'singulus' meaning 'unique'. This chapter stands alone, and really is unique, whereas all the other chapters are part of the Doctrines and Treatises. In other words, the Singular Chapter has its own rare excellence. Unlike Galen, Guy defined Surgery more than simply a method of treatment. He makes it a part of Medicine. He blames Avicenna and the physicians after him for their disdain of surgery. He praises William of Saliceto and Arnold of Villanova as shining lights in the faculties of medicine where they performed both as physicians and surgeons. After Guy, however, the separation between Physicians and Surgeons was even more accentuated.
In this Chapter Guy provides a brief and interesting history of Surgery, and he offers us the gift of his erudition, a review of the books that existed in his epoch, and he shows us the methods of his study. He provides a masterful and honest description of the conditions faced by the true surgeons. At the end of the chapter he outlines the plan that he follows in composing the book. As an aside, he tells us something abut himself. He says that he practiced at Lyons for a long time, during which he period he operated at many placed (EN). This Singular Chapter appears in many mss and printed editions. Nicaise describes them all in detail, and I shall not reproduce that bibliographic material (LDR).

the other measures, which are food, beverages, and restoration of a good life-style (ie and the applications of medicines). Therefore we agree to define Surgery as follows: *Surgery is the science that teaches the methods and the arts of closing wounds, making incisions, and performing other manual operations for curing people whenever that is possible.*[4]

The science of Surgery is part of the general therapeutics, and no one can deny that it is called an Art in many places. The word *Science* has a broad connotation that is not limited to pure Medicine. The mind considers them together, and the term covers both of them.

Indeed, there are two kinds of Surgery. One is academic, and it deems itself alone to deserve the term 'Science', and that kind of surgeon need never to use his hands. The other is surgical practice and is what commonly is called Surgery, the handiwork that deserves the term Art. That person may know nothing except how to operate. That kind of Surgery was included in Aristotle's category of Mechanical Arts. Galen, in Book 1 of his book *On Diets* said, "Someone cannot become a seaman or have another similar career simply by reading book. Only by diligent practice can we become adepts and artisans, etc. etc." We must agree that his statements are true.

Then we should add, "for treating people when that is feasible", because, as my Master Raimond of Montpellier said, nothing is absolute; while some things are quite certain, a physician cannot always offer relief or achieve a cure. To demand certainty from a physician is like asking one who stammers to deliver a sermon, both use imperfect instruments. The subtle doctor (Averroes) told us to act as our art dictates.

That is why the Art commands us to strive for a cure, with three exceptions: 1. When the malady is known to be incurable, as is leprosy. 2. When the malady is curable but the patient will not accept the recommended treatments or he cannot tolerate the suffering caused by them, as in the treatments for a necrotic ulcer on a limb (ie requiring amputation).

And 3. When the treatment itself will engender complications that are worse than the primary malady, such as inducing a virulent fever (ie mal mort) or by over-treatment of chronic hemorrhoids (ie mild bleeding or discomforts). Hippocrates taught that treating such may result in hydrops or mania.[5] Galen said the same in his *Therapeutics,* Book 4. Good treatments should not cause pain or suffering; they should preserve and not destroy; they betoken a good physician rather than a bad one. In Book 12 of the same he wrote that one cannot promise the impossible simply to obtain a fee. Avoid harmful treatments and false promises, lest you incur a bad reputation.

The word *Surgery* derives from *cheir,* meaning hand, and *ergeia* meaning operation. So it is that Surgery is the science of manual operations.[6] Let us proceed:

Surgery includes opening the body to treat a malady that surgery alone may cure. And it can prevent an illness and preserve one's health whenever that is possible. Those are its goals.

---

4 Joubert's own definition: "Surgery is skill or a science adopted by someone who usually or occasionally is a physician. He is responsible for teaching not only surgeons, but also apothecaries, each of whom has his own particular skills for providing what a physician orders. Surgery, narrowly defined, is what a surgeon does, but in a broader sense, yet what he does is a physician's responsibility." (Joubert)

5 Mild bleeding from hemorrhoids was accepted as a form of phlebotomy, a kind of prophylaxis that taps off the humors that could cause ascites. Hemorrhoidal veins were thought to be emunctories of the liver; they could be dammed back and even offend the brain. (LDR).

6 Nicaise notes that Guy knew no Greek. In his Latin Ms he wrote *ciros* and *gygos,* which are Arabic versions. (EN).

The Parts Of Surgery And The Operations

Surgery, according to Joannitius (ie Honein) has two parts: treatment of soft tissues and of hard. In action it does five things: operations on swellings (ie aposthems), treatments of wounds and ulcers (ie unhealed wounds), the restoration of fractures and dislocations and a miscellany of maladies for which it is suited. There are three types of procedures: The separation of continuity (incisions), the restoration of continuity, and the riddance of redundancies. Phlebotomy and scarificatioin are in the first category. Closure of wounds and the reduction of fractures and dislocations are in the second. Ablation of tumors such as aposthems and glands are in the third.

A Surgeon's Instruments

The surgeon's actions vary. Some are routine and others are special to a case at hand. The common measures involve what the physician routinely employs, and the special measures may require metallic tools. The medical treatments include attention to general regimens: foods, beverages, phlebotomy and leeches, ointments, plasters and powders The metal instruments are for cutting: scissors, razors and lancets; those used for removing things: large and small forceps. In addition we use cauteries (olivaries, cultelaries); tools for probing: sounds, and tubes; and catheters, dilators, and needles. And there are special instruments for trephining the cranium, and scythe-like lancets for operations at the anus.

That list tells you that a surgeon's work is artificial.[7] He should always have at hand five kinds of ointments: the Basilicon to wall off an abscess; the Apostles' to mondify; the White Oinment to consolidate; the Golden to generate flesh; and the Dialthea to soften the scar. His portable equipment should include five or six instruments: scissors, forceps, probes, razors, lancets and needles.

A well-armed surgeon should be able to perform useful operations, provided that the patient has been informed as to the nature of the procedure. Galen (*Therapeutics*) said that the surgeon should first treat things that are contrary to Nature, then go after Natural things and the Non-Natural with their annexes.[8] Galen also said (*Therapeutics,* Book 2) that we should begin our treatments by attacking the primary ailment and then go after the secondary ones that derive from the primary, and persist until we reach your goal of curing the malady. We follow those principles: first make a diagnosis of the malady and assess its nature, and then proceed step-by-step until we know everything, the obvious and the obscure.

Next, after determining the indications as stated, Galen said that we should determine what we should do, and what is or is not achievable. Then decide how to attain our goal. He continued (at the end of Parts 3 and 7) noting that if our goals are not unlimited yet are consistent, as for treating an ulcer or an uncomplicated wound, our choices will be easy. But if they are manifold and contrary, as for treating an undermining sordid ulcer or an aposthem in noble region, we must be aware of complications.[9]

---

7 Artificial meant art-ful, the work of an artisan with special skills (LDR).

8 The seven Natural things are a person's innate endowments: According to Guy they were: the elements, the temperaments (ie complexion), the humors, the limbs and body parts, the virtues (ie faculties), the body-functions, and its spirits. Four things are Annexed to the Naturals: age, color, dietary habits, and sex.

The six Non-Natural things (not part of the body) (hygiene) are important for health, and health will suffer if they are not considered next: air, food and drink, exercize and rest, sleep and wakefulness, excretion and retention, and emotions. The five Annexes to the non-natural are the temperature (ie weather), the season, the geographic region, coitus, personal habits (bathing, etc.)

The three things Contrary To Nature (ie the pathology) destroy the Natural dispositions disease, their causes, their symptoms. (EN)

9 Joubert's Note: An ulcer is a double malady: it is an excavated wound, and it may be a triple-threat if it is sordid or sloughing, or it may be inflamed (a fourth element). You must begin your treatment by cleaning away the slough, and finish the

First determine if the patient's life is threatened. Then find the causes for the threat and determine that it is impossible to treat the (ie the primary cause) first because the threat is imminent; it is a time for a quick decision. When we decide that our treatment should aim at the ailment, so be it. In other words determine the order in which we should deal with the problems. As Galen put it in Books 3, 4, and 7 of his *Therapeutics,* and he said that it in all three places search for a cause, or find the reason sine qua non, or what is most urgent[10] At times the need for haste is such that you must treat the threatening complication first as when a nerve has been pierced, or a vein is hemorrhaging or a muscle has been torn or a displaced bone appears in an ulcer.

How To Perform An Operation With The Instruments Cited Above

Arnold of Villanova said that there are four considerations. 1. The operating surgeon should know what operation is to be performed on a human's body. 2. What good reasons lead him to an operation? 3. Is an operation necessary and feasible? 4. How does one perform it?

The first is answered by considering all of the operations as described above and selecting the correct one. The second is answered by faith in the surgeon who dares to operate on a human, that he will know that what he is doing, that he will be successful, and that he will be confident of its safety. The third considers the operation as it affects the various parts of the body. The fourth is knowing that the operation will be tolerated by the body, that is, if it is done well and is acceptable to the patient, and that the surgeon has experience in performing it, and in preparing the patient before and caring for him afterward.

As an example, when we wish to eliminate the water of ascites (hydrops), we should decide that an operation is necessary, and we decide that among all the methods available that we should use the knife. Then we consider why we should operate and we agree that surgery is a good way to treat ascites: at least it will relieve the discomforts. Third: is an operation necessary? We say, "yes", because there is no other way to treat real ascites. Can the patient tolerate the operation? Yes, if he not too debilitated and we do not drain all the fluid at one session. Fourth: let us consider the technique. We shall lay the patient supine, to expose the skin of the abdomen below the navel, on the right side if the patient's discomforts are mostly on the left, and on the opposite side if the symptoms are on the right. We will pinch up the skin (ie and panniculus) and incise it (ie simply a nick) where there are no exposed blood vessels. Then we will thrust in a cannula and drain as much fluid as the patient tolerates. We withdraw the cannula and release the skin that will cover the opening in the abdominal wall and stop the leak. When you wish to tap off more fluid, repeat the maneuvers and abide by the patient's tolerance. So be it.

A History Of Surgery

I shall describe in order all the surgeons whose works I have studied, and have cited in my book. I think that is a better way to distinguish each from the many others.

First came **Hippocrates** who towered above all the others. He was the first Greek to bring Medicine out of obscurity, as Macrobius and Isidore wrote in their *Etymologies,* and as is quoted in the prologue of Rhazes' *Continent.* Medicine had been dark during the five centuries after **Apollo and Aesculapius,** they

---

treatment by promoting the closure of the defect by cicatrisation. In the 'triple' case you begin by allowing the ulcer to fill with granulation tissue. Galen describe all of them at length in Books 3 and 4. (J).

10 Mingelausoux explained this passage: that Guy referred either to a direct complication of the malady, or to a separate threatening accident that demanded treatment first (M).

who invented the art. Hippocrates lived for ninety-five years and wrote many medical works as are decribed by Galen in Book 4 of his *Therapeutics* and elsewhere. I believe that Galen preserved Hippocrates and many others from obscurity.

Galen was the disciple who farmed the seeds taken from Hippocrates, and he added to the crops. He wrote many books in which Surgery is mixed with Medical topics, especially in his *Book of Tumors Contrary-to-Nature* where a summary of Surgery appears, and in the first six books of his *Therapeutics.*[11] In the last two he deals with aposthems and other maladies that require manual operations. Seven other books which made up the *Catageni* listed and classified the medications; I regret that we retain only a summary version. Galen was the premier scientist during the reign of Marcus Aurelius Antoninus, about one hundred-fifty AD. He lived to age 80 as testified in *The Lives and Conducts of the Philosophers.* According to **Avicenna** in Book 4 of his *Fractures,* and in glosses of the same, the long interval between Hippocrates and Galen lasted three hundred-twenty-five years,. But a truer chronology measures the interval at five hundred-eighty-six years.[12]

After Galen, we cite **Paul of Aegina** who made much of Surgery. He devoted his entire Book 6 to it, which was used by **Rhazes** in his *Continens* and by **Halyabbas** in his *Royal Dispositions.*

After them we meet **Rhazes, Albucasis** and **Alcaran.** The claim that all three names represent one person is not born out by the *Almansor* and its Divisions[13], by Albucasis in his *Divisions, Surgery),* and by Halyabbas, who described them as separate persons. He quotes Rhazes often, from his *Continens*—also called Helham in Arabic—in which he collects all the works of his predecessors. However, the exact citations are not stated; and a tedious and thankless search through that long Helham now seems unnecessary.

Halyabbas was a great Master, and his 'seed' is in his *Royal Disposition,* in which he devoted the ninth part of the Second Sermon to Surgery.

Avicenna came next, the honored 'Illustrious Prince'. The fourth book of his *Canon* is a nicely arranged surgical text, as are all of his works.

We know that before Avicenna all medical practitioners were physicians as well as surgeons. After him, however, whether due to timidity or to the increased complexities of treatment, Surgery was separated and relegated to the hands of 'mechanics'. The first to appear in Europe were **Roger, Roland** and **The Four Masters.** They wrote books entirely devoted to surgery and included much that was empirical (ie Anecdotal rather than Methodistic). Jamier followed: a brutal surgeon full of meaningless twaddle. All of them followed Roger's lead In most matters.

Then came **Bruno** who very carefully provided a summary of what he had learned from Galen, Avicenna, and Albucasis, even though he did not have a complete translation of Galen's works. He completely omitted anatomy from his book.

Theodoric followed. He plagiarized Bruno and added some fables, about **Hugh of Lucca** who was his Master.

William of Saliceto was a valuable resource; he produced two treatises, one on Medicine, the other on Surgery. I consider them both well made.

11 Wounds, ulcers, and fractures are discussed in Books 3, 4, 5, and 6, but not in Books 1 and 2 (EN).

12 Joubert claimed that the numbers were added to one of Guy's mss. He placed the correct figure in his Venetian edition of 1559. It is not in the Montpellier Ms, but it appears in several earlier Venetian editions (EN)

13 'Almansor' is the title of Rhazes' great work, it does not name a person, However, Al Mansour was a highly respected mathematician at Cordova. In his General Introduction Nicaise implies the Rhazes named his book to honor the Second Caliph of Bagdad who antedated Rhazes by at least one hundred-fifty years. The name Mansour means 'victorious' and it may have been a boast by Rhazes rather than a tribute (LDR).

Lanfranchi also wrote a work which included many of the things he had learned from William, although his book is arranged differently.

In the same era **Master Arnold of Villanova** flourished in another Faculty.[14] He wrote many fine books.

Henri de Hermondaville began to write a very powerful treatise at Paris and was noted for his melding of the methods of Theodoric and Lanfranchi. His premature death prevented him from completing the work.

During that era **Nicolas of Reggio** worked in Calabria and being proficient in Latin and Greek, he worked at the behest of King Robert, and translated many of Galen's books with which we now are endowed. They are the best and most elegant translations, better than those that had been made from the Arabic versions.

Finally, I shall mention a faded English Rose that had been sent to me and which I scanned; where I had hoped to find a delicate aroma, instead I found fables from Spain, from Gilbert and from Theodoric.[15]

In my day I have met good practicing surgeons; Master Nicolas Catalan of Toulouse; Master Bonet, Lanfranchi's son from Montpellier; Masters Peregrin and Mercadant of Bologna; Master Pierre de l'Argentiere of Paris; Pierre Bonant, a veteran practitioner at Lyon; Master Pierre of Aries; and my associate Jean of Parma.

Last, I list myself, Guy de Chauliac, both a surgeon and a physician. I come from the border of the Auvergne in the diocese of Mende. I am a chaplain and a physician and a friend of our Noble Pope. I have witnessed many operations and I have read treatises by the old masters, especially those of Galen which I have in translations. I studied them diligently and at length at the many places where I have found them. Now I live at Avignon in this year 1363, during the first year of the Papacy of Urban V. In this year I have completed the assemblage of this work, with the help of my friends, and with the good will of our Lord.

The Sects

Two chief sects of operating surgeons: persist to this time: the Logical or Rational[16], and the Empirics, of whom Galen disapproved in his *Book of Sects* and in his *Therapeutics.*

There have been five groups of the Empirics. The first group included Roger Roland and the Four Masters. They believed that suppuration was important in all wounds and aposthems, and they used poultices and bouillies based on what they read in Book 5 of the *Aphorisms* where it says, "The Gentle is Better and the Harsh is bad."[17]

---

14 This is Guy's first mention of a French surgeon. And the first to be titled 'Master', that is, one who was the product of a University, and the first from Montpellier. Guy tips his hat to an alumnus of his own school (LDR).

15 The reference is to John of Gaddesden's *Rosa Anglica*, full of mystical nonsense, ca 1310 (LDR).

16 A few commentators have read 'Laics' for 'Logicals', and they are wrong, because the laics were the empirics, with no rational (ie book-taught) bases. Many of them are illiterate. The physician-logicians (ie the rationals) were declared the best by Galen (J).

17 They used plasters which today are called cataplasms made from flour, roots, leaves, fruits, seeds, and flowers, all cooked, peeled and strained through cloths to make the pastes. A poultice-bouillie has the consistency of a cataplasm, but is made of wheaten flour wet with some liquid and thickened while heating and stirring to become what we call bouîllee d'armotte. We surgeons call it a triarpharmac mol when it is composed of wheaten flour, water and oil (J).
Much of this and the ensuing paragraphs is an almost verbatim transcript of what Malgaigne wrote in the Introduction to his edition of Pare. (See pp. xxxix ff). I cannot say who came first: Guy, Joubert or Malgaigne. Certainly Nicaise followed Joubert nearly always and did not compare him with Malgaigne word for word in making this edition (LDR).

The second group included Bruno and Theodoric who tried to treat all wounds without pus, using wine as the only substance. That method also was Galenic (*Therapeutics)* where he stated, "The dry is healthy, not so the wet."[18]

The third sect included William of Saliceto and Lanfranchi who tried to steer a middle course, using ointments and soft plasters based on Galen's *Therapeutics:* he advised following his simple dogma: treat safely and cause no pain.

The fourth sect are the Teutonic Knights and policemen, and other warriors. They treat all wounds with magic potions, with oil, wool-fleece, and cabbage leaves, believing that the Lord endows words, herbs and minerals with curative powers.

The fifth sect are the women and the idiots who relegated all sick persons to Saints. Their only treatment was based on this prayer: "The Lord giveth as he pleases, and he deals with me as he pleases. Bless His Name, Amen."

These sects will be refuted in the text that follows, and I will not carry on with it here.

However, I am amazed that people follow leaders like cranes in flight; they repeat what someone else has said. I cannot decide if it is fear or love that makes them listen only to what they are accustomed to and has been approved by some authority. They misinterpret what Aristotle wrote in Book 2 of his *Metaphysics* where he demonstrated that when there is a choice between two approaches to the truth, one should ignore biases and fears, and even if Socrates and Plato are our friends, the truth is even more a friend.[19] Truth comes first, it is holy and honorable. That characterizes the Dogmatic Doctrines of Galen as expressed in his *Book of Sects* and especially in the *Therapeutics* which is entirely a composite of reason (ie logic) and experience, where one seeks the facts and ignores words. The same is taught in the epilogue of Chapter 7 of his *Constitution of the Dogmatic Method;* he said it again in Chapter 10 of his *Natural Faculties:* "He who will be ahead of others in knowledge cannot become so of a sudden. He must be born intelligent and be well taught from the first lessons on. When he reaches boyhood and then puberty his restless spirit will love the truth. He will study diligently night and day and he will learn everything that was taught by the most renowned Ancients, and when he reaches full manhood he will be endowed with the ability to judge for himself what he examines at length and with due care, and accordingly he can advise what he agrees with and what he rejects." He added, "I hope what seems relevant to me will avail the Reader. However, to some it may seem superfluous, or a fable told to a fool."

I do not claim to have experienced everything that is written here. Galen wrote in many places that there are two sources from which to make a decision. Yet, there is a third source, other than what is based on personal experience and logic (ie reason). It is dependence on what others have witnessed. He said (early in Chapter 3 of the *Therapeutics*), and in the *Miamir* or *The Compositions According To The Places),* that one increases his faith in what he reads if he has confidence in the authors. And that is why he repeated all the medications that he took from the works of expert physicians. And I will do the same here, with God's help.

The Requirements For All Surgeons

Now I shall discuss the conditions to be met by all surgeons who use their art on human bodies, and I will describe how to operate. Our forefather Hippocrates commented with this subtle conclusion to his

18 Malgaigne wrote: "One makes a serious error in attributing this to Bruno and Theodoric (who copied Bruno). Bruno cited the Aphorism "Laxa bona" and credited it to Roger. This is not meant to detract from Guy." (Malgaigne ibid) (EN).

19 I interpret this passage as a reflection of the disputes between the Platonists and the Aristotelians in France, especially at Paris at that epoch, as influenced by Thomas Aquinas et al. (LDR).

introduction of *The Aphorisms:* "Life is short, Art is complex, The Time and the Occasion may be demanding and occur suddenly, and experience may be misleading and perilous, and judgment difficult. Your actions should involve not only your own experience in such actions, but also the consideration of your patient, your assistants, and your control over the external circumstances.

According to Arnold of Villanova, that eloquent Latinist, there are four sets of requirements: One set involves the surgeon, a second involves the patient, a third deals with the assistants, and the fourth concerns the externals.

The four requirements for the surgeon are: 1. His education. 2. His skills. 3. His ingenuity, and 4. His personality and conduct. Therefore the surgeon must be well educated, not only in the principles of surgery, but also in the theory and practice of medicine.[20]

As to Theory: he must know the Natural things and the non-natural and the contrary to nature things. Of the Natural Things, Anatomy is the most important, a sine-qua-non for surgery, as will be seen in the text. Also, he should understand Complexion and know that the varieties thereof will affect his choice of medications (see *Versus Thessalus*[21], and in all parts of *Therapeutics).* The same holds for knowing the Virtue, which means the life-force (ie spirit).

The Non-Natural Things concern the Air, Foods and Beverages, etc, all of which affect the health of the patient. The Things Contrary-To-Nature are the malady itself which he intends to cure, and its causes, which he must know if he will treat it. His success will depend on that rather than on lucky guesses. He must be aware of the complications in order to attack their causes and forestall them and interfere with the treatments of the malady. Galen repeats all that in the *Glaucon.*

As to Practice: The surgeon should know how to manage the life-style (ie the regimen) as well as the medicaments, because operative Surgery is the third instrument of Medicine. Galen said that in his *Introduction.* The use of medicines (pharmacy), follows the properly managed regimen, and surgery comes third.

Therefore, the surgeon who operates should know the principles of Medicine and have some knowledge of the other arts. Galen (*Therapeutics*) said in opposition to Thessalus, "Physicians should know something about geometry, astronomy, and dialectics (ie rhetoric), and other good doctrines that will affect the conduct of the scrapers, carpenters, merchants, and others who would change their careers and take up Medicine.[22]

The second requirement for surgeons is Skill. He should be an expert when he operates. The wise Avenzoar quote, "Every physician should know things (ie been taught) and then learn from his own experience with them." Rhazes said the same in his *Almansor* (Book 4) and Halyabbas agreed (*Commentary on Hippocrates' Theory).*

The third requirement is Ingenuity and Common Sense. Haly stated (Book 3 of *Techni).* "The surgeon must have a good memory, common sense, proper motives, good vision, and be healthy". Later he added that the surgeon should be well-made for the job, with slim fingers, strong hands, clear eyes, and lack tremors.

The fourth requirement is a good Presence. The surgeon should be daring when the outcome will be assured, but he should tread carefully in face of peril, and he will avoid harmful treatments[23] and other such actions. He should be gracious with his patients and generous with his friends, and be wise with his prognoses. He should be chaste, sober, and be sympathetic with those who suffer. He should not

20 Arnold's term was 'Physic', meaning all of medicine (J).

21 Thessalus of Tralles, a Greek in Nero's Rome. He was a leading Methodist. See Sarton, Vol. I, p. 262 (LDR).

22 A bitter jab at the empirics and Thessalus (LDR).

23 Again we remind the Reader that 'harmful treatments' in general were open surgical operations (LDR).

connive and seek extortionate fees and he should willingly state in advance fees that are commensurate with his work and the patient's ability to pay, in view of the results of his treatments and in view of his professional status.

The three conditions required of the patient are: 1. He must follow the surgeon's instructions, much as a peasant obeys his feudal seigneur (Galen, *Therapeutics).* 2. He should trust the physician (Galen, *Prognostics)* and 3. He should be patient, because patience overcomes fearful thoughts (also Galen).

The four requirements for the assistants: Be gentle, be gracious (agreeable), be faithful, and be discrete.

In regard of the externals, there are many elements that must be arranged for the sake of the patient, as Galen wrote in his *Commentary on the Aphorisms of Hippocrates.*

How I have Arranged My Text

After this Singular Chapter, I will follow a plan which simply is what Averroes suggested, at the beginning of his *Colliget.* He wrote that every Artisan's practices should have three rules. 1. Know your subject. 2. Know what your goals are. 3. Know your tools and how to use them to obtain your goals.

Because our Art is practical and operative, the treatises must be at least of three sorts. However, in our book I have set them into seven Treatises, to cover the three parts described in the *Colliget).* 1. Anatomy, where maladies occur 2. Treatments and 3. Usage.

In summary: The seven treatises are: 1. Anatomy. 2. Aposthems. 3. Wounds. 4. Ulcers. 5. Fractures and Dislocations. 6. Other surgical maladies, and 7. The Tools, including the Antidotary.

Each Treatise will describe two doctrines, and each doctrine will have about eight chapters. Each chapter will have three parts, as in Galen's *Therapeutics,* which will refresh the physicians who wish to follow the Dogmatic methods. 1. The malady and its causes. 2. The symptoms that will lead to your diagnosis and to decisions about treatments and curability 3. The treatments: why and how to operate. That is the order I will follow throughout the book, with God's help.

HERE BEGINS THE MAIN TEXT OF THE MAJOR SURGERY TREATISE I THE ANATOMY

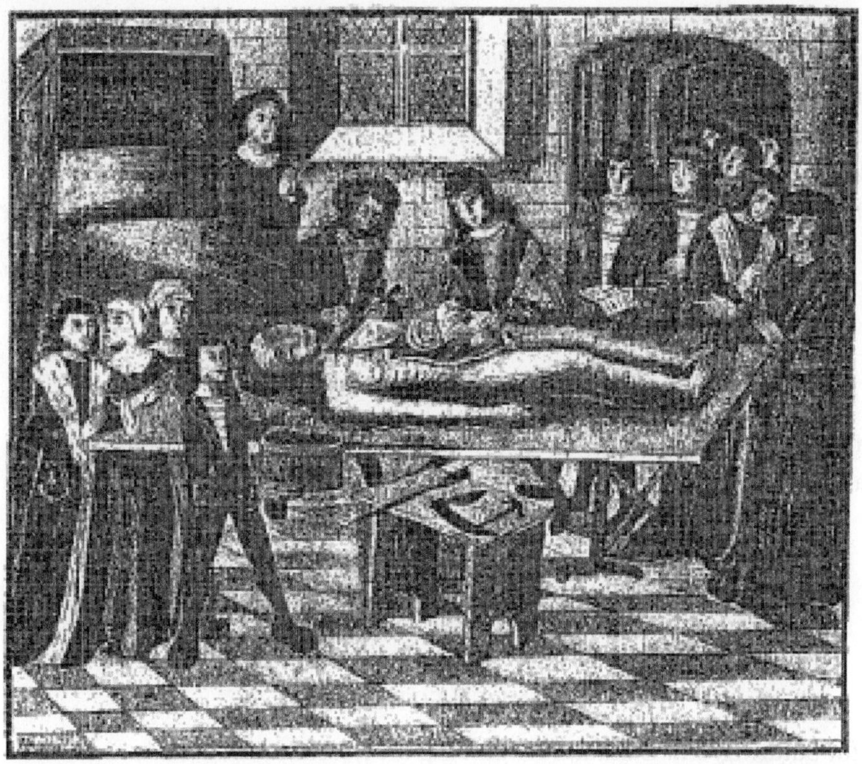

Figure 3. AN ANATOMICAL DEMONSTRATION IN THE 14 C A Reproduction of a Miniatuer in a 14th C French Manuscript of Guy's Treatise of Anatomy Ms 184, Library of The Faculty of Medicine at Montpellier. Courtesy of The Surgeon General's Library, Washington, DC. Copyright in the Public Domain.

APPENDIX II: SURGICAL INSTRUMENTS

Nicaise's (Translator's) Note

Guy used many instruments. He listed his armamentarium for removing foreign items from wounds, for trepanation, for operations for hernias and bladder stones, for operations on the eyes and the ears, for fumigation and for dental work. He mentioned many more, but he left no drawings, unless some had been inserted in lost manuscripts. The only illustrated surgical treatise before the invention of printing was that of Albucasis. The first printed edition that contained illustrations of instruments was by Brunschwig. I have reviewed the books that show instruments used by the ancient surgeons, as they were found at Herculaneum and Pompei, and many books printed after the 15th C. Here I will use simple line drawings to illustrate the brief descriptions of what Guy used. My sources are:

H. Brunschwig, 1497, *Das Buch der Chirurgia.* Strassburg

A. H. Gersdorf, 1542. *Das Feld buch der Wundartzney,* Strassburg, dela Croix, 1573. *Chirurgiae universalis,* Venise, 1573

Scultetus, 1672, *Armamentarium chirurgicum*, Amsterdam

Arneman, 1796, *Instrum de chirurg.* Gottingen

Rudtorfer, 1817, *Instr. De chir.*, Vienna

P. Savenko,1821, *Note sur la chirurgie dans les premier ages.* In Rev. Med Hist.

Vulpes, 1847, *Illustrazione de tulligli strumenti chirurgica scavati In Ercolane e Pompei,* Naples

J. Sichel, 1866, *Nouveau recueil de pierres sigillaires,* Paris

Schoutetten, 1867, *Hist. des instrument, de chir. etc.* Paris

Translator's Note

The instruments are named, followed by brief comments. The numbered items are pictured in the five Plates, as I,#l. Others are described without numbers.

The Instruments

INDEX FOR PLATE I

Needles for Suturing, and Cannulas for guiding the needles *I, #1, 2, 3, 4.*
Lead Needle for use in nosem mouth, anal fistula, etc. *I, #5*
Cataract Needles. *I, #6, 6a.*
Urethral Cannulas, with stents. *I, #7, 7a*
Crossbow for Removing embedded arrows. *V, #1*
Apparatus for Reducing and Splinting Fractures. *V, #2*
Metallic Cap to protect an injured fingertip
Truss to Protect the Lower Abdomen.
Cannulas:
- Cannula to direct a needle (see above)
- Fenestrated Cannula to accept a sharp chisel to snip off an excrescence caught in the window. *I, #8, 8a*
- Cannula to introduce a caustic for application only at the uvula, which is trapped in the window. The caustic is applied on a tuft at the end of a piston.
- Bronze or silver cannula fro draining ascites. *I, #9*
- Cannula for draining ears of children *I, #10*
- Cannulas for fumigation. Can be attached to tubes for introduction into the vagina, etc. *I, #11,12*
- A solid 'catheter' or sound with a rounded tip for probing wounds

Cauteries: These may be solid hot metal, boiling oil or a wooden stick with a burning ember at the tip. The potential cauteries are caustics, called emptors. The Ancients had many varieties, whereas Guy named only six.
- The Cultellary: With one cutting edge, the Dorsal, *I,#14*
- With two cutting edges, the Ensal *I, #15*
- The Olivary, named for the shape of its tip. I, *#17*

The Dactilary. Its tip shaped like a date-pit, is longer and heavier than the Olivary *I, #17b*
The Punctual. A slim rod with a rounded tip to destroy a node or polyp. Its depth is limited by a lateral pin. It is applied through a perforated plate. *I, #17 and 17.*
A narrow rod-cautery is applied through a cannula to reach a deep spot and protect the surrounding tissues. *I, #18,18a, 18b*
Guy used some very thin, wire-like silver cauteries for insertion into dental caries, or he used a red-hot silver or bronze probe.
A Seton Cautery: This was a long, hot or cold, cutting-edge needle passed through perforations in apposed blades of a forceps that gripped a fold of skin. The needle was armed with a tough ribbon or cord which remained as drain when the apparatus was removed. *I, #19, 20, 21, 22, 23.*

PLATE 1

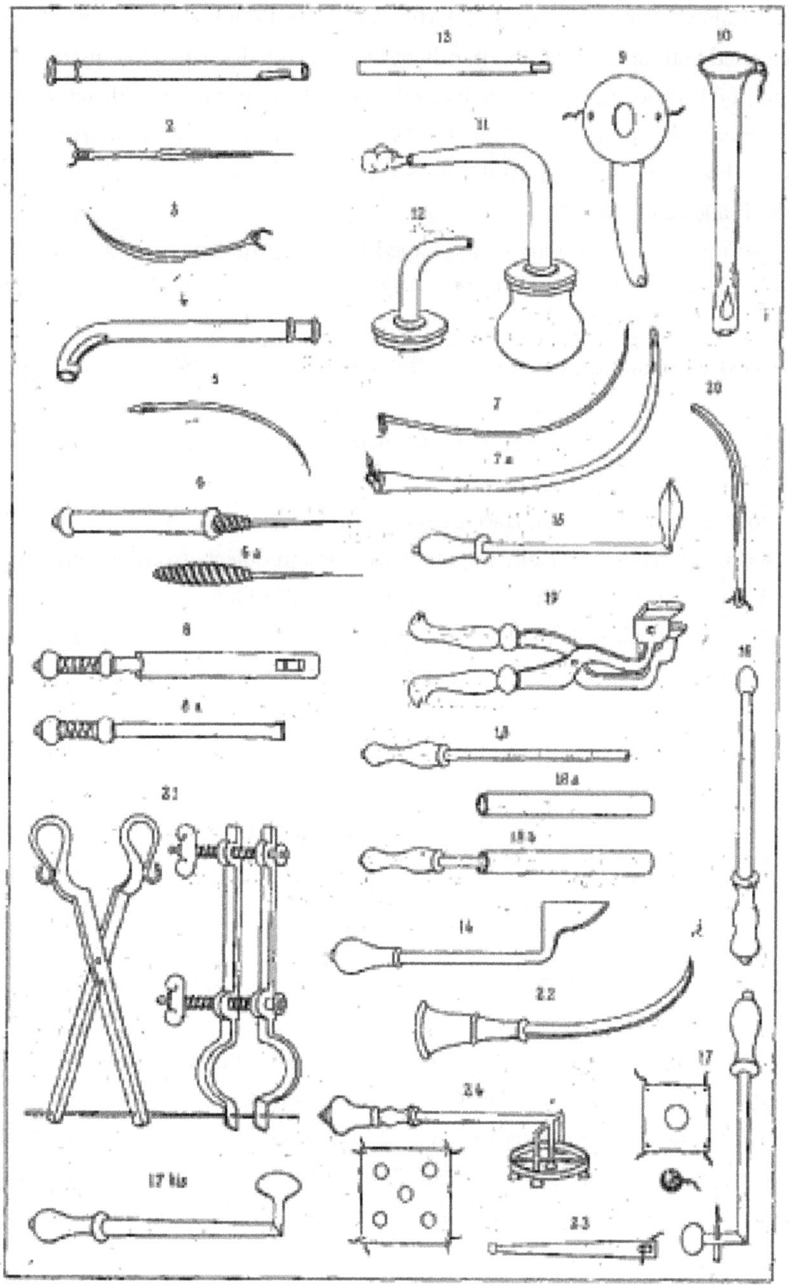

A Circular Cautery: has five buttons or points attached to the undersurface of the ring, to burn a node or other lesion at five places simultaneously. It was applied through a perforated plate *I, #24*

INDEX FOR PLATE IV

1. Described them but provided no drawings. Celsus had described his own as straight, as are the materials found at Herculaneum and Pompei. *III, #65, 66 (not included here)*.
2. Rasps for scraping: Guy used one for removing teeth. There were many shapes and sizes,. Guy described one that was hollowed, as a gouge.
3. Saws: Amputations were rare events, and saws were seldom mentioned. *III, #81 (not included here)*.
4. Setons: see clysters above. The term was used in different ways, both before and after Guy's era, with different types of devices, used both in humans and in other animals. Guy described his instruments and how he used them to drain scrotal hydrocoeles, and to reduce edema in the upper body with setons in folds of the skin of the nape and the axillae. His practice was adopted by Pierre Franco and by Gatinaria. *I, #19, 20, 21, 22, 23*
5. Guy used a grooved probe for treating fistula-in-ano. The trough guided a cultellary cautery. That instrument was improved by Franco and Pare.
6. Spatulas: blades to mix medicines. Guy's was shaped like a myrtle-leaf. He also used it to apply medicines on the eye. Those from Herculaneum and Pompei had a usable tip at the handle: a button, olive, curette, or elevator.
7. Speculum: Guy used several kinds. One exposed the inner vagina: *IV, #82*. Another depressed the tongue, *IV, #84*.
8. Traction Apparatus for reducing fractures. *V, #2*, (drawing from Gersdorf). The device was used by Guy.
9. Taste: see Probe. The taste was a flat wood or metallic blade (resembling a tongue depressor in the 21st C) The surgeon used it to flatten an irregular surface before incising it. *IV, #85*.
10. Forceps: Guy used many types, especially for removing foreign objects from wounds. Avicenna's had curved blades with teeth. Albucasis used them to crush the head of a dead fetus. *IV, #86*
11. Albucasis' (another) had 'bird-beak' blades with teethe. He used them to remove arrows. Some were used to extract teeth. *IV, #87, 88, 89, 90, 91*.
12. Forceps with gouged blades were used to remove barbed arrows. *IV, #92,93*
13. Guy described a forceps with long curved blades for removing foreign objects caught in the throat *IV, #94*. He used a long narrow forceps to extract small stones trapped in the penile urethra. He used a small forceps to extract teeth. It resembled the clamps used by coopers to tighten the bindings on barrels. *IV, #95, 96*.
14. Tents: Guy used them in many ways: to apply detergents, to prevent early closure of a wound, to enlarge an opening, to promote drainage from wounds and abscesses. Sometimes he used perforated cannulas of silver or bronze.
15. *IV, #104, 105*. He used similar tents of wood or lead to prevent re-adherence of a dissected prepuce, or to dilate a hymen.
16. Tracheotomy: Guy inserted a cannula between two tracheal rings, thereby distinguishing it from laryngotomy (he called it epiglottis). He intubated the larynx through the throat.
17. Trepanation: I will not repeat the material presented inTreatise III, Doctrine, II, Chapterl, or what was discussed in the Biographical Section of my (Nicaise) Introduction. Guy described three trepans: Galen's with a chaperone pin. *IV, #97* The Parisian with a variable pin, *IV, #98*, and the Bolognese with a tapered lancet-cutter, *IV, #99*.

PLATE IV

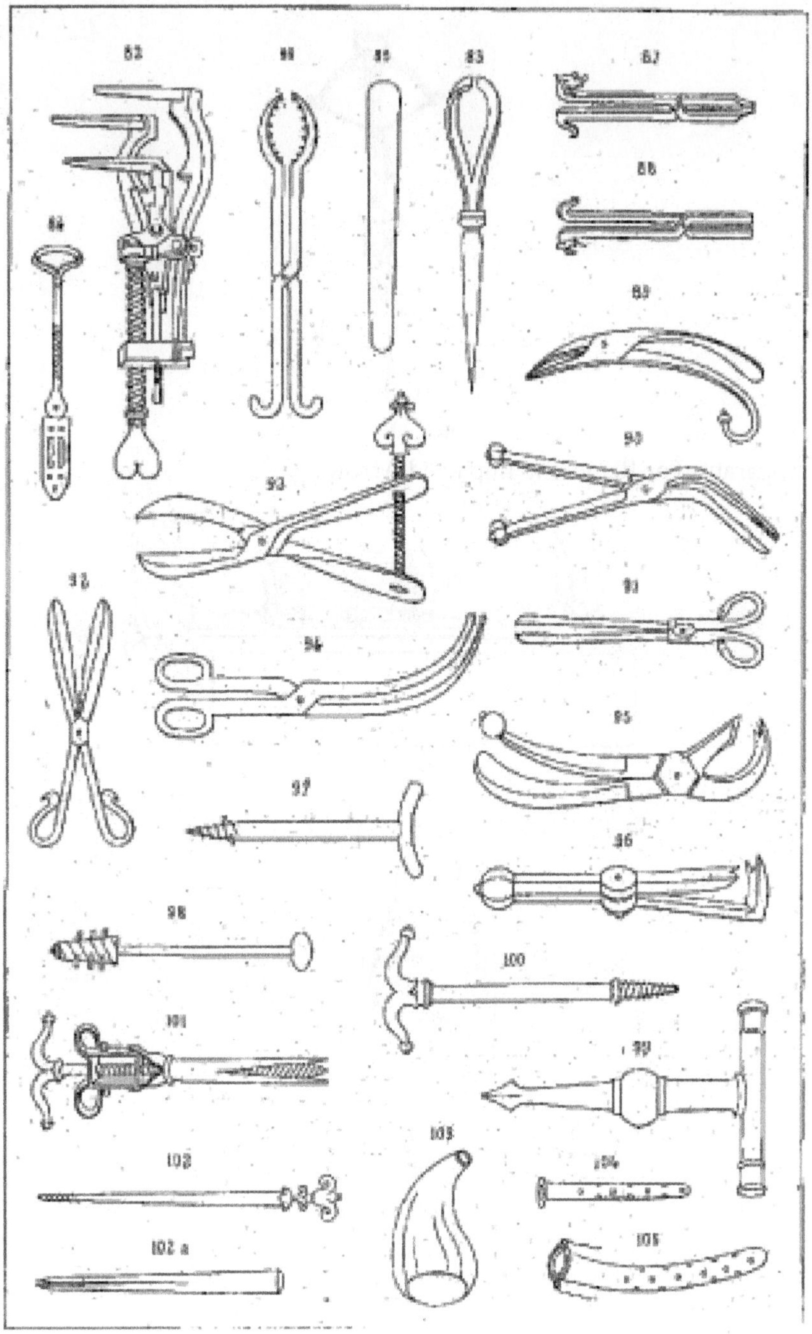

Guy used a borer-drill (tarrier) to enlarge the opening in a bone in which an arrowhead was embedded. *IV #100, 101*

Other Tarriers: A slim one to enter a stone trapped in the penile urethra either to remove it or to break it. *IV, #102, 102a*

Pipes: short tubes to tighten the splints around a fracture. *V, #2*

Cups: made from ivory, copper or glass, with or without openings for suction *IV, #103.*

PLATE V

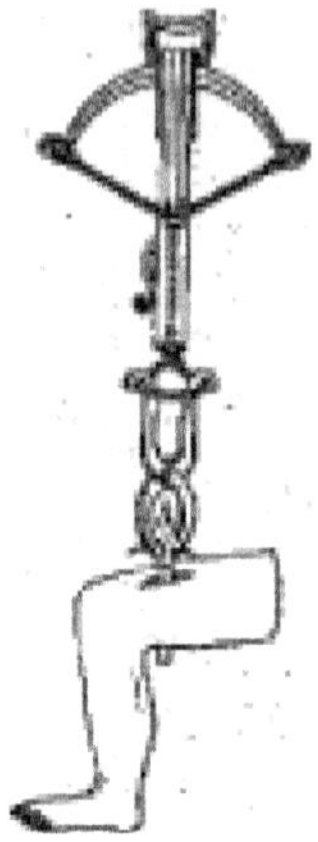

Strong-bow Apparatus For Removing Impacted Arrows

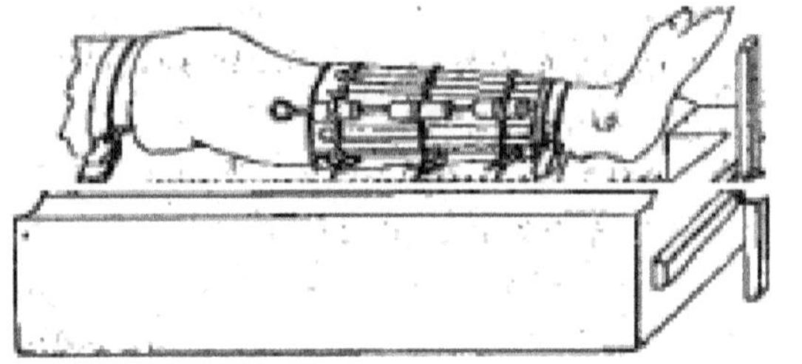

Windlass Box For Reducing and Splinting Fractures

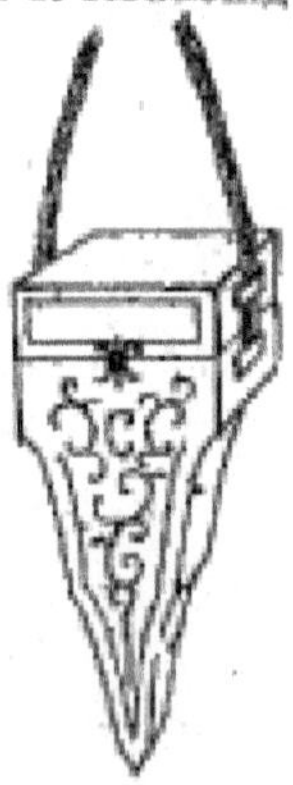

Portable Case (Pennarol) For Surgical Instruments

Chapter 7

Leonardo da Vinci: *Anatomical Notebooks* (1519)

HISTORICAL HIGHLIGHTS

- Leonardo da Vinci (1452–1519)
- Born at Vinci near Florence, Italy
- Educated as artist under Verochio
- Recognized as universal painter
- Was a Renaissance polymath, painter, architect, and sculptor, among few
- Became well-versed anatomist
- Examined 30 human corpses
- Performed anatomical studies from 1472–1513
- Defined importance of heart, its four cavities and contraction of the ventricles
- Many anatomical discoveries passed by his genius drawing pen
- His anatomical drawings remained hidden at Windsor Castle until 1796

Editor's Note: Text that appears in italics throughout this chapter is original to Leonardo da Vinci. The remaining text was written by Charles D. O'Malley and J.B. De C.M. Saunders. We have utilized O'Malley and Saunders' excellent writings on Leonardo da Vinci to explain the anatomical contributions of the master of Vinci.

THE WRITINGS OF O'MALLEY AND SAUNDERS AND LEONARDO DA VINCI

Anatomical Illustration Before Leonardo

If it may be said that the fourteenth century ushered in a new period of civilization, for convenience called the Renaissance, then it may be remarked that anatomy in that new age was long to remain mediaeval, at least insofar as it was reflected in medical illustration. Prior to this new era the teaching of anatomy had been based largely upon the dissection of animals, but in the thirteenth century even this limited procedure of direct observation was largely superseded by the Arabic influence which led to efforts to

Charles D. O'Malley and J. B. De C. M. Saunders, from *Leonardo da Vinci on the Human Body: The Anatomical, Physiological, and Embryological Drawings of Leonardo da Vinci.* Readings selected and historical highlights written by Luis Horacio Toledo-Pereyra.

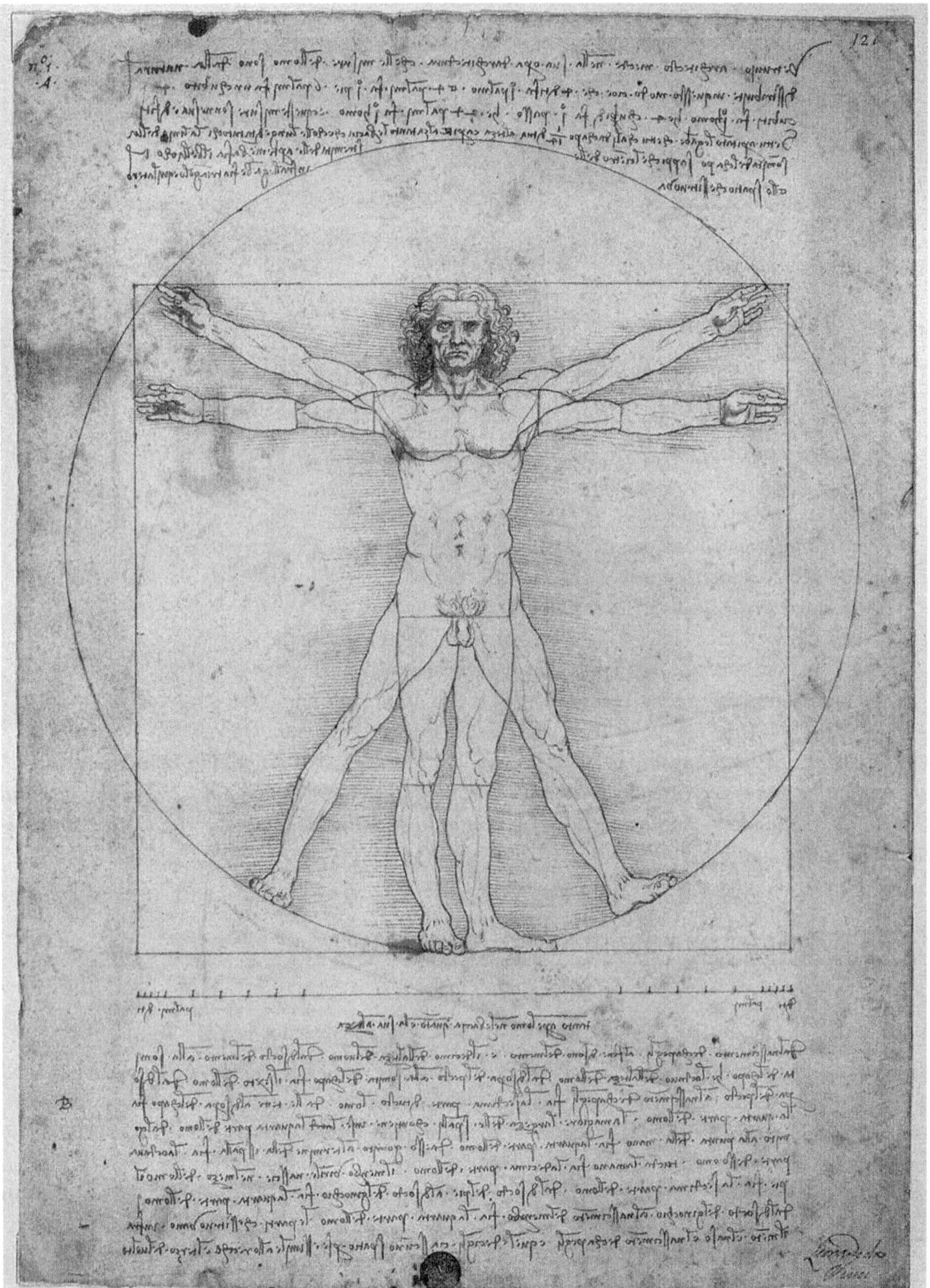

The Vitruvian Man (c. 1485)
Academia, Venice

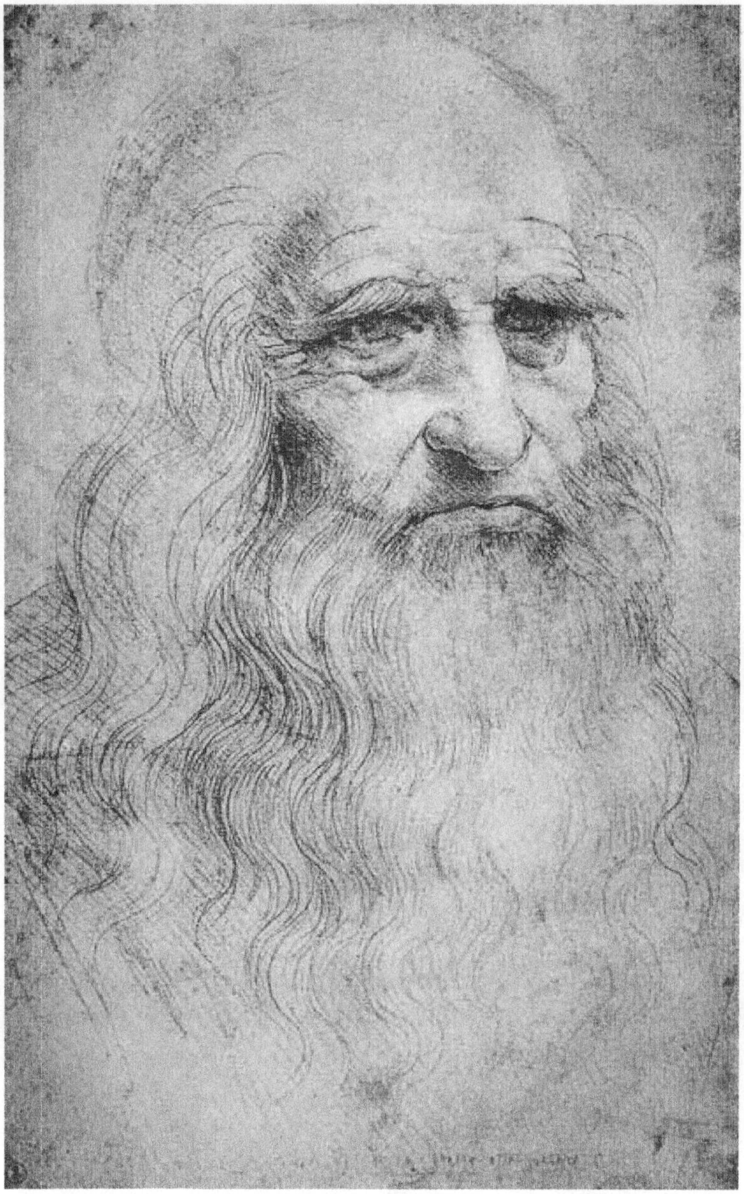

Self-portrait by Leonardo da Vinci, chalk drawing (1512). Located at the Palazzo Reale in Turin, Italy.

teach anatomy wholly from textbooks. Although the Arabic influence was to be cast off eventually, yet anatomy was still to suffer from strictures arisen from a misunderstanding of the position of the church. In 1300 Pope Boniface VIII had issued a bull, *De sepulturis,* which proclaimed excommunication for any who should follow the practice of boiling the bones of persons, in particular crusaders, in order to make their storage and transport easier for burial at home. This bull was frequently and incorrectly interpreted, even by anatomists, as a prohibition against dissection. Partly perhaps as an outgrowth of this situation and partly as the result of too literal religious views there was also considerable popular opposition to dissection of the human body for fear of the consequences upon resurrection.

Despite such obstacles there was a limited knowledge of anatomy, partly traditional, partly the outgrowth of surgical experience and very likely from time to time the reflection of surreptitious dissection.

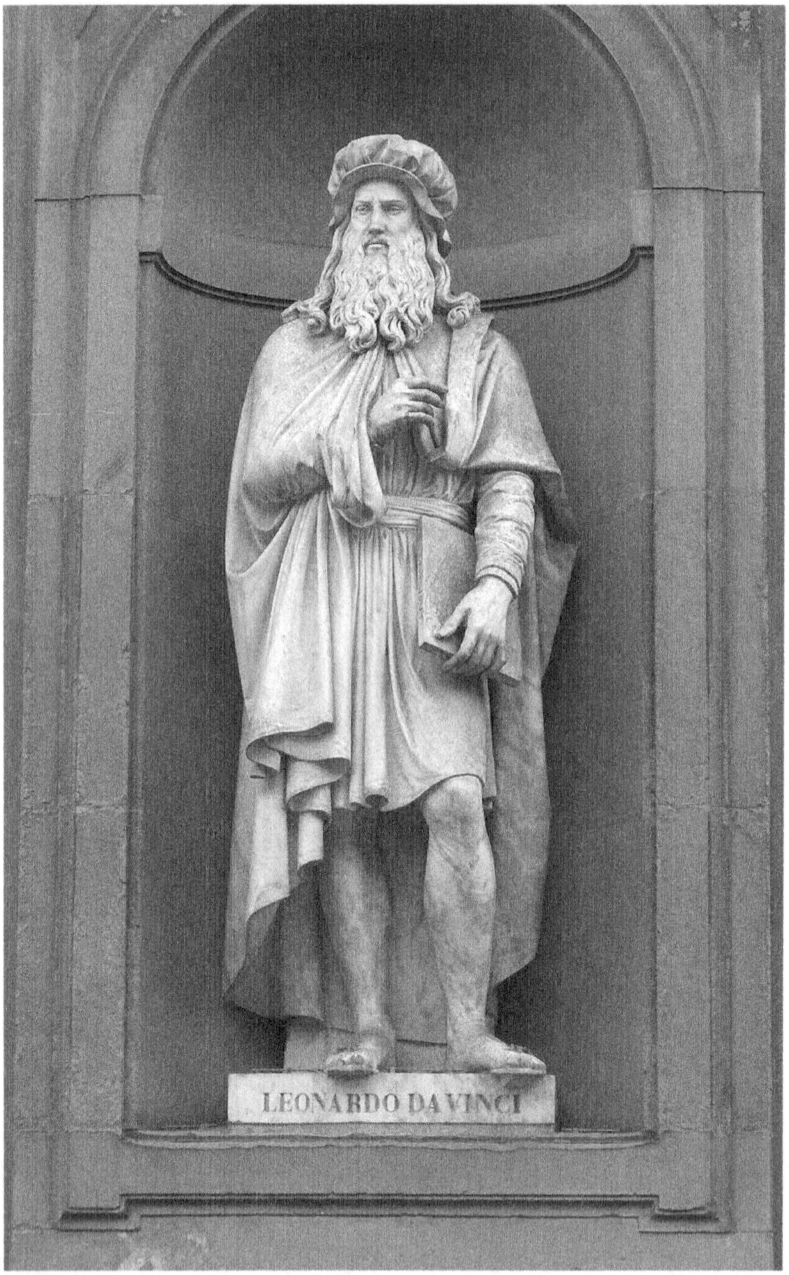

Statue of Leonardo da Vinci standing outside Galleria Uffizi in Florence, Italy

The first open mention of dissection was of one performed in Italy in 1286. However, it was nothing more than a post-mortem examination of a victim of a pestilence then raging and was for the purpose of attempting to find the cause of death. There is a more formal account of an examination performed in 1302 in Bologna to ascertain the cause of a death which had occurred under suspicious circumstances. The account does not suggest the procedure as unusual and presumably post-mortem examinations as legal devices had previously been performed. Yet such examinations would yield little anatomical information since normally the procedure required little more than the opening of the thorax and an examination of the contents.

With the appearance in 1316 of the *Anothomia* of Mundinus (c.1270–1326) we enter upon what might be called the non-mediaeval rather than the modern period of anatomy. Moreover, it should be emphasized that in this period anatomy was considered to include both a knowledge of the structure and of the function of the human body. Mundinus' book is the first devoted entirely to this subject, and although the Arabic tradition is still strong, yet it is obvious that Mundinus incorporated the results of dissection and, indeed, performed the dissections himself. From the time of Mundinus the medical school at Bologna was to become the centre of such anatomical knowledge as there was. There dissection was officially recognized by university statute in 1405, to be followed in 1429 by a similar recognition at Padua. However, permission did not necessarily imply opportunity, and cadavers were only very infrequently at the disposal of the schools. Furthermore, the successors of Mundinus for the next century and a half did little more than echo and confirm what he had already propounded, and this is not to be wondered at in view of what passed for dissection.

This limited interest in anatomy is supported by text and illustration, although the situation is more precisely defined in the former since it was not until the sixteenth century, and even then far from unanimously, that physicians came to look upon correct anatomical drawings as having any pedagogical value. Indeed, many physicians up to this time decried the employment of anything which might tend to distract the reader from the text. Under such conditions, it is not astonishing to find that illustration displayed no development. Such as there was remained traditional, often having no immediate relationship to the text and frequently merely a kind of symbolic decoration. Thus to judge the anatomical knowledge at any given time from such illustrative material would be wholly misleading.

The major tradition insofar as anatomical illustration is concerned was one which is said to go as far back as the time of Aristotle who in his *De generatione animalium,* I:7, speaks of the teaching of anatomy through "paradigms, schemata and diagrams". Thereafter the Alexandrian anatomists such as Herophilus and Erasistratus are said to have continued the employment of such sorts of illustrative materials in their teaching.

While it is impossible to say precisely what these illustrative materials were, nevertheless there is fairly general support for the belief that what Karl Sudhoff called the "Five Picture Series" represents a portion of them. These five views, representative of the bones, muscles, nerves, veins and arteries, and displayed in crude human figures, invariably in a semi-squatting position, have been found not only in Europe and Asia, but also in the western hemisphere. The similarity of pose—with full anterior view of body and face, the latter completely rigid—suggests a long-standing tradition which Sudhoff considers as indicating characteristics of early Egyptian and Greek sculpture and therefore supporting a Hellenic and Alexandrian origin.

Through successive centuries the tradition appears to have remained constant with the exception that occasionally a sixth figure was added, either a view of the pregnant woman or depiction of the generative organs, either male or female. However, the anatomical content of the series passed on to successive centuries without change despite the fact that anatomical texts indicate gradually increasing knowledge. It is not astonishing therefore that as anatomical knowledge increased, notably at the end of the fifteenth century, this series of five or six crude figures is less and less associated with the physician and becomes a device to assist the unlearned barber-surgeon in his activities, especially that of bloodletting. Nevertheless the pedagogical aspect of the tradition associated with the figures continued in regular medical circles. Thus the *Tabulae anatomicae* of Vesalius (1538) are the result of this influence although the new pose of the figures, the superior draughtsmanship and far more nearly correct anatomy represent a novelty.

If therefore the traditional anatomical drawings became less and less a true representation of the state of anatomical knowledge with the passing centuries, there is another sort of anatomical drawing which does more truly represent the situation. This is the miniature which is to be found on manuscripts from about the fourteenth century, depicting dissection scenes. While it is true that the extent of knowledge is not indicated in these miniatures, yet the dissection scenes are revealing. Human dissection, it is apparent, was once again being practiced, and in the course of time such dissections would inevitably lead to an increase of anatomical knowledge. It is true that the dissection was still an occasional affair and indicated as such by its ceremonious nature. It is also true that the actual dissection was delegated to assistants, and the physician-teacher lectured from a book with little profit to himself or to his students. Yet inevitably and gradually, knowledge would be acquired. From our advantage of hindsight it may be said that the appearance of the dissection miniature meant the eventual banishment of the traditional anatomical series from academic medical circles.

While it can be said with considerable correctness that from the fourteenth century on the physician looked with more and more scorn upon anatomical illustration—possibly in some degree because of its useless character so long as it remained traditional—about this time the professional artist was becoming interested in the study of anatomy as an auxiliary to a more naturalistic portrayal of the human body. In recent years (1916, 1919) a study of this was made by E. C. Streeter, and while certain of his conclusions are tenable, unfortunately too great enthusiasm for his thesis and certain incorrect interpretations have distorted the picture. These errors were then compounded and strengthened by the affirmation and support of F. H. Garrison (1919, 1926). However, a thorough study of the anatomico-artistic career of Leonardo da Vinci suggests certain revisions in what might be called the Streeter-Garrison thesis.

According to Streeter, Florentine painters were accustomed to purchase their pigments in the apothecary shops, and as a result tended to become acquainted with physicians who were also patrons of such establishments. The result of such contact produced a certain fellow-feeling which led the artists to apply for admission into the guild of physicians and apothecaries (1303). This condition was to remain for "more than two and a half centuries" and consequently led to a considerable exchange of interest and information. Thus Masaccio was to join the guild as an apothecary (1421) but decided to continue his membership as a painter (1423). In addition to such changes of interest there developed a number of close friendships between physicians and painters such as that of Giotto with Dino del Garbo and Luca della Robbia with Benivieni. The presumption here is that along with the artist's desire for greater naturalism in painting he was further fostered in this direction through his association with physicians. Here it might be interposed that such association, like a double-edged sword ought to cut both ways, yet we have no evidence that the physician was influenced to an appreciation of the role which art might play in medicine.

However this may be, it appears that from the time of Giotto onwards the movement was toward greater anatomical realism, and it was Giotto's assistant, Stefano, who was called "the ape of nature" because of the skill he acquired in the depiction of the superficial veins in the human body. Indeed, the story is that barber-surgeons studied his pictures before opening a vein. This story, needless to say, has a certain apocryphal ring to it, since in view of the prevalence of bloodletting the barber-surgeons would have had through experience even more knowledge of the position of the superficial veins than Stefano, while the appearance of the veins on the surface of the body would make it unnecessary, if study were required, to resort to paintings. Finally, it is rather difficult to imagine the barber-surgeons of that era, in view of their general character, taking such pains over anything so common as a matter of venesection.

Through the close contact of artist with painter it is related that in their pursuit of naturalism the artists perceived the advantage to them of anatomical study through dissection, which had been authorized at the Florentine university in 1387, and began to attend and then to assist their guild colleagues, the physicians, at such dissections. Thereafter these artists began to dissect for themselves, the first who undertook such scientific study of anatomy being apparently Donatello (1386–1466), who has left us a bronze tablet "The anatomy of the miser's heart" in commemoration of his interest. The weakness in this otherwise fascinating thesis is the fact that dissection as it was performed provided very little anatomical knowledge, certainly no more than was already available in Mundinus, while such studies, particularly that displayed by Donatello, would be of little or no value to the artist who naturally would be interested in the more superficial structures and certainly for his purpose not in the contents of the thorax.

Further consideration of the artist as anatomist rests upon the anatomical correctness with which he has painted the human body and the various accounts given by Vasari, an authority who, be it noted, is frequently unreliable. Of Antonio Pollaiuolo (1432–1498) Vasari has written: "He understood the nude in a more modern way than the masters before him; he removed the skin from many corpses to see the anatomy underneath". A recent judgment of Pollaiuolo's "Battle of the Ten Nudes", in which perhaps his anatomical knowledge is best portrayed, declares him the great anatomical student among artists before Leonardo. Without criticism of the latter judgment, it should be noted that Vasari's statement suggests both truth and error. It is quite within reason that the artist "removed the skin … to see the anatomy underneath", that is, his interest was mythological, while the dissection as performed in the medical school would have no particular value for him. To call an artist whose interest is only in such structures as would be reflected in the surface features of the body a student of anatomy is to distort the meaning of the term, especially in the Renaissance sense of anatomy and physiology. Finally, Vasari's reference to the "many corpses" which Pollaiuolo flayed suggests a legendary growth, in view of the great difficulties that confronted the medical schools in obtaining, cadavers, and the relatively few specimens that Leonardo obtained a century later.

In the case of del Verrocchio (1435–1488) it is said that as a student under Pollaiuolo and Donatello he displayed a like scientific interest. Moreover, as the teacher of Leonardo it has been assumed that he initiated his great student into anatomical studies; hence he himself must be a student of anatomy. While del Verrocchio did not paint many nudes, yet, as it has been stated, in his drawings there is no question of his anatomical studies, as for example, his representations of the surface muscles in bodies from which the skin has been removed. Again Vasari has been cited, regarding del Verrocchio's restoration of the limbs of an ancient torso of the flayed Marsyas:

> [Lorenzo de'Medici] gave it to Andrea to restore and finish, and that artist made the legs, sides and arms that were lacking. … This antique torso of a flayed Marsyas was made with such skill and judgment that some slender white veins in the red stone came out, through skilful carving, in the proper places, appearing like small sinews, such as are seen in natural figures when flayed, and this rendered the work most life-like.

Here once again it must be noted that del Verrocchio has displayed not much more knowledge than might have been gained from a flayed cadaver and from close observation of a very lean, but living subject. And in view of the fact that Leonardo recommends precisely this latter sort of study for knowledge of superficial structures, it is entirely possible that much of the anatomy of artists of the time was gained in this fashion.

No doubt the artists attended the public dissections at the medical schools, as indeed did also a great many of the townsfolk both lay and ecclesiastical. It is in regard to such dissections that Vesalius has remarked in his *China Root Letter* (1546): "As for those painters and sculptors who flocked around me at my dissections, I never allowed myself to get worked up about them to the point of feeling that I was less favored than these men, for all their superior airs". But to use this remark as indicating a high degree of anatomical knowledge among artists is to misunderstand the case. It is true that Vesalius has been the victim even in the twentieth century of certain hasty and ignorant conclusions as to his true position in the history of anatomy, but to men of his own day who were competent to judge, such as Cardan, Columbus and Fallopius, there was no question as to his primacy. If it is true that "a little knowledge maketh a fool", then such would be Vesalius' opinion of at least some of the artist spectators, well-acquainted with certain of the superficial structures, and probably therefore authoritative in their attitude about such things, wholly ignorant of everything else and finally and most important, completely unsystematic in whatever anatomical knowledge they possessed. Even Leonardo, who eventually passed from the superficial structures to a study of the deeper parts, never overcame this defect.

What then is the precise position of the artist in relationship to the development of anatomical knowledge. A tempered judgment suggests first that he was interested in anatomy only insofar as it would assist him in a more naturalistic portrayal of the human body. For this purpose he studied living subjects, preferably lean ones in whom muscle contours, tendons and certain superficial blood vessels could be identified. Then possibly certain artists went a step further by flaying cadavers, when obtainable, for this even better mode of studying the surface muscles. Yet cadavers for such purpose were seldom obtainable, and more frequently such study was piecemeal. Thus Luca Signorelli (1442–1524) is said to have visited burial grounds in search of parts of bodies. The purpose of all such studies was not anatomy *per se*, and the result was that the artist never achieved a systematic knowledge of the subject and made no contribution to the advance of anatomy. The one exception to much of this was Leonardo, who, always primarily the artist, yet came to recognize anatomy as more than merely a subject auxiliary to art. It was this attitude which led him to pursue it beyond the point of need for his major interest as an artist. Nevertheless Leonardo was never an anatomist since he, too, unsystematically followed only those aspects which interested him. However, he represents the closest approach of art to anatomy.

Meanwhile it has become fashionable to suggest that artists were the true anatomists and had better knowledge of the subject from approximately the period of Giotto to Leonardo. This belief arises from a study of their paintings and certain statements made by Vasari together with a liberal dash of enthusiasm. It also bases itself upon the traditional medical illustration such as the "Five Picture Series" mentioned above. Rather conveniently it overlooks the fact that the traditional illustrations were retained by medical writers purely as traditional and that frequently there was no relationship with the text, and, moreover, that among very many of the medical writers any illustration was frowned upon. Among artists the important thing was detail; among anatomists it was system. The artist from observation could draw superficial muscles correctly; the anatomist might be well acquainted with them and far more capable of relating them to the rest of the human structure, but he was incapable of good draughtsmanship. The drawing can be observed readily, the textual description is in difficult Latin. Leonardo at times unwittingly emphasizes the distinction when he fails in his efforts to draw from memory some structure which he can draw superbly from direct observation. If we follow the anatomist from the superficial to the deeper structures it is possible to point out many errors, but here it is impossible to make any comparison with the artists since with the exception of Leonardo who, be it remembered, thought of anatomy as a separate discipline, none of them pursued the study this far. Indeed, Leonardo represents the greatest heights reached by the artist-anatomist. Thereafter and gradually the anatomist asserts superiority in this combination of disciplines. Gradually the pedagogical value of correct illustration was recognized although only after a struggle with such conservative forces as Jacobus Sylvius who even as late as the mid-sixteenth century frowned upon the contamination of text by illustration.

He was, however, fighting a losing battle. With the publication of Vesalius' *Tabulae anatomicae* in 1538 and the *Fabrica* in 1543, the employment of anatomically correct and naturalistic illustrations produced under the direction of the anatomist and carefully related to the text became an important adjunct to the further advance of anatomical studies. Thus the final integration was achieved of these two arts which had first become acquainted in the apothecary's shop in fourteenth century Florence.

Leonardo's Anatomical Achievements

To bring Leonardo da Vinci into proper historical perspective it is essential that his biological contributions be viewed as a whole. It is not enough to examine his illustrations alone, but if we are to understand this extraordinary figure as a unified personality and historical phenomenon, it is necessary to study the many notes and observations which accompany the drawings. We may excuse the incompleteness and disorganization of his writings on the pounds of their haphazard informality, and we can make allowances for the uncertainty which surrounds their chronological sequence, but we cannot ignore them and the imperfections which they reveal without gravely distorting the true historical picture. Without the notes it would be impossible to perceive beneath the genius of his art the groping of his mind as it sought emancipation from a debased mediaeval Aristotelianism, through a corrupted Galenism to the achievement of a position of relative scientific independence. We would fail to see him as part of the contemporary growth, and we would lack an appreciation of the difficulties which he had to surmount. It has been this failure to consider the notes and illustrations as one which has been responsible for the many specious and unjustifiable claims that have been made on his behalf such as the all too frequent assertion that Leonardo had knowledge of the circulation of the blood.

Moreover, it needs to be emphasized how slender were Leonardo's resources in human dissection material, and it should be pointed out that the word anatomy does not necessarily mean a human dissection. He uses the term in its literal sense as a dissection and applies it when he is definitely referring to the dissection of an animal or a portion of an animal. Despite various assertions which have been made regarding the numerous dissections—presumably human—which Leonardo performed, the only evidence of human dissection which can be drawn from the note-books seems as follows: (1) a human head and neck dissected during the first Milanese period; (2) dissection of the centenarian and Leonardo's statement of having dissected a child of two years, during the Florentine period; (3) dissection of a human foetus c.7 months; (4) the dissection of the series in Fogli A which seems to have been that of an elderly man (cf. 45), and perhaps the body of a younger individual, cf. facial features (36, 56); (5) perhaps a leg. Undoubtedly Leonardo was a spectator at other dissections.

Osteology

Leonardo's representation of the skeletal system is one of the outstanding features of his work, but all the evidence seems to suggest that at no time did he ever possess an intact skeleton* Around the year 1489 he acquired, possibly from an execution, a human head, and from the dissections of this were made the series of magnificent illustrations of the skull found on plates 3–7. However, the accompanying notes display his Aristotelian position and the fact that he was more interested in the materialistic psychological implications than in the osteological system as such.

In his examination of the action of the bones as levers and especially in the mechanism of pronation and supination of the forearm, Leonardo turned his great knowledge and deep interest in mechanics to excellent account.

Fairly late in his career, c.1509–10, he acquired a copy of Galen's *De usu partium*, a work which must have appeared to him as a revelation, and thenceforth Leonardo became essentially a Galenist. It is from this period on that most of his studies on the skeletal and the myological systems date. His great powers and imagination in illustration are best seen in the series on the foot, but here again the misarticulation of the tibia and fibula with the tarsal bones of the opposite side indicate the incompleteness of his skeletal material.

Leonardo's greatest difficulty was with terminology which was then in a very confused state, most of the terms being of Arabic origin. As late as 1510 we find him reminding himself of the origin of the word *acciaiolo* (11). Indeed, he seems to have depended upon the physicians for his terms for on plate 214 he reminds himself to enquire about "the vein which was searched for in the lungs on Sunday". Despite the many imperfections, Leonardo's standard of osteological illustration is immeasurably superior to that of his predecessors and is, together with a large part of the myological section, one of the few systems in which his illustrations are based on human dissection.

Myology

For accuracy of representation Leonardo's figures on the muscular system are among his best drawings. However, his interest is primarily that of an artist concerned with the influence of the superficial muscle masses on surface modeling as indicated by the large number of illustrations which treat of this aspect, and seldom does he penetrate very far below the surface. This initial interest is later extended to the action of muscles and physiological problems.

It is noteworthy that almost all the dissections are dated between 1505–10, and that the great majority of the material is human. We suspect that most of the drawings are based fundamentally upon the dissection of the centenarian.

Leonardo's early dependence upon spare living subjects led him to the conception that muscles such as the deltoid, pectoralis major, etc., are compound or multiple muscles, and this explains his division of these muscles in dissection into multiple fasciculi. Logically he extends these ideas to the production of cord diagrams.

While it is true that the presentation of muscles, as in the case of the series on the upper extremity, viewed from every aspect, is indicative of his very considerable imaginative skill, yet in the representation of the abdominal muscles Leonardo is still relying upon tradition.

As mentioned above, almost all the studies of muscles are from the period 1505–10, and it was during this period that he had come into possession of Galen's *De usu partium.* We suspect that Leonardo derived much profit from this work, especially as regards his consideration of muscle action and the action of antagonistic muscles, and it may have been the cause of his very considerable preoccupation with the problems of respiration and the action of the intercostal muscles.

It is extremely difficult to attempt any comparison between the treatment of muscles by Leonardo and contemporary physicians since myology was at the time one of the most poorly understood aspects of anatomy. Among the difficulties plaguing any study of the muscle structure was the lack of any proper myological nomenclature. Few of the muscles were specifically named, and the result was constant confusion of identity which bothered Leonardo no less than the medical fraternity.

Comparative Anatomy

Leonardo has been called the first comparative anatomist since Aristotle, but this statement cannot be accepted without many reservations. Like Galen, Leonardo dissected many forms and like Galen, he made the fundamental error of supposing that the structure of man was essentially the same as that of most animals, differing only in relative proportions. Consequently in a large number of his drawings it will be found that he has transposed observations made on animals to the human body, distorting the proportions to fit the outlines of the human figure, or combining observations made on both. Nonetheless, he was aware that in many cases certain animal structures differed from the human. It was his interest in proportional differences which enabled him to draw correctly such comparisons between the bones of the lower limb of man and the horse as found on plate 58. His comparative anatomy was thus an extension of his interest as an artist in body proportions. It is therefore quite impossible to separate altogether Leonardo's observations in comparative anatomy from his major interest in the anatomy of the human body without creating a false impression. It is only when he makes a faithful and accurate drawing of some animal part such as his dissections of the bear's foot or the wing of a bird that it is possible to segregate his studies on animals. Unlike Aristotle, Leonardo's interests are directed towards the structure of the body in relationship to its workings, and here the structure of animals had much to offer.

Cardiovascular System

At the outset it should be stated that Leonardo had no knowledge of the circulation of the blood and that his views on the function of the heart were in a continual state of flux. Prior to 1500 he appears to have derived his opinions entirely from Mundinus or other contemporary sources and to have had little or no experience of the cardiovascular system based on dissection (cf. 116). Consequently illustrations from this period reflect a debased Galenism in which the emphasis lies on the liver as the source and origin of the vascular tree. Later he was to adopt a mediaeval-Aristotelian position in which primacy is placed in the heart, and thereafter reverted once more to a modification of the Galenical theory on the flux and reflux of the blood. However, it is extremely difficult to provide a connected account of Leonardo's final concepts on the movement of the blood since not only do his ideas vary over a very short space of time, but he makes no complete statement. His earlier observations are quite sporadic and desultory, but c.1513 he began to study the heart and its action more intensively, and the great majority of his drawings and notes on the cardiovascular system date from this period. However, these later observations are made almost exclusively upon dissections of the heart of the ox.

As has been mentioned, Leonardo's views on the motion of the blood were largely governed by the Galenical theory of its flux and reflux. Piecing together Leonardo's theory as well as possible, his views may be briefly stated as follows: Right ventricular diastole is initiated by the active contraction of the papillary muscles which open the tricuspid valve and the active dilation of the ventricle itself which creates a vacuum. Blood is simultaneously forced into the ventricle by active contraction of the right auricular appendage and the passive elastic recoil of its previously dilated walls. Owing to the action of these forces the right ventricle is filled with great impetus, creating frictional currents and eddies among the interstices of the irregular muscular walls of both chambers which heat and thin the blood. Excessive expansion of the ventricle is prevented by the moderator band. In the meantime, the left ventricle has contracted so that right ventricular diastole occurs with left ventricular systole.

Right ventricular diastole is followed by its systole which forces the blood in three directions. That portion of the column of blood lying in the tricuspid orifice and between its valves is returned to the right auricle which is passively dilated. A second portion is driven through the pulmonary orifice into the lungs for their nutrition. A third portion is forced through the pores of the interventricular septum into the left ventricle. The passage of the blood through the septum is facilitated by the simultaneously active dilation of the left ventricle which has established a vacuum creating a *vis a fronte* and by the loss of viscosity of the blood due to its frictional heating, The septum thus acts as a filter removing impurities which are left behind in the right ventricle, and the subtilized blood becomes the vital spirit of the left heart. Thus, as Leonardo puts it, "the right ventricle has a double loss", to the lungs and to the left ventricle. This loss "is paid back by the liver, the treasurer", but the amount of the loss is very small, being calculated, by means unknown, as seven ounces per hour.

Diastole of the left ventricle occurs simultaneously with right ventricular systole at which time not only does the left ventricle receive the minute quantity of blood which passes through the septum but also that forced into it by the contraction of the left auricle. On the other hand, blood escapes in two directions on left ventricular systole, a part returning to its auricle and the pulmonary veins by way of the mitral valve and a part being expelled into the aorta. Owing to the flux and reflux of the blood and the greater thickness and power of the left ventricular wall, the blood is heated more on the left than on the right. This heat subtilizes and vaporizes some of the blood and converts it into gas which is carried with the blood on systole to the lungs to escape into the bronchi. At the same time the blood is cooled and refreshed prior to its return to the left heart. The blood which escapes to the aorta is lost to the tissues and is apparently made good by that which sweats through the septum so that the greater quantity of blood participating in the ebb and flow movement on the left side is that which passes through the mitral valve to the pulmonary veins.

The cycle of events between two beats of the pulse is thus right ventricular systole, left ventricular diastole, left ventricular systole or as Leonardo puts it, "Between one and the next beat of the pulse, the heart closes twice and opens once". Likewise systole and diastole of the auricles alternate on the right and left sides.

It is thus apparent from the above outline that Leonardo's opinions on the movement of the blood are no more than a speculative extension of the Galenical ebb and flow theory. The most important modifications are the attempt to supply a mechanistic explanation of the ancient mystery of the source of innate or vital heat and the application of dynamic principles in an attempt to understand the mechanism of closure of the valves. Neither of these problems could be solved without the discovery of oxygen centuries later and without a knowledge of the circulation.

As to the distribution of the vessels, Leonardo's descriptions are very incomplete, confused and uncertain. Again we find a curious mixture of findings based on observations made from dissections of animals and the appearances found on inspection of the superficial veins in the living human subject. His supply of human cadavers was too small to accomplish his purpose and the only human dissection carried out with any degree of thoroughness to uncover the human vascular arrangement was that made on the body of the centenarian at Florence, c.1504–06.

Nervous System

Leonardo's treatment of the central nervous system, based upon traditional materialistic psychological notions of mediaeval times, is vague and confused. In his earlier figures he attempts to illustrate these primitive ideas as he drew them from Avicenna or Albertus Magnus by means of schematic sketches. Leonardo's outstanding contributions were the introduction of an injection technique to obtain casts of the cerebral ventricles and his physiological experiments on the nervous system of the frog from which he concluded that the spinal cord was the center of life. The vast majority of his observations were made on animals, almost all his work on the distribution of the peripheral nerves of the extremities being based on dissection of the monkey with the findings distorted to fit the contours of man.

Later he comes more and more under the influence of Galen and begins to make excellent independent observations on the arrangement of the nervous system. The point of departure can be traced to the dissection of the centenarian, and all his best drawings are derived from this specimen, cf. 148–50, 156–8, 167–8.

Respiratory System

Leonardo's observations on the respiratory system, the majority of which are very late, c.1510–13, are based exclusively on animal material. His opinions on the physiology of respiration are almost entirely Galenical with few or very slight modifications. As a musician he was especially interested in the larynx, which he considered the essential organ of the voice and of phonation. He was, of course, far astray since he failed to recognize the vocal cords. The trachea was compared to an organ pipe, and by its length and diameter the pitch of the voice was correspondingly altered.

In respect to the mechanism of respiration, Leonardo was initially confused by his acceptance of the Galenical statement that the pleural cavities contain air; later, however, he became dubious of this statement. While he granted that the function of the lungs was to cool and refresh the blood, this was not by any direct communication with the pulmonary vessels. On the special action of the diaphragm and abdominal muscles in the forcing on of the food through the alimentary tract, see below.

Alimentary System

Leonardo's considerations on the alimentary system are very incomplete. Pre-Leonardine illustrations can only be regarded as pure conventionalism, and this conventionalism is also to be seen in Leonardo's early drawings where the alimentary tract is shown diagrammatically and with no pretence to accuracy. The great change came with the dissection of the centenarian in Florence, 1504–06. Almost all the best drawings of the digestive organs, insofar as accuracy and realism are concerned, seem to have been derived from this dissection, cf. 183, 185–6, 188–9.

Leonardo's main interest is in the physiology of digestion, and this physiology is primarily Galen's, but whether he derived his notions of Galen indirectly from Mundinus and Avicenna or directly from the *De usu partium*, which he was beginning to read about this time, is difficult to say. He devotes considerable attention to the mechanism by which the alimentary contents are passed on from one segment to another, and here his observations and theory are original. However, the wave-like contractions of the intestines which we call peristalsis were quite unknown to him, and, indeed, he specifically denies that the stomach contracts to expel its Contents (177). Instead he theorizes that it is the rhythmical contractions of the diaphragm and abdominal wall in respiration which force the food onward, while the flexures prevent reverse movements of the contents. It is noteworthy that he does not accept the Galenical idea that the longitudinal and circular fibres of the intestines are responsible for the retention and expulsion of the contents.

Genito-Urinary System

There is not much that can be said on the urinary apparatus beyond that which is contained in the notes to the illustrations. Almost all Leonardo's studies on the kidneys were carried out on animals. He says very little regarding the physiology of the kidney, and his views are very primitive—as, indeed, were the theories of his contemporaries. He was most interested in the mode of entrance of the ureter into the bladder and in the mechanism which prevents reflux of urine from the bladder into the ureters.

The reproductive organs of the male and female are treated with a curious mixture of fact and fancy.

Most of the figures have some objective basis which is, however, overlaid by traditional theories on function. Again, as is common in Leonardo's drawings, the earlier figures reflect primitive mediaeval theories of generation which later on are replaced by drawings and text in which Galenical ideas are predominant.

embryology

To avoid repetition of what is expressed in the notes to the plates, we shall here merely note the chief points of Leonardo's belief.

He started out as an Aristotelian, probably having derived his ideas from Albertus Magnus. Eventually he became a follower of Galen. This is all discussed on plate 201.

There is positive evidence that he dissected a to man foetus of c.7 months.

The remainder of his observations are drawn from animals, and since he knew nothing of the foetal coverings of the human, he added those of the 01 cf. plates 210–11.

DaVinci's anatomical treatise

Vasari's detailed but misleading statement has led to a widely held assumption that Leonardo had written a treatise on human anatomy in collaboration with Marcantonio della Torre and that long since this treatise was lost. This belief has been fortified by quotations from Leonardo's writings in which he speaks of a "Treatise on Anatomy" as though the work had been completed. However, it is now abundantly clear that Vasari's statement is a highly colored and inaccurate reference to one or other of the existing note-books and that Leonardo's mention of a treatise on anatomy reflects his intention, never fulfilled, and not unlike similar remarks regarding other contemplated works such as that "On Waters". Nonetheless, Leonardo had established a plan for such a treatise as early as his first Milanese period, and c.1489 he began to jot down a rough outline of its contemplated contents to which he later (c.1500) added a terminal paragraph.

On the order of the book

This work should begin with the conception of man and describe the nature of the womb, and how the child lives in it, and up to what stage it dwells there, and the manner of its quickening and feeding, and its growth, and what interval exists between one stage of growth and another, and what drives it forth from the body of the mother, and for what reason it sometimes comes forth from the belly of its mother before the proper time.

Then describe which are the members which grew more than the others after the child is born, and give the measurements of a child of one year.

Next describe a grown male and female, and their measurements, and the nature of their complexions, color and physiognomy. Afterwards describe how he is composed of vessels, nerves, muscles and bones. This you will do at the end of the book.

Then represent in 4 accounts 4 universal conditions of man, that is, joy with various modes of laughter and represent the cause of laughter; sorrow, in various ways with its cause; strife, with various acts of slaughter, flight, fear, ferocity, daring, murder, and all things which pertain to such cases.

Then represent labor with pulling, pushing, carrying, restraining, supporting and the like.

ATTITUDES

Then describe attitudes and movement.

EFFECTS

Then perspective through the office of sight; and on hearing. You will speak of music and treat of the other senses.

SENSES

Then describe the nature of the 5 senses.

We shall demonstrate the mechanical structure of man by figures of which the first 3 will be on the ramification of the bones, that is, one from in front which shows the latitudinal position and shape of the bones; the 2nd will be seen from the side and will show the depth of the whole and its parts and their position; the 3rd figure will be a demonstration of the bones from behind. Then we shall make 3 other figures in similar views with the bones sawn across in which one will see their thickness and cavities. We shall make 3 other figures of the intact bones and of the nerves which arise from the medulla and in which members they ramify; and 3 others of the bones and vessels and where they ramify; then 3 with the muscles; and 3 with the skin and the proportions of the figures; and 3 of the female to show the womb and the menstrual veins which go to the breasts. [Clark 19037V/FB 20v: c.1489; last paragraph c.1500].

To the above could be added innumerable other notes of approximately the same period modifying or, more usually, extending Leonardo's grand plan to encompass every phase of the normal and abnormal anatomy and physiology of the human and animal body. But a single example, typical of his restless and inquiring mind, must suffice.

Represent whence catarrh [i.e., the phlegm supposedly from the pituitary gland] *is derived. Tears Sneezing. Yawning. Trembling. The falling sickness* [epilepsy]. *Madness. Sleep. Hunger. Sensuality. Anger, where it acts in the body. Fear, likewise. Fever. Sickness. Where poison injures. Describe the nature of all the members. Why lightning kills man and does not wound him, and if man blew his nose, he would not die, because it injures the lungs. Write what the soul is. Of Nature which, if necessary, makes the vital and active instruments of suitable and necessary shape and position. How necessity is the companion of Nature. Illustrate whence comes the sperm. Whence the urine. Whence the milk. How the nourishment proceeds to distribute itself through the veins. Whence comes intoxication. Whence the vomit. Whence the gravel and the stone. Whence "pain in the side"* [pleurisy or dolor lateralis as it was called]. *Whence dreams. Whence frenzy resulting from sickness. Whence it happens that by compressing the arteries a man falls asleep. Whence it happens that when pierced in the neck, the man falls dead. Whence come the tears. Whence the turning of the eyes, so that one draws the other after it on sobbing* [Clark 19038r/FB 21r:c.1498].

Nonetheless, keeping in mind that art theory had gone scientific, a careful reading of the description of the contemplated work makes it apparent that at this period Leonardo's conception was that of an artist to which had been grafted the universal outlook of that period. Thus in attempting to classify his drawings it is at times difficult to determine whether a particular drawing was intended to be a scientific or a purely artistic production. It is equally clear that despite the formulation of his thought, no particular plan had as yet jelled, and hence his plans remained in a somewhat nebulous state. Gradually the formlessness of his notes and drawings began to dawn upon him. By c.1509 their mass was so great as to cause some concern, and in reference to those on physics he wrote in the beginning of that collection known as the Arundel Mss. (B.M.1r):

Begun at Florence in the house of Piero di Braccio Martelli, on the 22nd day of March 1508. This makes a collection without order, taken from many sheets which I have here copied hoping to arrange them later, each in its place according to the matters of which they treat. I believe that before I make an end to this I shall have to repeat the same things many times, for which, O reader, do not blame me, for the subjects are many and the memory cannot retain them, and say, "This I do not need to write because I have written it before". If I wished to avoid falling into this error, it would be necessary in every instance when I desired to copy, that I should read over all that had gone before so as not to repeat myself, and especially so since the intervals of time between one writing and the next are long.

About this time, Leonardo may have made some attempt to arrange his anatomical notes, for a memorandum written c.1507–09 (Clark 19070V/Q I 13V) reads: *Have your books on anatomy bound,* which, if carried out, would of necessity have required some sort of ordering of the many loose sheets.

Leonardo had high hopes of completing the work while at Milan during the *winter of 1510* (Clark 19016r/FA 17r), but these hopes were never to be fulfilled. However, he began to compose at a later period, c.1513 a series of more connected and finished passages (Clark 19061–67/Q I 2–8), obviously intended for incorporation in the projected book. Among these is an introductory chapter outlining in more definite fashion his latest plan of arrangement. Because of its importance this passage is given in full.

ORDER OF THE BOOK

This my depiction of the human body will be shown to you just as though you had a real man before you. The reason is that if you wish to know thoroughly the parts of an anatomized man, you must either turn him or your eye so as to examine him from different aspects, from below from above and from the sides, turning the subject around and investigating the origin of each member, and in this way, satisfying yourself as to your knowledge of the actual anatomy. However, you must realize that such knowledge will not leave you satisfied on account of the very great confusion which results from the combination of membranes intermingled with veins, arteries, nerves, cords, muscles, bones, and the blood, which of itself stains every part the same color. The vessels which discharge this blood are not perceptible owing to their minuteness. The continuity of the membranes is inevitably destroyed in searching for those parts enclosed within them and as their transparency is marred by staining with blood, this prevents recognition of the parts covered by them, owing to the similarity of their sanguineous color. You can have no knowledge of one without confusing and destroying the other. Therefore it is necessary to make further anatomies, three of which you will need to acquire a complete knowledge of the veins and arteries, destroying everything else with the utmost care; three others to acquire a knowledge of the membranes; three for the cords, muscles and ligaments; I three for the bones and cartilages; and three for the; anatomy of the bones which must be sawn through I to demonstrate which are hollow and which are not, which are medullary, which are spongy, which are thick from without inwards, which are thin. And some are extremely thin in one part and thick in another, and in other parts hollow or full of bone or of marrow or are spongy. Thus it may be that all these conditions will sometimes be found in one and the same bone and there may be a bone which has none of them. You must also make three of the female body in which there is a great mystery owing to the womb and its foetus

Therefore through my plan every part and every whole will be made known to you by means of a demonstration of each part from three different aspects; for when you have seen any member from the front with what nerves, cords or vessels which j arise from the opposite side, the same member will be shown to you turned to the side or from behind, f just as if you had the same member in your hand and went on turning it gradually until you had a complete understanding of what you wish to know. And so, similarly there will be put before you in three or four demonstrations of each member from different aspects, in such a way that you will be left with a true and full understanding of all you wish to know of the human figure.

Consequently, here will be shown to you in fifteen entire figures the cosmography of the Microcosmos in the same order as was adopted before me by Ptolemy in his Cosmography. Likewise, I shall then divide each member as he divided the whole into provinces, and then I shall describe the use of parts from every aspect, placing before your eyes a knowledge of the entire form, and habit (valitudine) of man, insofar as it has local motion by means of its parts. And might it so please our Creator that I be able to demonstrate the nature of man and his customs in the way that I describe his figure.

I would remind you that an anatomizing of the nerves by means of bodies macerated in running water or in lime-water, will not give you the position of their branchings nor into what muscles they ramify, because, although the source of their origin may be discerned without, as well with water, their ramifications tend to unite under the influence of running water, just as flax or hemp combed for spinning becomes tangled all in a bundle, so that it is impossible to find out again into which muscles, with what, or with how many ramifications, the nerves are distributed into the aforesaid muscles.

In the margin of the same page Leonardo describes, as an example, the manner in which he hopes to demonstrate certain portions of the body, such as the hand.

ON THE HAND FROM WITHIN

When you begin the hand from within, first place all the bones a little separated from one another so that the true shape of each bone on the internal aspect of the hand may be readily recognized, and further, the real number and position of each. Prepare some sawn through the middle of their thickness, that is, longitudinally, so that you can show which are hollow and which are full. Having done this, place these bones together properly articulated and draw the entire hand, fully open, from within. Then set down the figures of the first bony joints. The next demonstration will be that of the muscles which tie together the rasetta [carpus] and the pettine [metacarpus and phalanges]. The fifth will demonstrate the cords which move the first joints of the fingers; the sixth, the cords which move the second joints of the fingers; the seventh, those which move the third joints of the fingers; the eighth demonstration, the nerves which provide sensibility. The ninth will demonstrate the veins and arteries. The tenth will show the intact hand, complete with its skin, and its measurements, which measurements should also be made of the bones. And whatever you do for this side of the hand, you will also do for the other three aspects, that is, from the internal side, from the dorsal side, from the external side and the side mentioned above. [Clark 19061r/Q I 2r:c. 1509–13] From time to time Leonardo proposed numerous other plans from the traditional scholastic arrangement from the head to the feet, to a consideration of the body from the surface to the deeper structures, almost always extending his plan until it would have reached such encyclopaedic proportions, and illustrated with such prodigality that he could not hope for its completion or expect its publication.

History of the anatomical manuscripts

On 10 October 1517, Leonardo, then living at Cloux, was visited by Cardinal Louis d'Aragon and his secretary Antonio de Beatis. The artist, partially paralyzed and almost at the end of his life, displayed his drawings and note-books to his visitors, and Beatis, recording this visit in his journal, remarks:

> [Leonardo] has compiled a special treatise of anatomy with pictorial demonstrations of the limbs as well as of the muscles, nerves, veins, joints, intestines and whatever can be imagined in the bodies of men as well as women, such as never have been made before by any person. All this is what we have seen with our own eyes. And he said that he had dissected more than thirty bodies of men and women of all ages.

Such is the only account of the intact collection of Leonardo's anatomical drawings during the lifetime of the artist.

In 1519 Leonardo died, and by his will all his drawings and note-books were inherited by his faithful disciple Francesco Melzi and remained in his possession until his death in 1570. Melzi brought them to his villa in Vaprio near Milan where they were inspected from time to time by visitors. There is record of a visit paid to Melzi somewhere between 1537 and 1545 by the person known today only as Anonimo Gaddiano who has left a description of the collection. Presumably the mathematician and physician Girolamo Cardano, a native of Milan, also saw the collection. His remarks are of considerable interest because of their relationship of Leonardo to Vesalius. In his *De subtilitate,* after remarking that a painter is at once philosopher, architect and dissector, he continues, "for proof there is that remarkable imitation of the whole human body which [I saw] many years ago, by Leonardo of Vinci and of Florence, which was almost complete; but the task required a great master and investigator of nature such as Vesalius". Apparently Cardano the physician immediately recognized the non-systematic nature of the work. Leonardo's treatise on anatomy is also mentioned by Biondo in his *Eulogy of painting* (1549).

Still later (1566), Vasari paid a visit to Melzi, and in his record of it propounded the troublesome thesis of the proposed collaboration of Leonardo and Marcantonio della Torre:

> In this attempt Marcantonio was wonderfully aided by the genius and labor of Leonardo, who filled a book of drawings in red crayon, outlined with the pen, all copies made with the utmost care dissected by his own hand. In this book he set forth the entire structure, arrangement, and disposition of the bones, to which he afterwards added all the nerves, in their due order, and next supplied the muscles, of which the first are affixed to the bones, the second give the power of cohesion or holding firmly, and the third impart that of motion. Of each separate part he wrote an explanation in rude characters, written backwards and with the left hand, so that whoever is not practised in reading cannot understand them, since they are only to be read with a mirror. Of these anatomical drawings of the human form, a great part is now in the possession of Messer Francesco da Melzi, a Milanese gentleman, who sets great store by these drawings, and treasures them as relics. ...

Vasari's statement is incorrect in respect to the order in which Leonardo made his drawings, but nevertheless it does suggest that they may at the time of his visit have been arranged in some such order. He would have had neither the anatomical knowledge nor the time to discover discrepancies in the chronology of the drawings and the varying states of Leonardo's knowledge of the subject. A theory is therefore possible that at some time, possibly after his removal to France, Leonardo had actually arranged the drawings into some sort of system. In view of a similar effort to reorganize some of his note-books during his Florentine period, an effort thwarted by a constantly roving interest, it is possible that in his latter years, less widely occupied, Leonardo did actually achieve some sort of arrangement. Moreover, any such arrangement of the anatomical drawings would naturally have strengthened Vasari's belief in the truth of the story of the collaboration of Leonardo and Marcantonio.

The final visit to the collection prior to the death of Francesco Melzi was that of the Milanese painter Lomazzo who mentions his visit some twenty years later in his *Idea del Tiempo della Pittura:*

> Leonardo is worth remembering as he taught the anatomy of the human body … which I have seen at Francesco Melzi's, drawn divinely by Leonardo's hand … but of all these works none was printed, existing only in his manuscripts which in great part have come into the hands of Pompeo Leoni, … and some also came into the hands of Signor Guido Mazenta, distinguished scholar who treasures them lovingly.

Lomazzo's account therefore not only continues the recognition of Leonardo's anatomical studies, but also it is the first notice of the dispersal of the drawings.

In 1570 Francesco Melzi died and his property passed to a relative, the jurist Orazio Melzi, who appears to have had neither interest in nor realization of the significance of his" inheritance. Our knowledge of this episode is derived from Ambrosio Mazenta, and recounted by him toward the end of his life, 1631–35. According to Mazenta, when he was studying law in Pisa in 1588, another student, Lelio Gavardi d'Asola, a nephew of Aldus Manutius the younger, showed him some thirteen note-books of Leonardo which he had filched during an earlier period when he had been employed as a tutor in the household of Orazio Melzi. It had been his intention to sell them to Francesco de'Medici, Grand Duke of Tuscany who, however, had died before Gavardi had been able to show them to him. Mazenta eventually persuaded Gavardi to allow him to return the note-books, but as it happened Orazio Melzi who already had a houseful of books and relics of Leonardo was not eager to receive any more. As a result the Mazenta brothers, Ambrosio and Guido, retained the drawings. Thereafter as the Mazenta collection was seen by artists and its source was learned, Melzi found himself under constant request for more of Leonardo's drawings. The person who appears to have been the most eager to acquire them was Pompeo Leoni (c.1533–1608), a sculptor and pupil of Michelangelo, and now in the service of the King of Spain. When he promised that Melzi would gain honors and privilege in Milan, then under Spanish control, if the drawings were presented to the King of Spain, Melzi suddenly recognized a value in his inheritance—hardly aesthetic it may be said—and besought the return of the note-books from the Mazenta brothers who returned seven of them which Melzi in turn handed over to Pompeo Leoni. Eventually the six note-books retained by the Mazentas were dispersed, three of them after the death of Guido Mazenta, coming into the hands of Leoni. It is also possible that he had meanwhile acquired even more drawings from Orazio Melzi. At any rate, Leoni took apart the original note-books and mounted the sheets in paper frames so that both sides were visible. Thereafter he assembled them disregarding any previous order and bound them in two large volumes.

One of these volumes Leoni took to Spain in 1591 where he sold it to Don Juan d'Espina. This volume may have contained the anatomical drawings which eventually found their way to England, although the route is not always clear. We do, however, know that Thomas Howard, Earl of Arundel, purchased the volume while travelling in Spain (1636). The Codex Arundel, representing a portion of the purchase, upon the urging of John Evelyn, was presented by its owner to the Royal Society in 1681 and thence was transferred to the British Museum in 1831. However, a large collection of drawings, including the anatomical ones, in some way or other, and exactly when is unknown, found their way into the Royal Library at Windsor. All that can be said about them is that they were in the Royal Collection as early as

1690 when Queen Mary showed them at Kensington Palace to Constantijn Huygens. Thereafter they appear to have been unnoticed until mention is made of them shortly after 1735 in an inventory of the prints and drawings "in the Buroe of His Majesty's Great Closet at Kensington". Again the collection seems to have been lost until 1778 when "Mr. Dalton, Royal Librarian, fortunately discovered it on the bottom of [a chest]". At this time the collection was said to number 779 drawings. However, when the drawings were properly mounted and cared for in the nineteenth century only 600 could be found Sixty-four pages had at some time been removed, but why and whither they went is today unknown.

The drawings, in particular the anatomical ones, are next mentioned by William Hunter, the celebrated physiologist, who speaks of them with enthusiasm and announces his intention of publishing them, a task from which he was prevented by his death in 1783, and the first selection of the drawings, including some of the anatomical studies was brought out by John Chamberlaine in his *Imitations of Original Designs by Leonardo da Vinci* (1796).

Once again these drawings were neglected until studies of them were initiated by Gaetanao Milanesi (1872) and by Gustavo Uzielli (1872). In 1878 an exhibit was arranged at the Grosvenor Gallery, at the instigation of the Prince Consort, of a large number of the drawings, not however including the anatomical ones, and in 1883 appeared the first thoroughgoing study, including the anatomical drawings, by J. P. Richter.

The first effort to make the anatomical drawings generally available through publication in facsimile was that of Theodore Sabachnikoff who published a selection of the drawings in 1898 under the title of *Dell' Anatomia, Fogli A*. The volume contains an introduction by Mathias Duval, then professor of anatomy at the Ecole Nationale des Beaux Arts, and a transcription of Leonardo's text together with a translation into French. In 1901 a second volume was published known as *Fogli B*. Regrettably the introduction by Duval displays more admiration for Leonardo's drawings than scholarship and a considerable lack of knowledge of the history of anatomy. Similarly the transcriptions are not wholly lacking in error, while the translations into French contain numerous mistakes arisen through misunderstanding and ignorance of the subject.

Meanwhile Sabachnikoff had continued the photo graphing of the remainder of the Windsor Collection and had deposited the negatives with Eduard Rouveyre, publisher of the *Fogli A*. Apparently with the intention of supplying a waiting market Rouveyre, without waiting for the transcription of Leonardo's text to be completed, published an edition of the photographs. While this unethical if not piratical action is said to have hastened the death of Sabachnikoff, it also meant that the work would eventually have to be done over again.

Between 1911 and 1916, the need for a proper edition of the remainder of the anatomical drawings, that is, those pirated by Rouveyre, was finally met by the appearance of the *Quaderni d'Anatomia* published in Oslo through the editorial efforts of C. L. Vangensten, A. Fonahn and H. Hopstock and contains an Italian transcription and translations into English and German. The facsimiles were carefully and beautifully made, but the volumes lack proper annotations, and the translations suffer frequently and woefully from error.

It is a curious fact that hitherto no editor has attempted to arrange Leonardo's note-books so as to indicate systematically what the extent of his anatomical studies was. This is now done, and the plates have been arranged according to systems. Within the systems, so far as possible, a chronological sequence has been observed to indicate Leonardo's growth and development as an anatomist. The text has been newly translated, and it is hoped that at least a few of the errors in previous translations have been removed. The sources from which the plates have been taken are indicated as follows:

FA *I manoscritti di Leonardo da Vinci della Reale Biblioteca di Windsor. DelV anatomi fogli A. Pubblicati da Teodoro Sabachnikoff* ... Parigi ... 1898.

FB [Ditto] *fogli B.* ... Torino ... 1901.

Q *Quaderni d'anatomia ... Pubblicati da ove C. L. Vangensten,* A. *Fonahn, H. Hopstock* ... Christiani ... 1911–16. 6 vols.

Clark, Kenneth. A *catalogue of the drawings of Leonardo da Vinci in the collection of His Majesty the King at Windsor Castle.* Cambridge, England, 1935. Clark's work indicates the number of each plate in the Windsor Collection, occasionally correcting errors such as the indications of recto and verso in Q. Clark has also attempted to date the plates, and while he has achieved considerable success in his efforts, nevertheless the anatomical content occasionally suggests an earlier or later date than he has ascribed.

Heart: superficial view

Originally this page was part of the same sheet as 87 on which similar drawings of the heart appear. The folded sheet was torn apart but is now mounted as one. The drawings belong to Leonardo's latest period and can be dated from fig. 179 with considerable accuracy as c.1513. By now Leonardo had begun to modify somewhat orthodox Galenical views on the fundamental mechanism of the heart. These differences will become apparent as the series of drawings and notes are followed. In the examination of the figures it must be borne in mind that almost all are based upon appearances in the bullock's heart and not that of man. The figures are not easy to interpret because of the displacement of the great veins which are pulled upwards.

fig I. The interventricular septum of the heart (p. 99).

For the technique employed to demonstrate the interventricular septum in this manner, cf. 104. The lateral walls of the ventricles have been displaced after sectioning the heart, thus exposing the septum. The interventricular septum was of great importance in the Galenical system since it was through its pores (cf. 91) that some of the blood which ebbed and flowed in the right ventricle passed to become refined or subtilized in the left ventricle as the vital spirits giving rise to the so-called natural heat of the body. The note accompanying the figure brings forward the Galenical system, but an ingenious attempt is made to explain the origin of the mysterious innate heat of the ancients on mechanical principles. Earlier Leonardo had paid little attention to the auricular appendages which he calls auricles or *additamenti,* terms borrowed from Mundinus, or the external ventricles, a term likewise derived, but by extension, from the statements of the same author. It is the mechanical stirring or beating of the blood in these appendages which helps to subtilize the blood. A great deal of confusion is avoided if it be remembered that up to the time of William Harvey (1578–1657) and beyond, the heart was considered as a two-chambered organ consisting of right and left ventricles. Thus following Mundinus, the ventricles are called intrinsic or internal. On the other hand, the atria were regarded as forming the stems of the veins, cava and pulmonary vein respectively, so that the auricles themselves were thought of literally as appendages to the venous stems and therefore *additamenti* or additions, external or extrinsic in position. Likewise, the heart muscle was divided into external and internal or extrinsic and intrinsic, the ventricular wall forming the first and the papillary and pectinate muscles, the second.

The blood is more subtilized where it is more beaten. This beating occurs through the flux and reflux of the blood which are generated in the two internal ventricles of the heart to the two external ventricles, called the auricles or additions of the heart. The latter are dilated and receive into themselves the blood driven from the internal ventricles and then contract to return the blood to the internal ventricles. The internal [papillary and pectinate] *muscles, capable of contraction, are of one and the same nature in the 4 ventricles, but the external muscles* [of the ventricular wall] *are solely for the internal ventricles of the heart and, for the external form only a single, continuous dilatable and contractable coat.*

fig 2. The ventricles of the heart divided at the inter ventricular septum.

This rough figure, now almost obliterated, shows the ventricles divided at the interventricular septum prior to the displacement of their lateral walls as in fig I above.

fig 3. Mechanical drawing to illustrate the function of the cardiac valves.

The figure is apparently designed to show the action of the muscular forces controlling the ventricular valves. The base of the triangle is supported by ropes passing over pulleys to which are attached the weights S f. At the apex of the triangle is another rope carrying a weight g. The triangle represents a ventricular valve, the base of which is stretched by the contraction of the muscle of the ventricular wall corresponding to the forces S f, and the valve closed. However, when this muscle is relaxed on

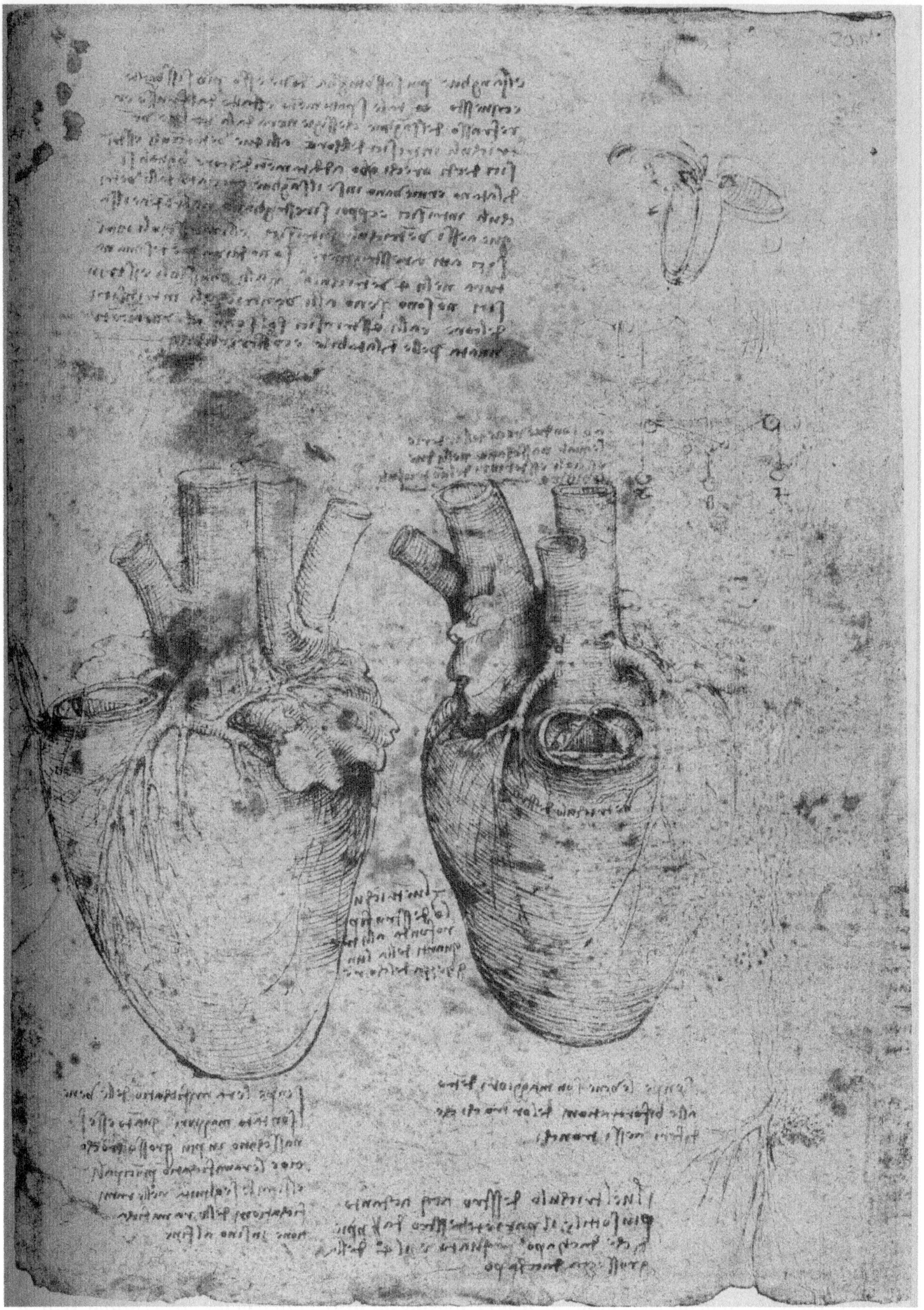

Figs I–6. Representation of the heart

diastole, the pull of the papillary muscle, represented by g, opens the valve. Thus Leonardo's theory was that the contraction of these muscles alternated in systole and diastole. In diastole, relaxation of the two ventricles and the contraction of the papillary muscle to open the atrio-ventricular orifice allows ventricular filling, while in systole the opposite closes the orifice.

fig 4. The heart from the left and posterior side.

In this figure of the heart, that of an ox, the root of the pulmonary artery has been severed and laid back to expose the root of the aorta giving rise to the left coronary artery. The left coronary is observed dividing into its descending and circumflex branches. A portion of the left auricle is displaced to reveal the branch to the roots of the great vessels. The aorta is also observed giving off a common brachiocephalic trunk. Behind and to the right of the aorta are the posterior vena cava pulled upwards and the anterior vena cava.

fig 5. The heart from the right side.

The same heart as in fig. 4 has now been turned to view from the right side. The root of the sectioned pulmonary artery has been removed to expose the pulmonary orifice and the medial, lateral and posterior semilunar valves guarding it. From the aorta spring the right and left coronary arteries, *a b, are two vessels* [coronary] *which arise from the two external openings* [i.e., aortic sinuses of Valsalva] *of the left ventricle.* Leonardo uses the term *usscioli,* openings, which is also employed for the valves themselves and for the cavities completed by the valves, forming what we now call the aortic sinuses of Valsalva. The distribution and branches of the coronary arteries are displayed with some accuracy, and the gradual diminution in calibre of these vessels as they pass distal is observed with the remark: *The branches of the vessels are always larger in proportion to their origin from larger trunk, that is, from the principal ramification, the same continues in the ramifications of the ramifications up to the end.*

On the figure, below the pulmonary artery, is written, *right ventricle.* In the interval between the two drawings, Leonardo notes that the right ventricle is less extensive than the left. *The right ventricle extends to a depth of three-quarters of the length of the heart.* He also notes the difference in thickness of the infundibulum of the right ventricle. *The right wall of the right ventricle is that much thinner at the base than at the apex as to be equal to a 4th of the thickness at the apex.*

Other structures identifiable are the brachiocephalic trunk from the aorta, the anterior and posterior vena cava, and the right auricle.

fig 6. Sketch of a coronary artery.

One of the coronary arteries, probably the right, is sketched to show the reduction in calibre of the vessel with each succeeding branch. The reduction in size is very evident in the case of these vessels as indicated in the note: *The vessels are always larger internal* [i.e., proximal] *to the bifurcation of their trunks than outside* [distal to] *these trunks.*

Other superficial views of the heart

The figures of this page are a continuation of the series found on 86 since originally the page was part of the same sheet which has become divided into two. The drawings belong to Leonardo's latest period, and like those of 86 the figures are all based upon dissections of the heart of the ox.

fig I. The heart from the right posterior aspect showing the distribution of the great cardiac vein (p. 102).

The dissection is that of an ox heart viewed from the right side and somewhat posteriorly. The posterior vena cava is pulled upwards, and at its root is the great cardiac vein or coronary sinus S G, receiving at S, the middle cardiac vein. The circumflex branch of the left coronary artery is lettered H. Of these vessels Leonardo states, S G, *is the vein* [great cardiac] *which encounters the artery S* G [left coronary], and that, the artery *is always beneath the vena nera* [cardiac vein]. The vessel lettered O is the anterior vena cava and, *p is the auricle of the left ventricle.* The apex of the heart is indicated with the letter T.

figs 2–3. The heart from the left anterior aspect showing the distribution of the left coronary artery.

The figures of an ox heart are said to be of, *the heart seen from in front.* In fig. 2 the words, *right side*, are written on the right ventricle, and above the letter N, we are told that this region is the left ventricle, by which is meant in Leonardo's terminology, the left external ventricle or auricle. Leonardo is confused. At M, is the left coronary artery dividing into r f, its interventricular branch and its circumflex branch associated with the great cardiac vein N. However, the left coronary artery springs from a vessel labelled the *vena arteriole*, i.e., pulmonary artery, which is undoubtedly the aorta shown giving off its brachiocephalic trunk. The pulmonary artery proper is roughly indicated displaced to the right of the specimen. This error is therefore found in the description of the left coronary artery. M, *a vein, arises from the vena arteriole* [pulmonary artery, in reality the aorta] *and is that which nourishes the substance of the heart.*

The interventricular vessels are described: *r f, a vein, and the front of the wall* [septum] *placed between the right and left ventricles of the heart. At S T, in the other heart* [fig. I] *are the vein and artery placed on the opposite side of the said wall, that is, on the back of the heart.* Improvements are to be made in the drawing, *Make the vein r /, more arched.* The great cardiac vein N, carries the notation, N, a vein, arises. Of figs. 1–3, Leonardo reminds himself, *Make these 3 demonstrations with all the vessels* [elevated] *from the heart upwards* [as in fig. 11].

fig 4. An abortive sketch.

The sketch lying to the left of the letter D, is now too badly rubbed and faded for its nature to be determined.

fig 5. The heart: right anterior aspect.

The *right ventricle* is so labelled just below the origin of the pulmonary artery. Behind the pulmonary artery the aorta gives off a brachiocephalic trunk as in the heart of the ox. The right and left coronary arteries are shown passing from the aorta to embrace the stem of the pulmonary artery. On the left is the posterior vena cava, pulled upwards, and the anteririor vena cava, and at their root, the lesser cardiac vein. The auricles have been turned back on either side. It will be noted that this, as well as several of the other drawings has an asterisk, formed by a circle with four lines running through it, placed above it. The significance of the asterisk is indicated by a note on 88 where we are told that such drawings are to be made enclosed by their capsule, i.e., the pericardium.

figs 6–9. Diagrams of the heart and coronary vessels.

The significance of these diagrams is revealed in the accompanying note in which attention is called to the crossing of the interventricular branch of the left coronary artery and the great cardiac vein as observed when the heart is examined from the left side and somewhat anteriorly as in the first, third and fourth of the diagrams. The second of this group of figures presumably shows the heart encased in the pericardium.

The heart seen from the left side will have its veins and arteries intersecting like one crossing his arms—and they will have above them the left auricle and within them the gateway [aortic orifice] *of triplicate triangular valves and the open gateway will remain triangular* [as shown in figs. 14–15 below].

fig 10. The heart viewed from the right and posteriorly to demonstrate the distribution of the right coronary artery.

The heart of the ox is shown as viewed from the right and somewhat posteriorly to reveal the extent of the right ventricle a b c, in relationship to the surface. The lateral wall of the right ventricle is indicated

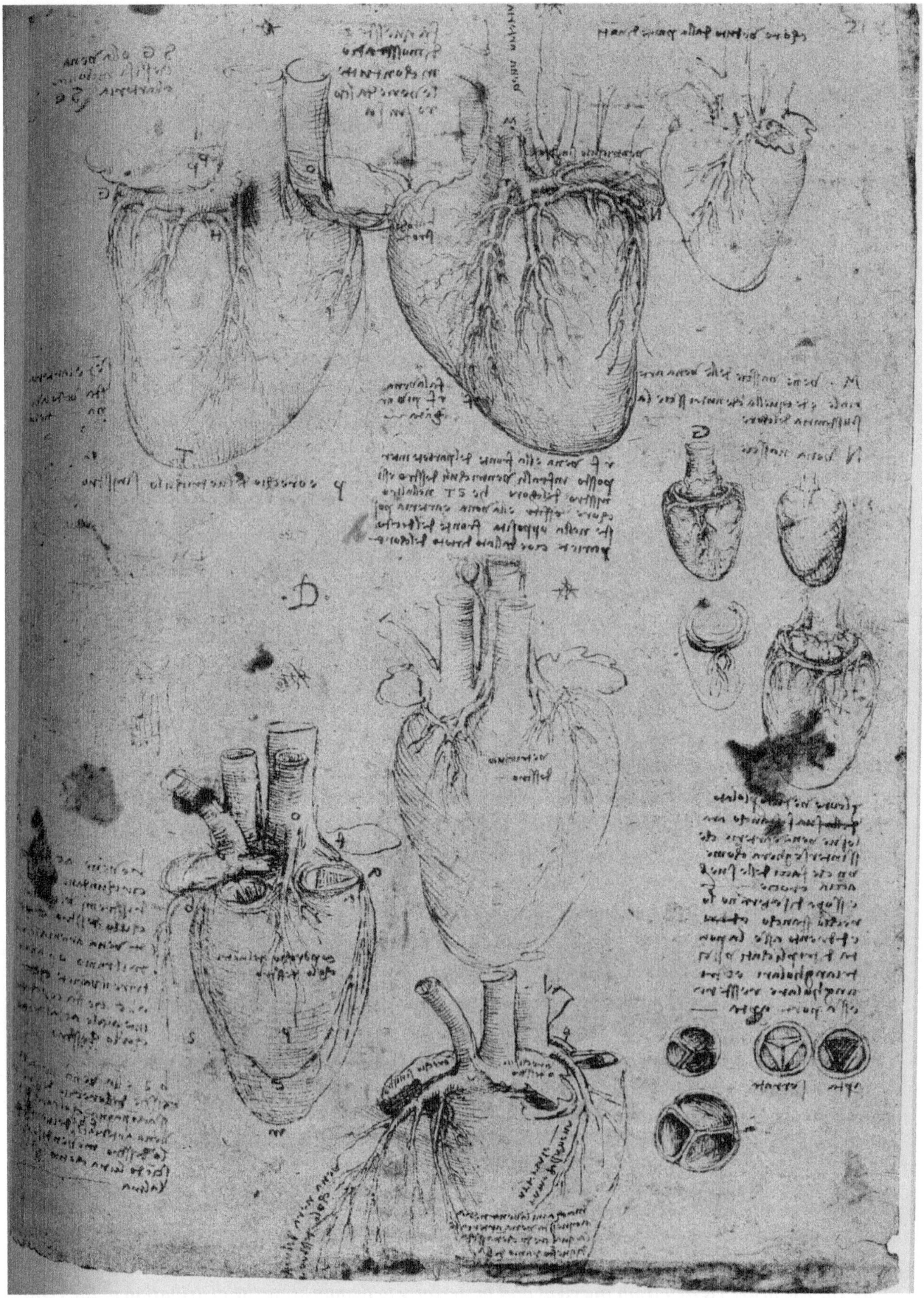

Figs I–15. Other views of the heart

by the words written on it, *The cover of the right ventricle.* The aorta, which has again been confused with the pulmonary artery in the notes, is shown giving off a brachiocephalic trunk and providing at o, the right coronary artery o p. The right coronary artery passes between the pulmonary orifice exposed by resection of the root of the pulmonary artery, and the right atrio-ventricular or tricuspid orifice which is revealed by division and displacement of the right auricle from its attachment to the region of the coronary groove. Above the right auricle are the roots of the anterior and posterior venae cavae, the latter being pulled upwards. Below the right auricle is the middle cardiac vein b s, dissected free and elevated from the inferior interventricular groove. The left auricle is lettered h and below it the course of the interventricular branch of the left coronary artery or great coronary vein is observed. The apex of the heart is indicated by m. The accompanying note discusses the distribution of the coronary vessels.

The vessels a c [anterior interventricular] *and b c* [inferior interventricular] *enclose the extremities of the right ventricle, and the vena arteriole* [pulmonary artery, in reality the aorta], *sends forth the branch o* p [ventricular branch of right coronary artery] *to nourish the wall a b c, which forms the entire covering of the right ventricle.*

b S, is the vena nera [middle cardiac vein] *which issues from the right auricle and is accompanied by a branch f b c* [i.e., o b c, circumflex and interventricular branch of right coronary artery] *of the vena arteriole of the right ventricle* [pulmonary artery, in reality aorta], *progressing and increasing opposite to one another.*

fig 11. The heart viewed posteriorly to show the coronary sinus and right coronary artery.

The heart is again that of an ox. The stems of the great vessels are from left to right of the figure, the posterior vena cava, the anterior vena cava and the aorta. The auricles are labelled respectively *left auricle* and *right auricle.* The great cardiac vein and coronary sinus have been freed and elevated with the notation, *Vena nera* [great cardiac vein] *of the right ventricle.* The right coronary artery is shown arising from the aorta, mistakenly called the pulmonary artery, and passing on the right side of the pulmonary orifice exposed by removal of the stem of the pulmonary artery. At f, is seen the stem of the left coronary artery. At the bottom of the figure Leonardo indicates the confusion resulting from his calling the aorta the pulmonary artery.

I lack the vena nera [small cardiac vein] *to this vena arteriole which I believe arises from the branch of the left vena nera* [great cardiac vein or coronary sinus].

figs 12–15. The pulmonary and tricuspid valves viewed from above.

The tricuspid valve is shown *closed* and *open.*

ON THE NAMES OF THE VESSELS OF THE HEART

fig I. The heart, interventricular septum and great vessels (p. 104).

A very rough sketch or diagram of the ventricles separated by the interventricular septum a b, through the pores of which Galenical physiology taught that some of the blood passed from the right to the left ventricle to be converted into vital spirit. Hence Leonardo notes that *a b* [interventricular septum] *is the sieve or common wall.* To the left is the vena cava receiving the hepatic veins below from the liver, indicated roughly by a circle, and entering the heart at a, the right atrio-ventricular or tricuspid orifice, since the heart was regarded as consisting of two ventricles only, and so the right atrium itself is part of the cava. The vena cava is named *vena del chilo,* i.e., vena chilis. Above the term vena chilis appear the words *The vein called the nourisher of the heart,* which have been deleted to be replaced with the notation on the right atrio-ventricular orifice: *a, the gateway of the vena chilis: the vein which nourishes the heart.*

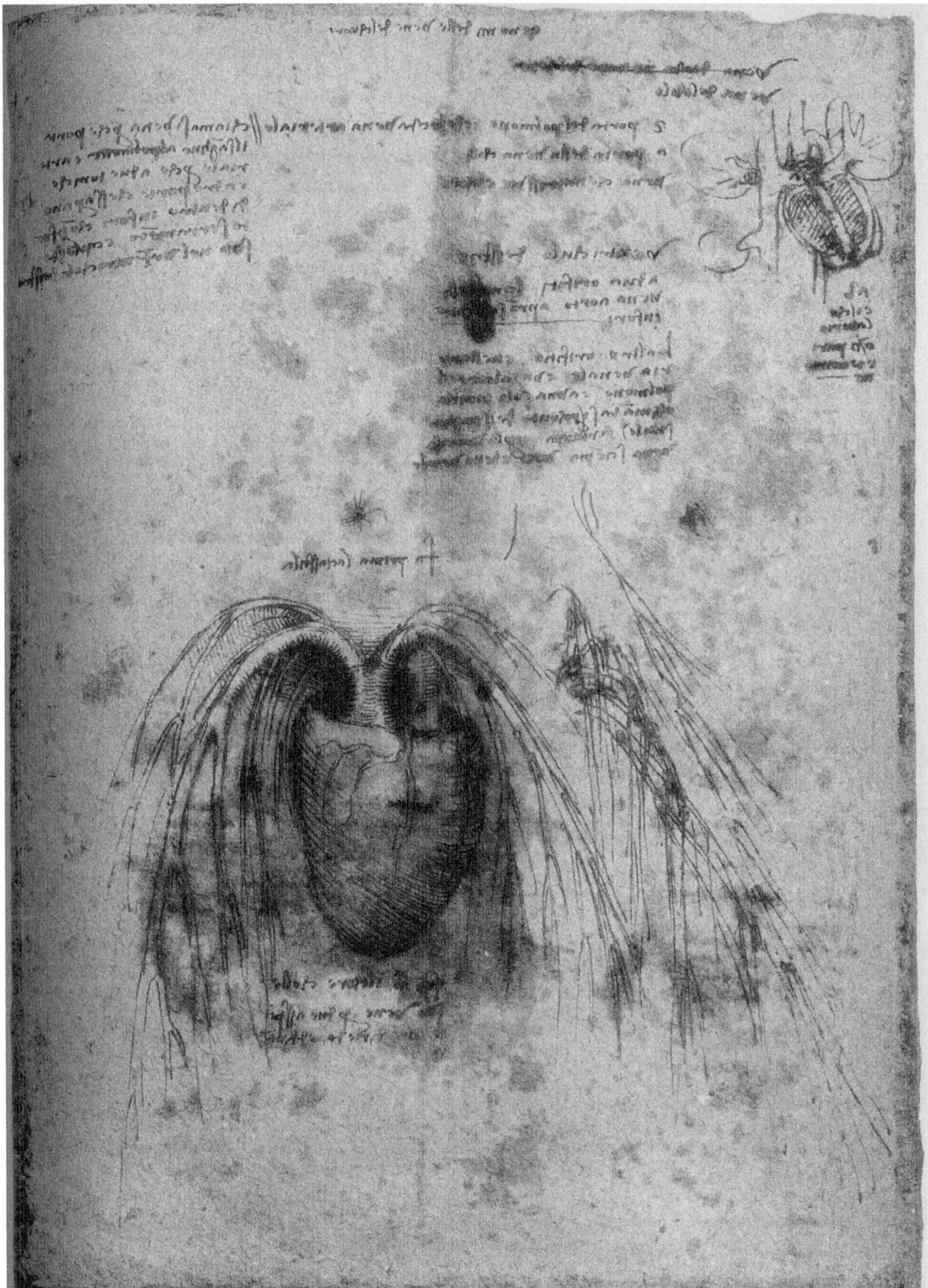

Figs I–3. Vessels of the heart

Above the heart is the arch of the aorta providing a single branch, the brachiocephalic trunk. The descending aorta may be followed to the region below the heart. On either side the lungs are roughly represented and passing to them the pulmonary arteries. The hilum of the right lung and right pulmonary artery is indicated by the letter S.

S, the gateway of the lung, and it is named the vena arterialis; it is called vena because it carries blood (to the lungs [deleted]*), and arterioles, because it has two tunics. It has three valves which open from within outwards with perfect closure, and these are in the right ventricle.*

The vena arterialis, i.e., pulmonary artery, following Galen's physiology, was necessarily part of the venous system although morphologically an artery. The information provided by Leonardo is to be found in all his sources. A further note discusses the left ventricle and its orifices.

The right [for left] *ventricle has two orifices at the aortic vessel (vena aorta)—they open within outwards—the other orifice is at the arteria venalis* [pulmonary vein-left atrium] *which goes the heart to the lung. It has a single tunic and is called arteria because of the spirituous blood and is named venalis through its being a simple vein.*

It is unfortunate that Leonardo has written "right" instead of "left" ventricle. This has given rise to much speculation. However, from the context it obviously a *lapsus calami*, as first pointed out by Boruttau (1913), and the substitution of right for left and vice versa is an error common in Leonardo's notes, doubtless due to his mirror-writing.

fig 2. The heart and pulmonary artery: posterior aspect.

fig 3. The trachea, right bronchus and its branches.

The above two figures appear to be preliminary stages of the drawing on 173 where the two figures are fused into one to show the distribution of the branches of the pulmonary arteries and bronchi in the lung.

On the heart is written the word *behind* for what is in reality the inferior or diaphragmatic surface of the heart, but the figure is somewhat diagrammatic. The absence of any indication of the left atrium is noteworthy. The vessel on this surface is presumably the right coronary artery providing interventricular and marginal branches, or perhaps the middle coronary vein. Above, the pulmonary artery is shown dividing into right and left branches, and thereafter subdividing in a purely fanciful or impressionistic manner. Behind and to the right of the pulmonary artery is the stem of the aorta. The right bronchus is likewise shown subdividing in a fanciful pattern. The drawing is marked by an asterisk below which is written: *First make the capsule.* Below the drawing is a memorandum reading: *First make the heart with its vessels from two aspects, that is, from behind and in front.*

Ventricles of the heart

fig I. The heart, great vessels and principal viscera (p. 106).

Both ventricles are opened exposing a series of moderator bands and the interventricular septum which contains the channels required in Galenical physiology for the transmission of blood from the right to the left side for the formation of vital spirits. The heart is regarded as consisting of ventricles only, but there is a suggestion of the left auricle. The branches from the aorta are presented as in ruminants. The right atrium is regarded as part of the vena cava, and reflecting Leonardo's highly speculative and traditional views at this time, the pulmonary veins open directly into the cava. The five-lobed liver of tradition is shown giving off the hepatic vein to the cava along which flows the new blood manufactured in that organ. Splenic vessels pass from the spleen directly to the liver and are supposed to carry the black bile. An umbilical vein extends to the porta hepatis. Other structures are easily recognized, but

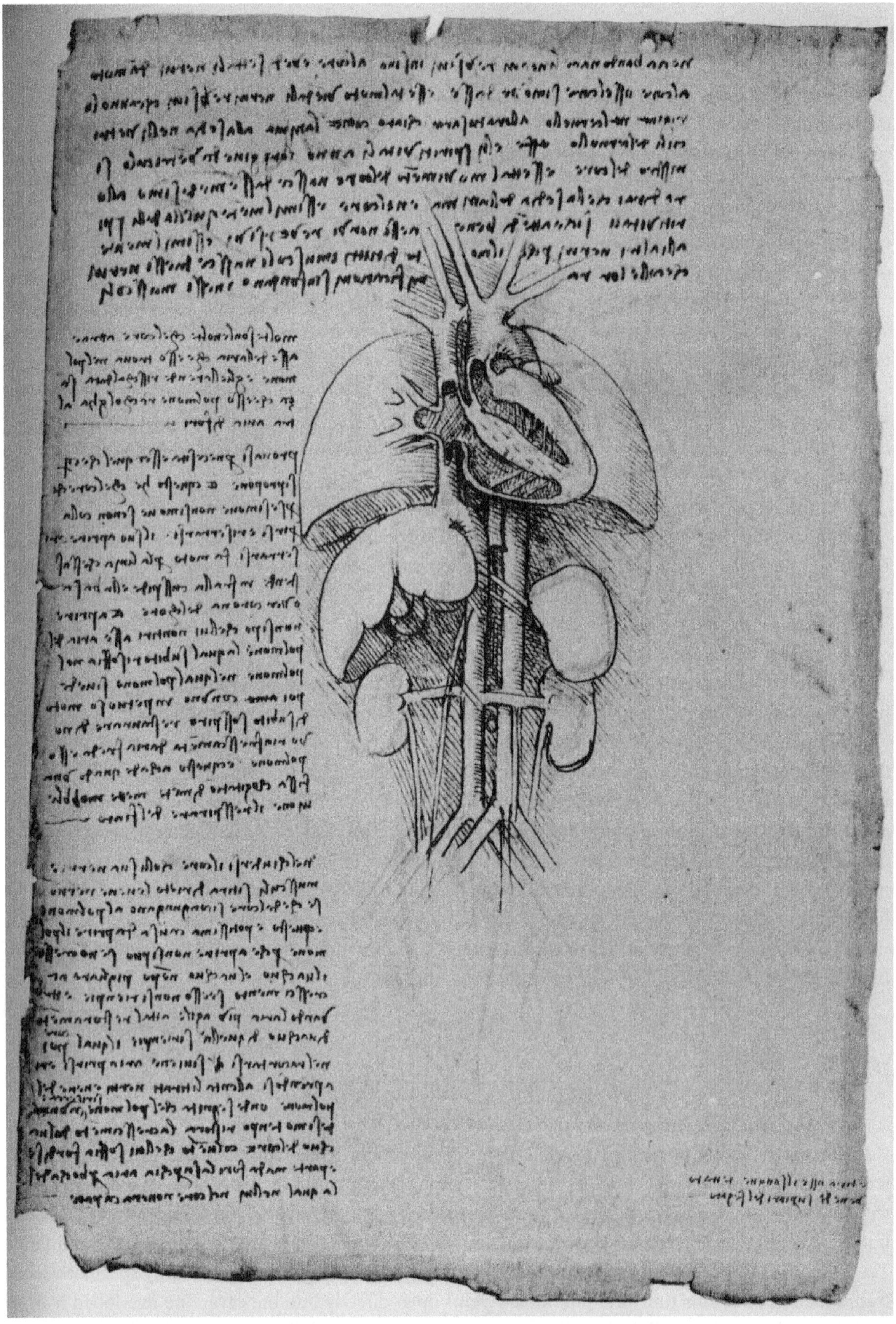

Fig I. Ventricles opened, intraventricular system, and the "pneuma" passing from the lungs to the heart

note the relatively correct arrangement of the spermatic veins especially the left. The discovery that the left spermatic vein drains into the left renal has been claimed for Vesalius, Berengario da Carpi, Achillini and many others.

The primary purpose of the illustration is to express in diagram the manner in which the so-called pneuma passed from the lungs to the heart. Leonardo's opinions are adapted from Galen, and how they differ will be discussed with the notes accompanying this illustration. The first of these notes brings to the fore the controversy between the Aristotelians and the Galenists. Primacy was placed by Aristotle in the heart which was also the seat of the intelligence or sentient soul. In Galen's scheme, held by the physicians, the vital spirit was carried from the left ventricle to the brain where it was transformed into the animal spirit which brought the nervous system into action through the supposedly hollow nerves. The vagus, since it gives off the recurrent, was commonly called the reversive nerve.

Do not leave the reversive nerves until the heart, and see whether these nerves give motion to the heart, or if the heart moves of itself. If its motion comes from the reversive nerves which have their origin in the brain, then you will clarify how the soul [i.e., animal spirit] *has its seat in the ventricles of the brain and the vital spirits have their origin in the left ventricle of the heart. And if this motion of the heart originates in itself, then you will say that the seat of the soul and similarly, that of the vital spirits, is in the heart. So you should attend well to these reversive nerves and likewise to other nerves because the motion of all the muscles arises from these nerves which with their branches are diffused through the muscles.*

In the Galenical physiology the basic principle of life was the pneuma, anima or spirit drawn into the lungs by the act of respiration. From the lungs it passed via the pulmonary veins to the left side of the heart to join with the refined blood which had passed through the interventricular septum to form the vital spirit distributed by the arterial system as the living force. Meanwhile, the blood in the right heart having picked up the impure exhalations from the organs, carried these so-called "sooty vapors" via the monary artery to the lung whence they passed to outer air. In this way the excess of heat general by the heart was dispersed.

Many are the times that the heart attracts to it the air which it finds in the lung, and after heating it, returns it without the lung taking in other air from without.

Leonardo attempts to relate the movements of systole and diastole of the heart to the transference of the pneuma and sooty vapors to and from the heart Respiration and the movements of the heart are coordinated except when one is voluntarily suppressed. The difference in rate is accounted for in part since he held that the ventricles contracted alternately thus producing two pulse beats in the cycle.

It is proved that of necessity it must be as here set forth. This is that the heart which moves of itself does not move except on opening and closing. Its opening and closing cause a motion along the line which extends between the apex (cuspide) and the base or crown of the heart. It cannot open without drawing into itself air from the lung which it immediately blows out again into the lung. In the lung it will then be seen that the lung is restored anew by the vigorous motion of sudden respiration of cold, refreshing air, and this happens when a fixed thought in the mind banishes into oblivion the respiration of the breath.

It is difficult to follow Leonardo's thought in the next passage. He attempts a mechanical explanation of how the pneuma and vapors pass to and from the heart and lungs. At a later period he comes to realize that there is no free passage of air to the heart and that the respiratory movements are due to the action of the muscles of the rib cage. Here, however, he seems to imply that respiration is fundamentally due to the movements of the heart which in diastole create a vacuum which by drawing out the air from the lung causes its collapse. With systole, the heart *pulls* the lung tissue open through the medium of its vascular connections which then creates a vacuum in the lung which is immediately filled by vapors from the heart. These ideas he later discards, indicating that these remarks are of early date.

In closing itself [i.e., in systole] *the heart with its sinews and muscles draws behind the sinewy veins* [pulmonary] *which unite the heart to the lung. This is the chief cause of the opening of the lung, because it cannot open if the vacuum does not increase. The vacuum cannot be increased if it is not refilled, and finding the air speedier for this restoration of the vacuum, it refills itself with it. The heart after contracting comes to open again and on reopening relaxes the drawn out sinews and vessels of the lung, from which it follows that the lung closes again and at the same time replaces the increases of the vacuum of the heart with the air which it blows out of itself. In part it sends out through the mouth the superfluous air for which there is no room either in it or in the heart.*

The liver being the blood-making organ, the heart by means of its diastolic vacuum sucks blood from it to make good that fraction supposedly expended in vital functions. *And it* [the heart] *draws to itself the blood sucked from the upper veins* [hepatic] *of the liver.*

The final note records an observation on the motions of a bird's wing in flight. The manuscript on the Flight of Birds is dated March-April 1505 which, with the internal evidence of the stage of his anatomical development, confirms the date of this study as c.1505. Between 1513–14 he again took up the study of flight, but the style and content of the present writing makes such a date out of the question.

Ionians used air, pneuma and wind synonymously, and the practice was continued by the pneumatist sect.

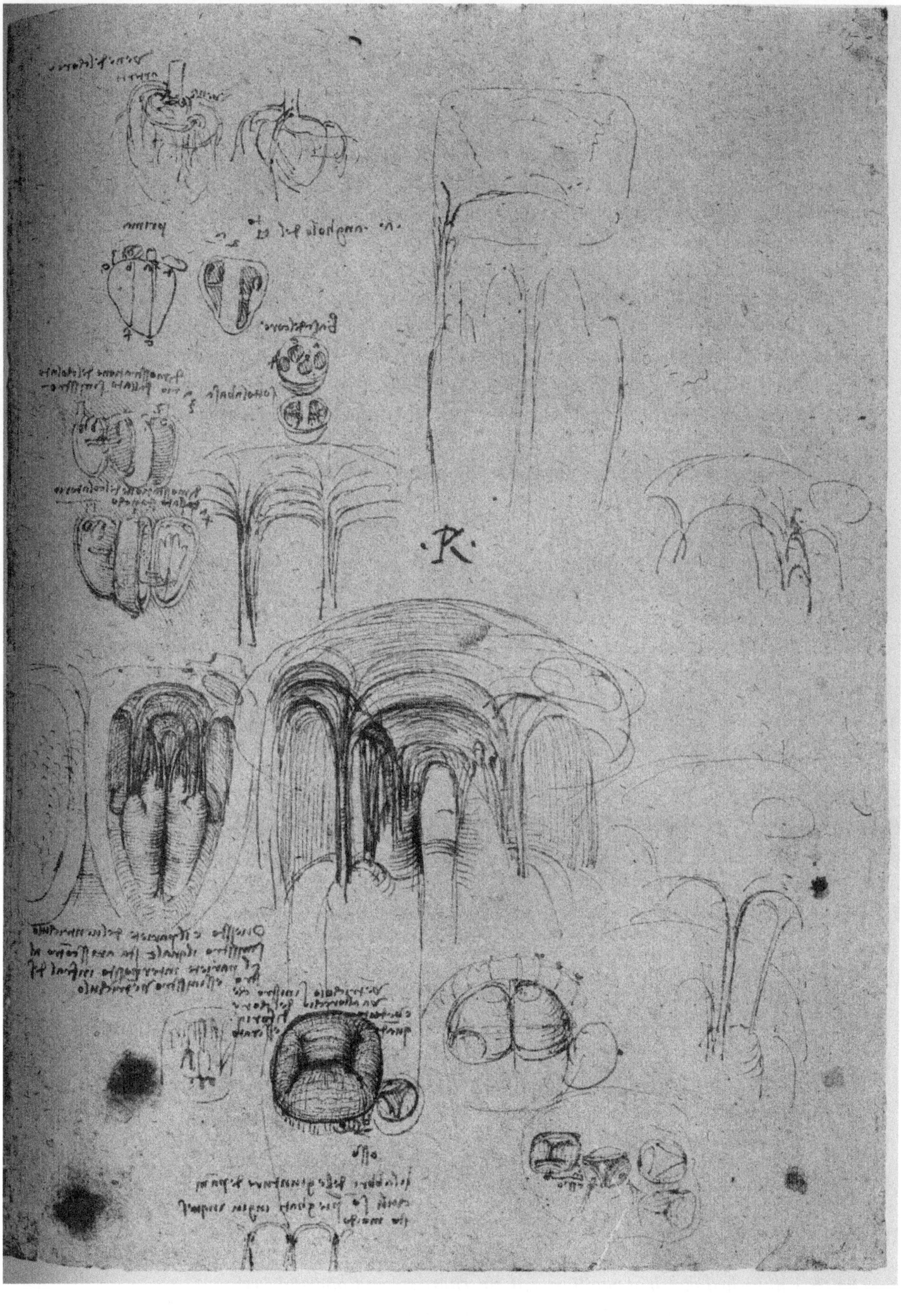

Figs I–18. Ventricles of the heart

Ventricles of the heart cont.

figs 1–2. Rough sketches of the heart and coronary vessels (p. 109).

Above the figures we read: *Vessels of the heart.* In fig. I, the two vessels arising from the aorta are indicated by the word *artery*, and that on the right as vein.

fig 3. Diagram of the heart with lines for section.

The lines for sectioning of the heart to expose the ventricles and interventricular septum as shown in the figures below are indicated by the letters a c, b c. The auricles are identified by the letters a c. This is called the *first* of the two contiguous figures.

fig 4. Coronal section of the heart to expose the ventricles and interventricular septum.

This figure is indicated as the *second.* Above it are the words *ay angle of the circumference* [?], which perhaps means that the section is to be cut from the point a, below the auricle on the left upper margin of fig. 3, in order to obtain the section as shown.

fig 5. Abortive figure of the papillary muscles and mitral valve.

fig 6. Transverse sections of the heart.

The upper portion of the figure labelled *base of the heart,* shows the four orifices, mitral, aortic, tricuspid and pulmonary, which carry the letters a b c d. The lower portion reveals the septum and the ventricular cavities, and the section is indicated as being *below the base.*

fig 7. Heart divided as in fig. 3, to expose the interventricular septum.

This is indicated as the 3rd figure of the series, and the legend reads *Demonstration of the sieve* [interventricular septum] *from the left* [for right] *side.* The moderator band is clearly shown.

fig 8. Heart divided as in fig. 3, to expose the interventricular septum.

The figure is indicated as the *4th* of the series. The legend reads *Demonstration of the sieve from the right* [for left] *side.* It will be observed that left and right are reversed which is not uncommon in Leonardo's notes and may be the result of his habit of mirror-writing.

fig 9. The chordae tendinae of a papillary muscle and the valve.

Leonardo here illustrates his belief that the chordae tendinae form the ventricular surface of the valve by spreading out as a connective tissue layer.

fig 10. Abortive figure of the papillary muscle and the valve.

fig 11. The posterolateral wall of the left ventricle hinged back to expose the mitral valve and its papillary muscles.

The technique is expressed thus: *This is the wall of the left ventricle which is opposite the wall* [septum] *interposed between the right and left ventricles.* Leonardo nowhere uses the term "mitral" which seems to have been introduced by Andreas Vesalius in 1543.

fig 12. Detail of the papillary muscles of the mitral valve.

fig 13. Rough, unfinished sketch of an atrio-ventricular valve.

fig 14. The mitral and aortic orifices: from above.

The legend reads: *The left ventricle which goes to the auricle of the heart is seen from without when closed.* Between and below the mitral and aortic orifices is written the word bone which points to the os cordis found in this position in the hearts of ruminants.

fig 15. Incomplete sketch of aortic orifice and valve.

fig 16. Unfinished sketch of papillary muscle, chordae tendinae and cusp.

fig 17. Diagram of mitral valve to illustrate closure of its cusps.

The junctional lips of the membranes are bent downwards in this manner.

fig 18. The four cardiac orifices.

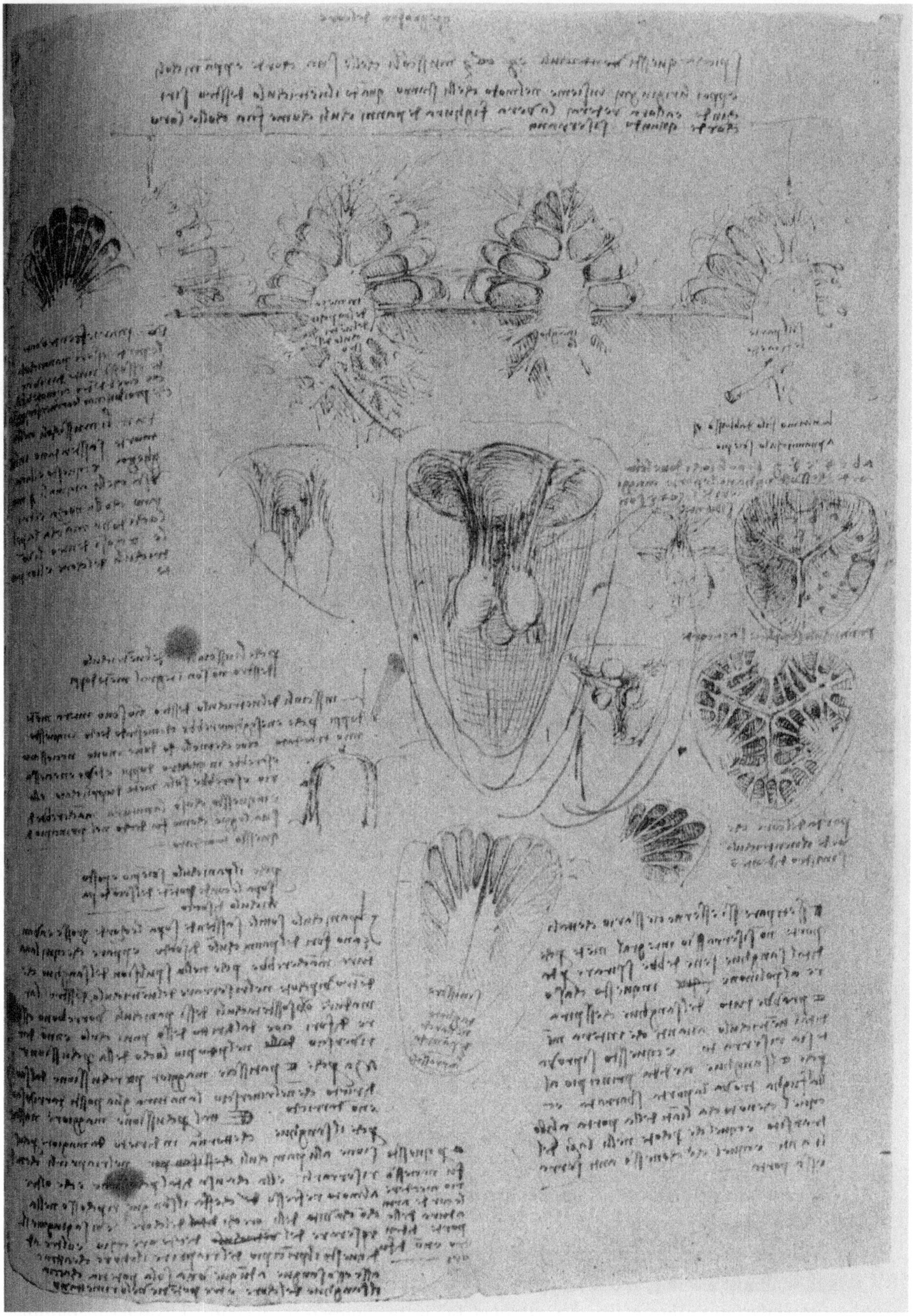

Figs I–10. Geography of the heart. Papillary muscle and tricuspid valve and right ventricle

The sketch clearly illustrates the nature and position of the mitral, aortic, pulmonary and tricuspid valves from left to right. Between the mitral and aortic orifices is the os cordis, labelled bone. In shape and position the os cordis once again indicates that the source of Leonardo's material was the ox.

GEOGRAPHY OF THE HEART.

fig I. A papillary muscle and its chordae tendinae (p. 112).

The chordae tendinae are shown expanding at their attachment to the ventricular surface of the valve. Leonardo held that the cusp consisted of two layers. The atrial surface is smooth and formed by the fleshy membrane or panniculus carnosus. The ventricular surface is "armed" or protected by a tendinous layer or panniculus nervosus established by the chordae tendinae of the papillary muscles.

In front [i.e., on the atrial surface] *the valves are found to be membranous and supported on the opposite side, that is, protected from within by threads* [chordae tendinae] *which prevent their flapping back. All the muscles stretch lengthwise in death, and this is the reason that animals die with the mouth, and other regions where the skin is lacking, [open], and so the interior of the ventricles of the heart and their valves* [are also open].

fig 2. The tricuspid orifice laid open to expose the papillary muscles and valves.

The three papillary muscles of the tricuspid valve are shown with their chordae tendinae extending to the margins of the cusps. The papillary muscle on the right is labelled *On the intermediate wall*, i.e., the septal muscle. The second is noted as lying *In the angle*, and therefore the inferior muscle. The third muscle at the left is said to occur *In the middle of the covering of the right ventricle*, and so is the anterior muscle of that wall. Below the papillary muscles on the right and on the left may be seen a moderator band which is shown divided in two. It occupies a position as commonly found in the heart of ungulates. Near the portion of the moderator band on the right are the words *The lowest filum of a simple membrane below*, which doubtless means that a second moderator band occurs below, as in the ox. The trabeculae carnae of the ventricle are also represented especially on the left. By including a portion of the right papillary muscle and its chordae on the extreme left, it will be observed that Leonardo has so designed the figure as to enable the reader to reconstruct the orifice. Attention is called to this in the note above the figure.

Cut out these 3 muscles with their cords and valves and then join them in the manner in which they exist when the right ventricle closes itself, and then you will see the true shape of the valves [and] *what they do with their cords when they shut themselves.*

The technique suggested in this note must be the first example of the use of paper cut-outs in the teaching of anatomy. The method became popular in the second quarter of the sixteenth century.

figs 3–4. The papillary muscles, tricuspid valve and right ventricle.

Diagrams to show the closure of the tricuspid valve when the wall of the ventricle has been removed.

fig 5. Tricuspid valve and the three papillary muscles from below.

The figure is badly faded but the outlines are still discernible.

fig 6. The ventricular surface of the tricuspid valve, chordae tendinae removed.

The points of attachment of the severed ch A tendinae are indicated on the upper cusp by the lett d c b a q f e, now almost illegible, and the note ab the figure reads: *a b c d e f g are the places where the chords which support the large valves of the heart situated.* Below the figure is the legend: *The simple membranes without cords.*

figs 7–8. The tricuspid valves, chordae tendinae and papillary muscles from below.

Leonardo's note adequately describes the figures: *The valves of the heart which the right ventricle sees from within.*

fig 9. Adjacent cardiac valves to illustrate the influence of margins on closure.

The area of overlap of adjacent cusps is indicated by a, the thinner margin, by c, and the apex, by b. The purpose of the illustration is to demonstrate that the margins of the cusp consist of a single layer, the panniculus nervosus, and the body of two layers, panniculus nervosus and carnosus, so that on closure the area of overlap will consist of two and not four thicknesses as described in 106. Thus nature's law that nothing is superfluous is demonstrated.

WHY THE CUSPS OF THE RIGHT VENTRICLE ARE NOT ENTIRELY DOUBLE.

The cusps (uscioli) of the right ventricle are not entirely double because it would follow, as has been said [106] *in this treatise of mine, that at the place* [contiguous margins of the valves] *where it is not necessary, it would be doubled to four* [layers] *and where it is necessary, it would be twofold only: and in this case Nature would be wanting in her law, as was said at the beginning of this treatise.*

fig 10. The mitral valve and left ventricle in longitudinal section.

The legend on the figure reads: *The left* [ventricle] *sectioned through the arch of the membranes in side view.*

Attention has been called to Leonardo's opinion that the valves of the atrioventricular orifices consist of two layers. The atrial surface is a layer of "flesh and thus, in the standard terminology of the times, a simple tissue. The ventricular surface of the valve is supportive and consists of "sinew" or "cord" established by the spreading out of the chordae tendinae to form this layer. An extensive note discusses the reason for this arrangement.

WHY THE SIMPLE MEMBRANE IS PLACED UPON THE POWERFUL CORDS OF THE SECOND LOWER MEMBRANE.

The thin membrane is stretched over the thick cords and extends on the outside [atrial surface] *of the lower membrane. It appears that Nature would fail here because on the expulsion of the blood which churns inside there* [in the atrium] *at the closing of the right, likewise when it returns the blood to the ventricle from which it was thrust, assisting the natural reflux somewhat with its contraction. The motion takes place more swiftly at the reflux of the blood in returning to the ventricle of the heart whence it was first expelled.*

The descent of the heart makes the same impulse as that created by the impetus of the motion which beats against the bottom of the lower ventricle. From here, during the time that it rebounds from the bottom, the heart contracts which increases the motion made by the blood at the second beat against the covering of the upper ventricle. If you should say that the beat made by the descent of the blood to the bottom of the lower ventricle is greater than that which beats against the covering of the upper ventricle [auricle], since one of these motions is natural and the other not, I shall here reply that a liquid in a liquid has no weight (except for the amount which the beat generates).

At one time part of a single sheet, now divided, the notes and drawings on this page continue to some extent the argument found on 96.

figs 1–2. Abortive sketches of the right atrio-ventricular or tricuspid valves (p. 114).

fig 3. The right atrio-ventricular or tricuspid valve of the heart opened out.

The three valves are indicated by the letters g f a, a b c, c d e, from right to left. The letter h, on the extreme right corresponds to d, on the left, the point of section. The letters n m o p q, mark the

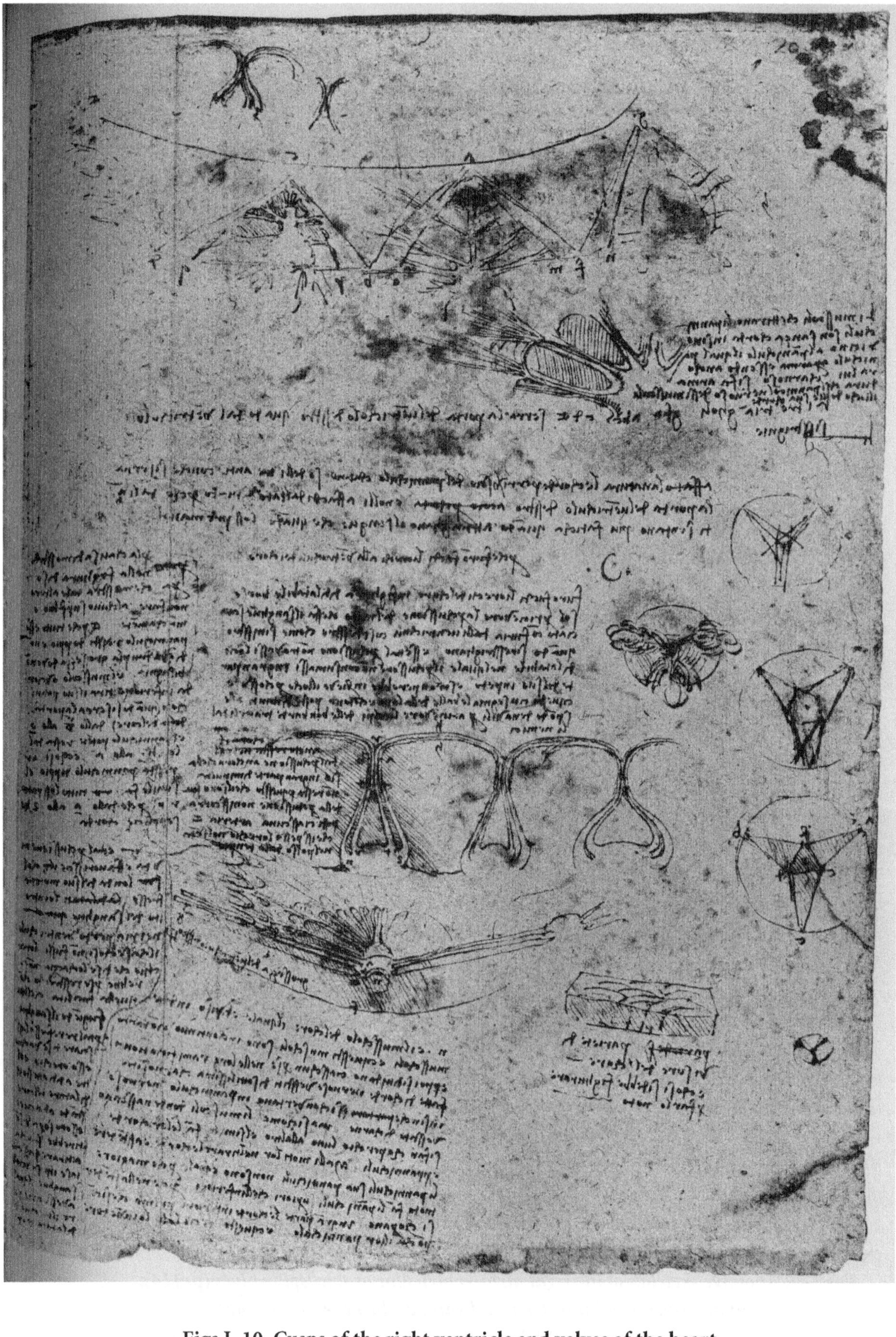

Figs I–10. Cusps of the right ventricle and valves of the heart

terminations of secondary lines outlining the valvular margins when stretched by the action of the papillary muscles shown with their chordae tendinae lying in the intervals between the valves. *The three triangles, g f a, a b c, c d e, shut the gateway* [tricuspid orifice] *of the right ventricle when that ventricle contracts.* A further note referring to this figure appears on 96, which became separated with the division of the sheet.

ON THE VALVES OF THE HEART.

On the shutting of the heart, the valves [mitral and tricuspid] *of the heart always give passage first to a quantity of blood before they shut from within outwards.*

And the valves [aortic and pulmonary] *which shut from without inwards return the blood to which they first gave passage. Those* [mitral and tricuspid] *which close from within outwards, before shutting completely, give passage to the impulse of that part of the blood which was within the lips of the opened valves c o* [in fig. 3]. *This part* [of the blood], *unobstructed, gives with its principal wave due nourishment to the vessels of the lung when, after being refreshed in the lung, it returns in large part to refresh the blood which was previously left in the ventricle where it was divided.*

The above note develops the Galenical theory on the flux and reflux of the blood. The portion of the blood which remains behind in the right ventricle is that which was supposed to pass through the interventricular septum to become vital spirits as explained on 96. A further note is a recapitulation of the function of the auricles in this process of reflux discussed at length on 96.

fig 4. A papillary muscle and its chordae tendinae.

The chordae tendinae of a papillary muscle are shown making a series of arches and spreading out to be attached not only to the apices and margins of a cardiac valve but also to its ventricular surface. Leonardo apparently considered a cusp to be formed of two layers. The first he calls the fleshy membrane and the second, which was established by the spreading out of the fibers of the chordae tendinae as a protective coat (armadura), he calls the sinewy membrane.

The [papillary] *muscles which draw the membranes are without cords until near the membrane, which membrane being also fleshy, forms for itself a protective coat which is the sinewy membrane of these muscles in place of their cords.*

figs 5–7, 9, 12. Diagrams of the right atrio-ventricular or tricuspid valve.

In fig. 6, the tricuspid valve is seen from below receiving the attachments of the chordae tendinae of the papillary muscles which are greatly foreshortened. In the other diagrams the valve is shown both open and closed. In fig. 9, the intervals between the cusps are lettered at their base a b c, and the apices of the cusps c d f. A note attempts to explain in terms of the theory of flux and reflux why the chordae tendinae are attached to the ventricular surfaces of the

Nature has made the chordae [to attach] *on the re verse side of the fleshy membrane of the three cusps with which the gateway of the right ventricle is shut She has not made them on the posterior aspect be* cause these cusps experience more effort when they draw the blood in than when they squeeze it out.*

fig 8. The tricuspid valve opened out to demonstrate formation of the margins of the cusps.

fig 10. Papillary muscle, chordae tendinae and cusp (greatly foreshortened).

To follow the accompanying note, figs. 8 and 10 must be taken together. In the first three illustrations the papillary muscle is shown giving off four chordae tendinae indicated by the letters s t v n, which blend to form the thinner margin of the cusp at a c, b d, over the interval of adjacent cusp contact r o, and at the apex of the cusp h h. Thus the margin of the cusp is formed by a single layer which Leonardo calls the *panniculo nervoso.* Since the margins of adjacent cusps overlap, on closure of the valve, the region of overlap consists of a double layer, each of which is formed by the extension of the connective tissue of the chordae tendinae. On the other hand, the remaining central portion of the cusp being thicker is said to be formed by a double layer, the *panniculo nervoso* on the ventricular surface and the *panniculo carnoso* on the atrial surface. It is necessary to recognize this distinction, which incidentally approaches the truth, to understand the note below.

In the second figure, a papillary muscle n, is shown attached to the overlying ventricular wall, labelled *The thickness of the right ventricle,* and also indicated by the letters f g. The papillary muscle blends with this wall at e, and two of its chordae tendinae are indicated by a b, at the muscle, and c d, where their fibres spread out to form the margin of the cusp and Leonardo's *panniculo nervoso.*

n [in fig. 10] *is the muscle of the heart which is divided into two muscles* [papillary, and muscle of ventricular wall]. *These muscles are in contact and continuous and then separate each by itself, into their branchings made up of sinewy cords* [chordae tendinae] *clothed by the thinnest of flesh* [endocardium?] *until they are converted into the sinewy membrane covered by flesh* [Leonardo's panniculo carnoso of the cusp]. *But just as the muscles* [of the ventricular wall] *from which they arise form a cover, one for the their cords do the same and* [form] *membranes. But their motions in pulling upon the cords and stretching the membranes are not equal because the upper membranes make a greater motion than the lower since on stretching they in large part cover the inferior cords before their membrane is formed. The Creator did this for the reason shown in the above illustration* [fig. 8] *which demonstrates that the Almighty makes nothing superfluous or imperfect. In order that the entire membrane remain double and not quadruple in thickness where it is not required, the [papillary] muscle or the inferior cords, pulls its membrane (when the gateway of the heart is shut) from r to o, and the strong membrane* [i.e., consisting of both the fleshy and tendinous layers] *remains from h to o. Thus a r [margin of cusps on overlapping] remains a double membrane and likewise does the entire interval r o, because from a to s, there is a simple cord* [i.e., single tendinous layer].

Aortic pulmonary valves

fig I. Diagram of the aortic valve and sinuses (p. 117).

The diagram is similar to that on 112. The centrally placed triangle a b c, is the aortic aperture. The larger semicircles about its three sides represent the aortic sinuses of Valsalva. Within them, the smaller arcs on the same base indicate the cusps, actually the thin lunules of the cusp, lettered r,r,r. From the center of the triangle d, pass five lines: d b, d c, to the base of the triangle: d e (like D) to the middle of the larger semicircle intersecting the cusp at r: and two other lines not lettered. Beside the figure is N to draw attention to the fact that this figure and note are inserted as a continuation of the discussion labelled N below. From the principles laid down in 112 on the behavior of liquids passing through a pipe, the meaning of the note is clear.

In the figure N below, placed here once more, is demonstrated how the blood, or the momentum, which moves backwards from the center d, along the line d e, has a much greater revolution than the momentum d b [since the latter is further from the center]. *Consequently its reflected motion has to turn further downwards to complete its circular motion than the blood d b.*

I doubt that all the principal orifices of animals open themselves because of death, that the orifice m o p h [aortic orifice, lettered in fig. 6] *does not open in the triangle a b c* [aortic aperture] *and whether, in* the *living, this orifice would close itself without the membranes a b r, a c r, b c r* [aortic cusps] *and swell like the flesh of the tongue or penis.*

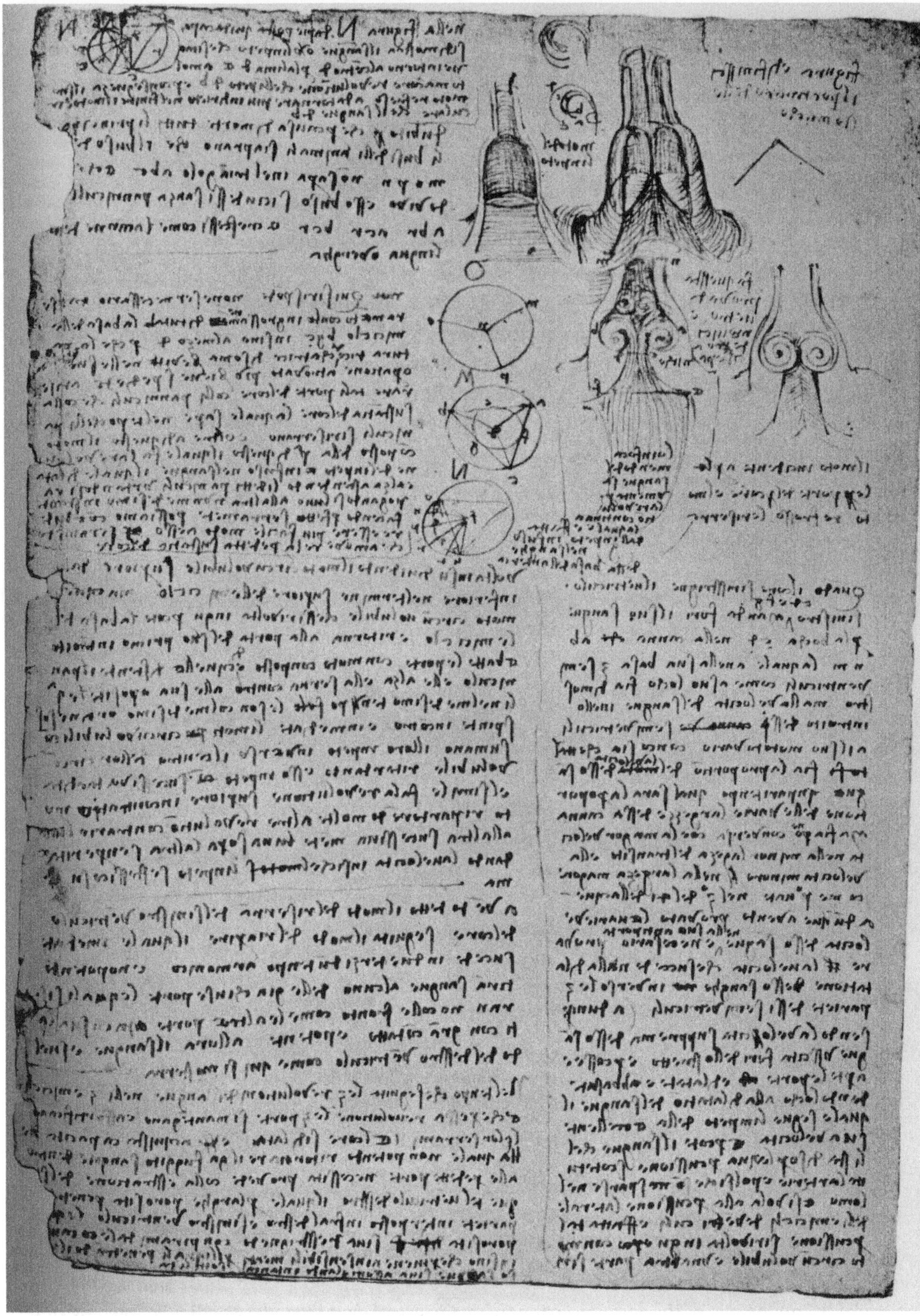

Figs I–8. Aortic valve. The motion of the impetus (of the heart)

In the above note he has in mind the possible action of the aortic vestibule of the left ventricle assisting as a sphincter (cf. 110) and reminds himself to *Draw and define the pyloris of the stomach.*

figs 2–3. Diagrams to illustrate formation of the aortic vortices of blood.

THE MOTION OF THE IMPETUS.

From the principles derived from observations made on the flow of water through a pipe described on 112, the formation of the vortices in the aortic sinuses is analyzed. In the second of the two diagrams, three streams a b c, lying successively nearer to the center of the orifice are shown. From fig. 1 on 112, stream b, intersects stream a, at e, since b, is nearer the center. From fig. 2 of the same page, stream c, rises higher than a or b, being still nearer the center but is deflected at the point d, where it comes in contact with the curved wall of the aortic sinus. This stream in consequence passes lateral to the others until curved upward by the curve of the cusp, thus causing the whole to revolve and form a circular eddy of blood as shown below.

figs 4–5. Figures of the aortic orifice, valves and sinuses to be made of glass.

On several occasions Leonardo mentions the making of a glass model of the aortic orifice and valves in order to study the closure of the cusps and the formation of blood eddies. While we do not know if it was ever constructed, these figures suggest such a model. Below the figure is a further note: *Make this trial in the glass* [model] *and move in it … the membranes.*

fig 6. Three diagrams of the aortic orifice and valves.

In O, the valve is shown closed by its three semilunar segments p n o, o n m, m n p. In M, the triangular aperture a b c, is added thus defining the lunules of the cusps a d b, a d c and b d c. The base of each cusp is looked upon as being part of the adjacent aortic sinus, and these are indicated by e f g. In N, the valve is open. Lines are drawn radially from the center of the aperture f, to the walls of the aortic sinus at o n p r t u. These lines intersect the base of the cusp at r o q s, and represent the various lengths of the blood stream which will be reflected from the walls of the sinus to roll back the cusp in closure of the valve. It is possible that these diagrams are in part related to the construction of a valve for the model illustrated above. In the accompanying note the reason for the presence of the thin lunules of the cusps is discussed in terms of Leonardo's law that Nature makes nothing in vain.

Here is replied: closure by means of the entire thickness of the base of the semicircle b g c [in fig. 6, N] *as far as the middle d, is not necessary, because Nature, seeking the greatest brevity in her operations, has found shorter expedients by closing the gateways of the heart with the membranes rather than with the substance of the heart which opens at the time that the membranes are closed. And besides, from the compound motion of the first thereof, which causes the revolution of the impetus introduced into the blood which expands and elevates while stretching the said membranes, clashing and opposing them against one another making a perfect closure, we can conclude is an easier way for this closure to occur than to move the aforementioned substance of the heart.*

fig 7. The left ventricle and aortic valve during systole.

fig 8. The aortic valve during systole.

These two figures are complementary. In fig. 7 the left ventricle e f g, is separated from the aortic vestibule c d f e, by the line e f. The aortic sinuses and cusps containing the primary blood eddies are lettered a b, and the rest of the aorta receiving the main stream and secondary eddies is noted by m n. On the ventric is the statement: *The heating of the blood is augmented by the continual revolution which is cause by the momentum introduced into the blood at t base of the artery.* Below fig. 8, we are once again informed that *The incident motion opens the valves the heart, and the reflected motion closes them.*

These notes are followed by a lengthy discussion on the formation and function of the vortices of the blood in the aortic sinuses following systole of the heart. The majority of Leonardo's observations on the flow of water are to be found in the Codex Atlanticus with several suggestions as to arrangement. But in the Leicester Codex is one of his latest notes on the order of the book, and therefore closely related in time to the present writing. Here (Leicester 15V) we learn that the third book carried the title libro 3° delle vene, that is, on the passage of water through pipes, which must be the work to which reference is made.

When the heart contracts, the left ventricle c def g [fig. 7], *sends out its blood through the opening c d, into the tube a b n m* [aorta] *which has 3 semiventricles* [aortic sinuses] *at its base as will be demonstrated in its place. However, the velocity of the blood at the entrance to these semiventricles has its motion varied owing to the fact that the proportional velocity of this blood in equal time will be equal to the proportions of the various dimensions of this tube* [cf. fig. 6,N], *but they will be inverse, that is, the greater velocity in the greater dimension as is proved in the 3rd* [book] *of the treatise on water.*

Therefore having proved the different velocities of this blood in its antechamber [aortic sinuses], *it is necessary to prove the velocity which follows upon the expansion of this blood toward the 3 walls of these semiventricles. Thus, when the highest velocity of this blood has issued from the narrows* [aortic vestibule], *it beats against and opens the valve. The dilated and lowered valve gives way to the expansion of the blood which follows the momentum of its rising velocity and beats against the blood which lies above it. This percussion throbs all the arteries and pulses distributed throughout man. It then turns to the lateral percussion of the semicircles of the ventricles and, having beaten against them, turns downwards with a circular motion. The other part [of the blood] revolves above, dividing the upper circular motion from the lower at the upper limit of the semicircle. But the circular motion which revolves below beats against the base of the semicircle and returns to the valve of its first entrance. It strikes the valve with a compound motion and distends its membrane, raising it and shutting it against its opponents, which at the same time with the same order are driven against it. Immediately the circular motions expend their momentum towards the centre of their circumvolution: the momentum slowing by successive steps. The upper revolution in opposite motion does likewise, giving birth to many other revolutions, opposed to one another, in succession one above the other, the velocity continuously slowing until the momentum expends itself.*

The statements in the final note are pure Galenism, and since the note was composed in his latest period, they completely destroy the fanciful notions of many that Leonardo possessed a knowledge of the circulation of the blood. Here we meet with the age-old theory of the passage of blood through the interventricular wall to form the vital spirit.

The manner of closure of the left ventricle of the heart having been described, there follows the manner of its reopening. This occurs immediately afterwards in two-thirds of a harmonic tempo and [the left ventricle] *not being able to draw any blood from the already closed [mitral] valves, which do* [not] *shut with their fronts like other valves, but with their sides by extensive contact and force, the blood is then sweated from the right ventricle as is here demonstrated.*

During the time which follows the 3 revolutions of the blood in the 3 semicircles [aortic sinuses] *and that the 3 valves maintain and strengthen their closure by these 3 revolutions, the heart is dilated and acquires capacity. The blood having already surged above the aforementioned valves and not being able to return into it* [left ventricle], *it is provided of necessity by the extraction of blood from the right ventricle. This penetrates through lengthy porosities the wall interposed between the right and left ventricles. These porosities proceed from contracting pyramidal cavities until they pass into imperceptible passages through which the viscous blood penetrates becoming subtilized to very great thinness.*

Owing to the number and arrangement of the drawings on this page it is easier to consider them in three groups enumerated in the usual manner from left to right within each group. This page, originally part of a larger sheet, the other half being 112–13, is also the verso although called recto in Q.

GROUP I. UPPER RIGHT CORNER.

figs 1–3. Diagrams to illustrate a note on the triangular shape of the aortic aperture (p. 121).

In fig. 1 the aortic orifice is shown closed by four hypothetical semilunar valves, one of which is lettered e h f, and its base w. In fig. 2 the aortic orifice, the customary three cusps are illustrated, and one is lettered cab, and its base S. In fig. 3 only two cusps fill the orifice. The accompanying note is explanatory.

Nature made 3 valves and not 4, because the pellicles which close such valves make greater angles, being 3 in number, as the angle cab [fig. 2] *shows,* [being greater] *than the angle formed by e h f* [fig. 1], *where there are 4 valves. Now for this reason the more obtuse angle is stronger than the right angle of the square* [valve], *inasmuch as the cathetus* [i.e., altitude of a triangle] *a s* [in fig. 2] *is shorter than the cathetus* [in fig. 1], *and the square aperture is more capacious than the triangular in one and the same circle. Consequently the membranes* [lunules] *of the 4 valves are weaker than those of the 3 valves because at their angles they are further removed from the base of their triangle than those of the 3 valves.*

fig 4. The aortic valve.

The cusps of the aortic and pulmonary valves were regarded by Leonardo as consisting of two parts. The membranes or pellicles corresponding approximately to the lunules of modern terminology made up one part and were attached, not to what we would regard as the base of the cusp, but to what he regarded as the base or continuation of the aortic sinus. The note below the figure tells us, as explained more fully in 113 that *It* [aortic valve] *opens itself through the incident motion and closes itself by the reflected motion.*

GROUP II. UPPER LEFT CORNER.

figs 1–4, 6. Sketches of the aortic valve and sinuses, many incomplete.

The largest of these figures shows the aortic vestibule, valve and base of the aorta to illustrate the vortex of blood in the sinus which it was believed closes the cusp. The mechanism is described in the note below and fully on 113.

fig 5. Diagram of aortic valve and sinus to demonstrate the formation of a vortex of blood.

In this diagram, the lower left member of the group, we are shown how a vortex or eddy of blood forms in the aortic sinus to assist in closure of the cusp. It will be noticed that the aorta is referred to as a conduit, tube or pipe. This suggests that Leonardo may perhaps be describing an observation made on the glass model, and the large fig. 6 may represent this.

When the blood n b m o a, revolves with a circular motion around its center of motion r, it wants to maintain its momentum along the line of the beginning of its revolving motion and tends to enlarge following the curvature of the beginning curve n b m. However by percussion against the wall m o [of the aortic sinus], *it becomes of lesser curvature and proceeds to follow the wall until it strikes against ay where is found the simple membrane of the valve a b. This momentum of blood would rupture it* [valve] *in a very short time, but sagacious Nature provided a very durable resistance at the lowest part of the circle of momentum by thickening the wall of the conduit* [aorta] *at 0 by the mass o a h L. Consequently, when from the motion of this blood its percussion is delivered against a resistant place, the revolving motion is suddenly turned upwards at the end of this wall at the point a where it encounters the membrane of the valve. The*

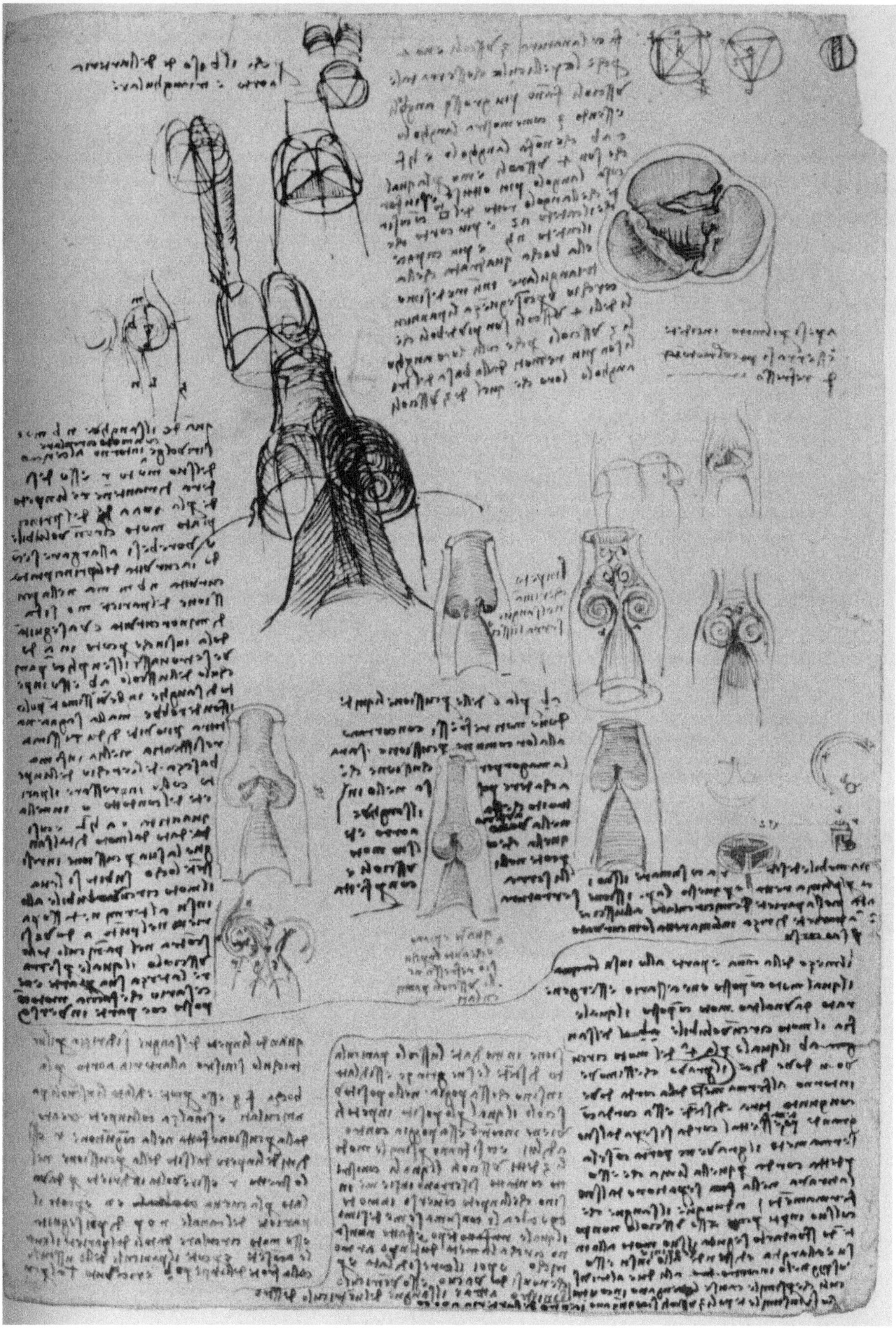

Figs I–4. (upper right corner) Aortic valve
Figs I–6. (upper left corner) Aortic valve
Figs I–13. (middle of page) Aortic valve

membrane, in order to close its third [of the opening] *necessarily must make a compound motion, that is partly towards the middle of the tube and partly upwards. This compound motion must be created by another compound motion which will be the revolving motion of the blood a by which according to the 4th* [book] *"on revolving motion"—where it is stated: The weight which moves around the attachment of a string, where it is joined, pulls and stretches this string with great force, and if such a string is severed from its attachment, the weight carries with it the said string along that line into which it was drawn at severance from its attachment. Therefore, the blood which beats against this valve with its momentum, being unable to rupture it, continues its motion upwards, enlarges and expands the fold* [lunule] *upwards, and drives it against the other two valves which, for similar reasons, advance to meet it. Thus, the 3 valves are joined together at the same time in the center of the aorta.*

GROUP III. MIDDLE OF PAGE.

figs 1–2. Abortive figure of aortic valve.

fig 3. The aortic valve shown fully opened at the beginning of systole.

To the right of the figure it is stated, *The momentum which remains in the blood closes the valve.*

figs 4–5. The aortic valve shown about to close at the end of systole.

The primary and secondary vortices discussed above are shown developing in the aortic sinuses and root of the aorta. In fig. 4 the aortic orifice is lettered a b, and discussed in the note where reference is again made to the treatise *On the nature of water, a b* [aortic valve], *according to the 6th* [book] *on the percussion of liquids, where* [it is stated] *reflected motion: combine to form a common percussion, will be the region of greatest percussion which can take place at the entrance which the blood makes into the aorta. It is this which by its motion beats against the valves and shuts them with perfect closure.*

fig 6. The aortic valve open at the beginning of systole.

The letter S on the right marks the figure as one of a series beginning with the diagram on the extreme right lettered O.

fig 7. The aortic valve closed during diastole.

The legend reads: *When it* [antechamber or aortic sinuses] *is full and the reflected percussion has been received by the membranous valves.*

fig 8. The aortic valve to show the fitting together of the lunules of the cusps.

fig 9. An aortic cusp showing the lunule of its free border.

fig 10 (below 9). The aortic cusps in closure.

This is figure U of the series.

fig II. Diagram on circular motion.

This is figure O and the first of the series. The diagram illustrates the manner of formation of the blood vortex and is similar to figs. 2–3 on 113. The blood stream is marked by the letters b d c, d being the point of reflection from the wall of the aortic sinus. Compare the accompanying statement to Newton's first law of motion.

Everything movable desires to expend its momentum along a straight line. And for this reason the percussion [of the blood] *delivered against the semicircular wall* [of the aortic sinus], *on leaving this wall, directs its first curved course in a straight line.*

fig 12 (below II). A diagram; significance unknown.

fig 13. Diagram of aortic valve and sinuses demonstrating the formation of a vortex of blood.

The lettering is difficult to read. Aortic orifice, f g; the blood stream at r, parts at e, to describe a circular eddy e a c, about a, center at b, in the aortic sinus n o p.

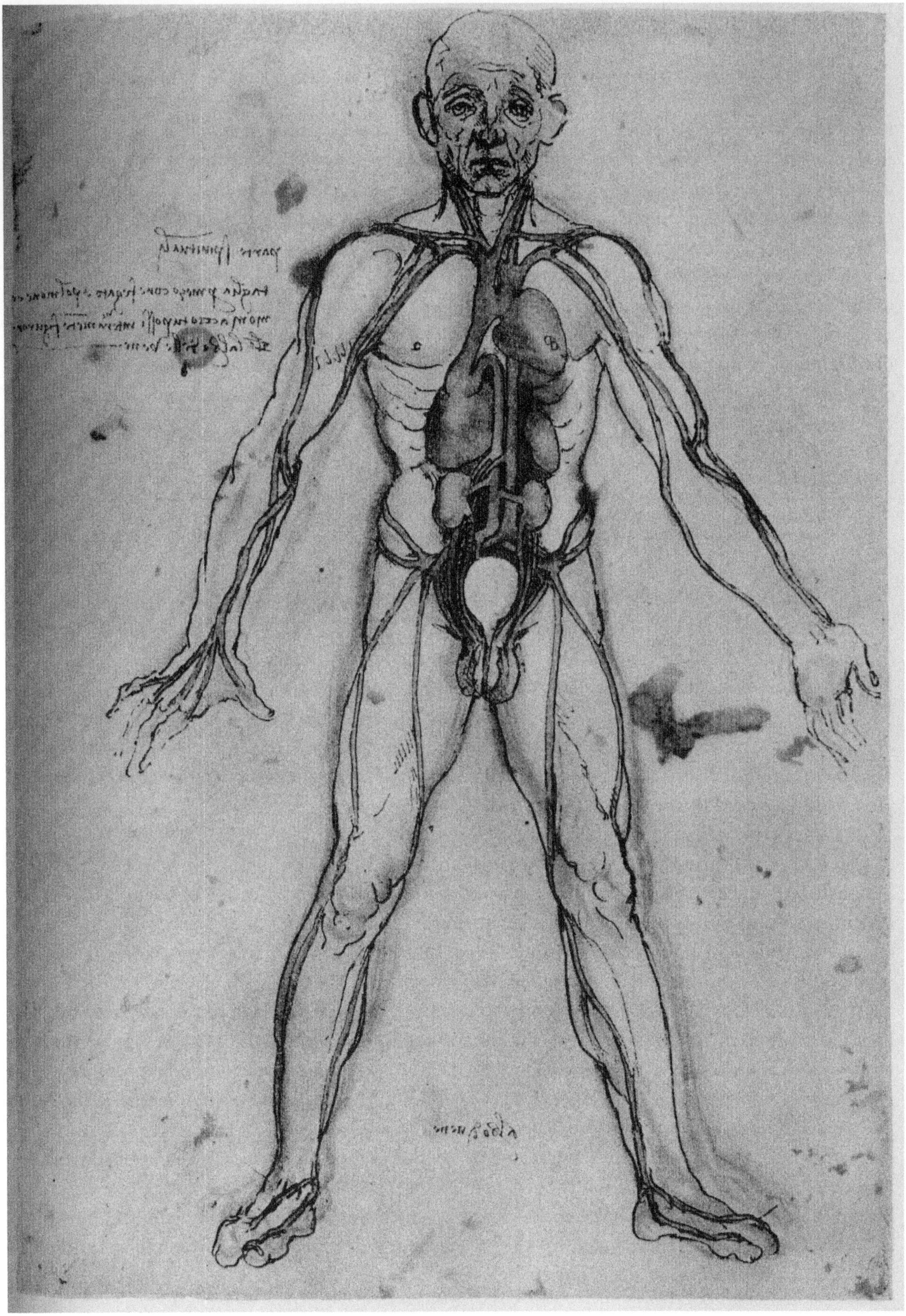

Fig I. Cardiovascular system, of the old man

When the momentum of blood is directed through the left ventricle to the aorta through the orifice f g, it beats against and dilates the membranous valves and ascends with the momentum created by the percussion occurring at the junction r. The momentum separates from the site of the percussion in the narrows r, and revolves backwards along the curve e n, and beats against the wall of channel n o p [aortic sinus]. *It then continues this circular motion imparted to it by the wall which yields, arid beats against the membrane of the valve with the front of the impetus b. Having received this percussion, the membranous valve immediately expands its folds and is dilated until it abuts against the opposite valve which through the opposed momentum advances to meet it and abuts against it. And so in a similar manner do the 3 said valves which shut together in close contact until the momentum, converted into a cochleariform motion, expends itself. In a healthy individual the time occupied is about half of a harmonic tempor. And then the heart is dilated, and since a vacuum cannot exist, this left ventricle attracts the blood from the right ventricle.*

Cardiovascular system

fig I. The vascular tree (p. 124).

To one side of the figure are the words *spiritual parts,* i.e., the Galenical vascular system carrying the natural spirits on the venous side and the vital spirit on the arterial. Below this is a reminder to construct a more elaborate picture of the vascular system such as that of 202. *Cut through the middle of the heart, liver and lung and the kidneys so that you can represent the vascular tree in its entirety.*

On the ureter is written *vena cilis,* possibly not in Leonardo's hand, since it is of course not the ureter but the vena cava, and this would be an unusual error for Leonardo judging from his use of the term even in his earliest period. Clark dates the figure as c. 1504–06 on stylistic grounds but admits that the pen and ink work as well as the rather ornamental writing look much earlier. In terms of the anatomical knowledge displayed we date the drawing c.1490–1500.

The ideas expressed in the figure appear to be based on a reading, possibly of Plato or of one of his commentators, possibly by way of translation from the Arabic version of the *Timaeus,* to which have been added findings derived from animal dissection and the surface inspection of the body. The caval system is represented as arising in the liver like the sprouting of a seed with roots extending downwards and the stem upwards. This is the Aristotelian conception which Leonardo later discarded in favor of the Galenical view that the venous system had its origin in the heart. No atria are shown, but the heart was regarded as a two-chambered organ consisting of ventricles only—a conception from findings in animals where the cava appears as a continuous vessel passing through the heart. The arch of the aorta and its branches show the ungulate arrangement, not the human. Leonardo had the support of Avicenna for this statement which he did not correct until the dissection of the centenarian, cf. 128. The superficial veins of the extremities show astonishing inaccuracies since they were open to surface inspection whereas the arteries of these members are portrayed in a manner to be expected from the reading of Mundinus and Avicenna. The arrangement of the kidneys is as in animals. Other structures recognizable are the spleen, right spermatic vessels arising from the inferior cava and descending aorta and the left spermatic, origin not shown. The bladder receives cystic branches from the common iliac veins, and the urethra has been laid open.

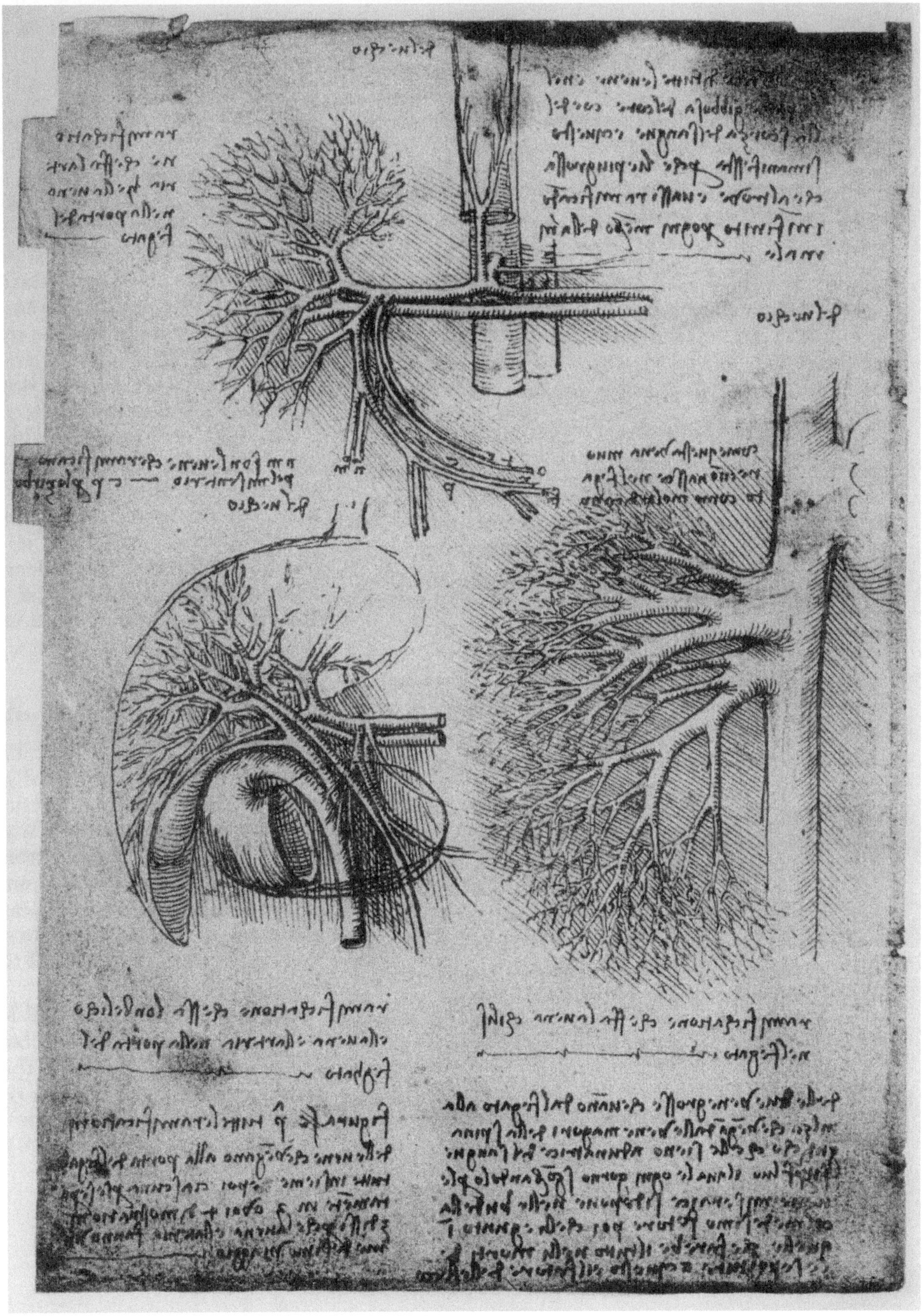

Figs I–3. The portal vein and coeliac vessels

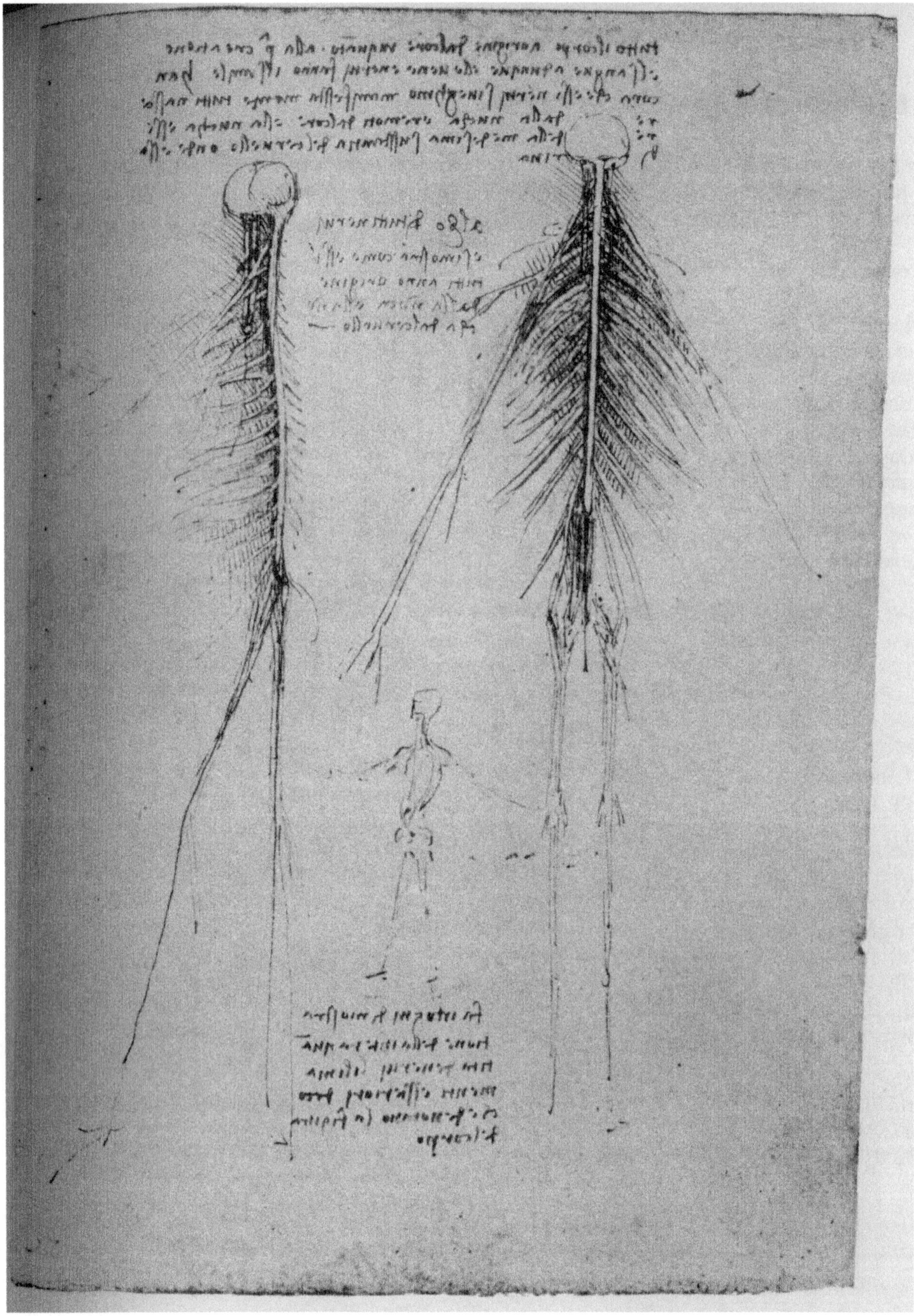

Figs I.2, 3, and I. Brain, spinal cord, peripheral nerves

fig I. The portal and coeliac vessels, of the old man (p. 125).

The oesophagus is cut short. Behind it the abdominal aorta is shown providing the coeliac artery from which the splenic, hepatic, left gastric, with oesophageal branches, and possibly the inferior phrenic arteries are given off. The hepatic artery provides the gastro-duodenal which is observed terminating in the superior pancreatico-duodenal at m, the right gastro-epiploic at p, and the right gastric at o. These vessels are accompanied by corresponding veins. However, Leonardo was somewhat confused as to the venous tributaries of the portal system. Below the branching coeliac artery is the splenic vein continuing as the portal to the liver. Leonardo regarded this as a single straight vessel. The vein n, must be intended as the superior mesenteric but he is very uncertain of this vessel. Concerning them he says: n m, *are the vessels which ramify through the mesentery, c p, through the omentum.*

The hepatic artery and portal vein after dividing into right and left branches are seen dissected out of the liver substance. He tells us (128) that the liver in this specimen was so desiccated as to crumble away exposing the ramifications of the vessels. Opposite these branches he writes: *Ramification which the artery and vein make in the porta of the liver.*

fig 2. The portal, hepatic and biliary vessels of the liver, of the old man.

The figure is in part the same as that above. The outlines of the liver and stomach are given. In addition, the gall bladder, cystic duct, hepatic ducts and common bile duct passing to the duodenum are amazingly portrayed. The third vessel, passing into the porta hepatis with the hepatic artery and portal vein, is presumably the umbilical vein enlarged owing to the cirrhosis of the liver. This is indicated in the legend: *Ramification which the artery and vein make in the porta of the liver.*

Future illustrations to be made are mentioned in a further memorandum: *Represent first of all the ramifications of the vessels which arrive at the porta liver, all together, and then each by itself in of the 3, or if you prefer, 4 demonstrations. I said 3 because the vein and artery take the same course.*

fig 3. The hepatic veins and the vena cava, of the old man.

On the right the cava is shown opening into the b of the heart. The atrium is a part of the caval system since the heart was regarded as consisting of the ventricles only. In the note above the drawing, Leonardo opposes the Galenical view that the liver is the source of the vessels and argues with Aristotle that the origin is the heart.

The root of all the veins is in the gibbous part of the hearty that is, the covering of the blood. And this is clear because it [i.e., the covering] *is thicker there than elsewhere and goes on to ramify infinitely through every member of the animal.*

Again the anti-Galenical position is indicated by the statement referring to the illustration of the hepatic veins: *How this vein* [the cava] *passes away and does not arise in the liver as many say.* In Mundinus, one of Leonardo's sources, the cava is called the *vena chilis,* meaning "belly-vein". Thus the second legend to the figure reads: *Ramification which the vena chyli* [cava] *makes in the liver.*

It was long held that the excess of black bile from the spleen was excreted into the bowel by way of portal radicles. This idea is expressed in the note below the figure.

Of the two thick vessels [splenic] *which go from the liver to the spleen [and] which come from the larger veins of the spine, I consider to be those which collect the superfluous blood. This, being evacuated every day by the mesaraic* [mesenteric-portal], *is deposited in the bowels causing the same stench when it has reached there as arises from all the dead in the sepulchres, and this is the stench of the faeces.*

At the top of the page is a note by Leonardo on the development of the nervous system in which he expresses the Aristotelian theory on the primacy of the heart.

The entire body has its origin from the heart insofar as the first creation is concerned. Therefore the blood, the veins and the nerves do likewise although these nerves are clearly seen to arise entirely from the medulla (nucha), remote from the heart, and that substance of the medulla is the same as that of the brain from which it is derived.

The term *nucha*, meaning spinal medulla or, more literally, marrow, is of Arabic origin and was apparently introduced into mediaeval Latin by the great translator Constantine the African at Monte Cassino and became the standard term until eventually displaced by the medical humanists in favor of medulla spinalis, first used by Alessandro Benedetti (1460–1525), author of an anatomy (1497) and Leonardo', contemporary.

figs 1.2. The brain, spinal cord and peripheral nerves in lateral and anterior projections (p. 127).

Leonardo describes these figures of the **general** rangement of the nervous system:

Tree of all the nerves; and it is shown how all these have their origin from the medulla and the medull from the brain.

The pair of nerves descending vertically from the brain are the vagi.

fig 3. Small diagram of a projected illustration on the nervous system.

The significance of this small diagram is made clear by the appended note. *In each demonstration* [above] *draw the entire extent of the nerves; the external outlines* [of] *which* [will] *denote the shape of the body.*

The illustrations and notes of this page contain some of the most important observations made by Leonardo on the central nervous system and its ventricles. Here, for the first time in the history of biology clear mention is made of the use of a solidifying injection mass to determine the shape and extent of a body cavity, cf. also Leonardo's remarks on wax injections of the heart, no. The history of anatomical injections has been traced in some detail by F. J. Cole (1921) who curiously omits Leonardo's contribution. Galen in his *De anatomicis administrationibus*, IX:ii, studied the distribution of the cerebral vessels by inflating them with air, and Alessandro Giliani of Persiceto (d.1326) is said, without confirmation, to have used solidifying injections of different colors to fill the blood vessels. However, it was not until the seventeenth century that the method came into general use and reached its apogee with Fredrick Ruysch (1638–1731) whose contributions were deemed, with perverse judgment, by the French Academy of Science to be of such merit as to warrant his being the worthy successor of Isaac Newton.

fig I. Wax injection of the cerebral ventricles: lateral view.

The vent-holes for the injection are observed at the base of the third ventricle. The method of injection and the figure are described thus:

Drawing of the *Sensus Communis*

Cast in wax through the hole n, at the bottom of the base of the cranium before the cranium is sawn through.

The lateral ventricles carry the word *imprensiva,* the perceptual centre. The third ventricle is labelled *sensus communis* or general centre for the special senses, and the fourth ventricle, *memoria.* For the origin of these notions of cerebral localization, cf. 142.

fig 2. Wax injection of the ventricular system as viewed from the base (p. 130).

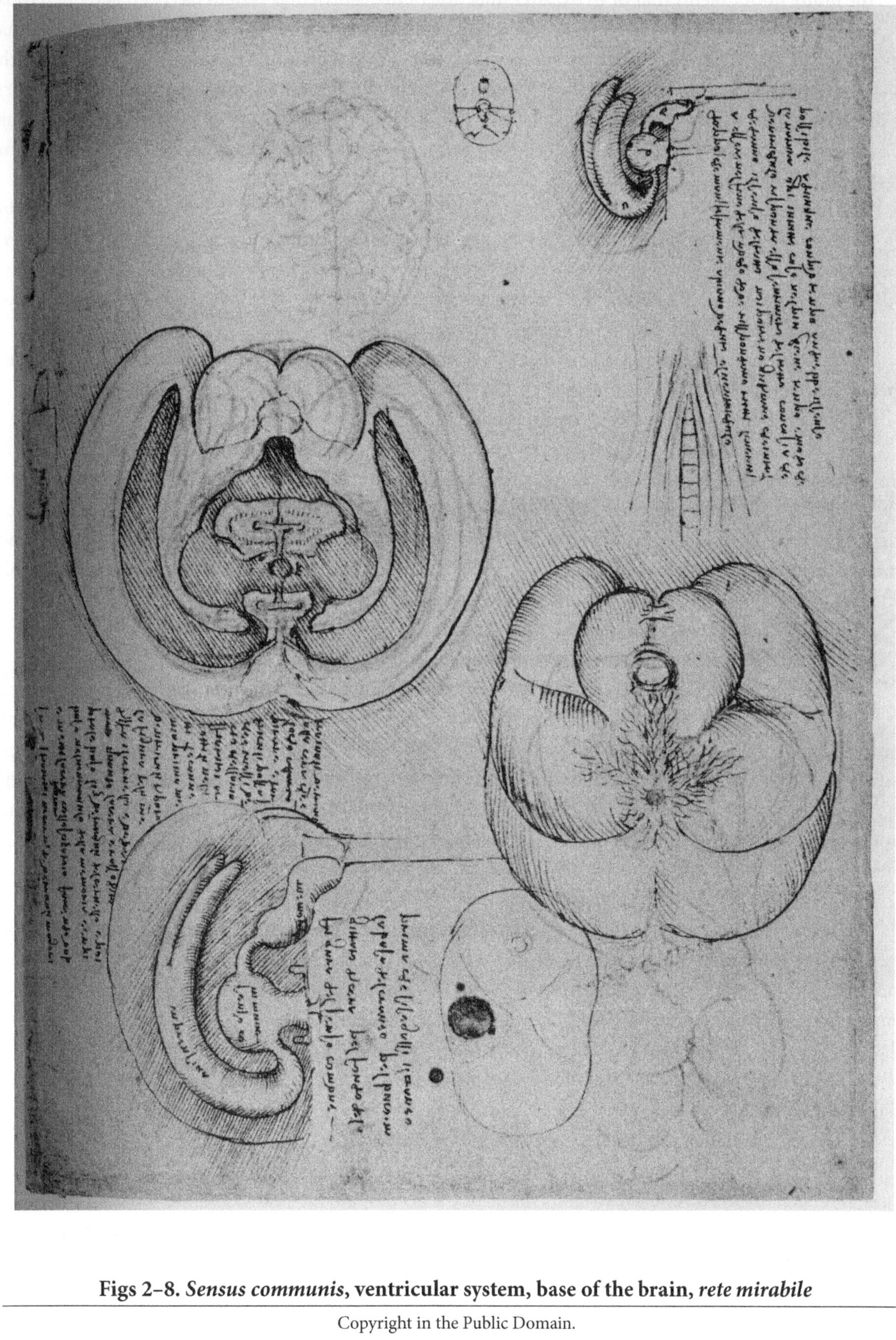

Figs 2–8. *Sensus communis*, ventricular system, base of the brain, *rete mirabile*

The brain, undoubtedly that of an ox, after injection of the ventricular system has been laid open thus exposing the connections of the lateral to the third ventricle by way of the interventricular foramina eponymously named for Alexander Monro primus (1697–1767) who minutely described them although they were well-known by Galen, Vesalius, Varolio and many others before him. The aqueductus cerebri is divided in two as it runs back to connect with the fourth ventricle, and named after Jacobus Sylvius (1478–1555) although it, too, was described long before his time. At m, the region of the infundibulum of the third ventricle, is the site of the injection described as follows:

Make 2 vents in the horns of the great ventricles and inject melted wax with a syringe, making a hole in the ventricle of the memoria [IVth ventricle] *and through such a hole fill the 3 ventricles of the brain. Then, when the wax has set, take away the brain* [substance] *and you will see the shape of the ventricles perfectly. But first put narrow tubes into the vents so that the air which is in these ventricles can escape and make room for the wax which enters into ventricles.*

The distortion of the ventricles as evident in the figures is to be anticipated in ventricular injection the unfixed brain.

fig 3. Dorsal view of the cerebral hemispheres.

This small pencil sketch shows the brain viewed from above. The longitudinal figure, sulci and gyri are indicated by scattered wavy outlines. On the assumption that the figure represents the human brain, McMurrich (1930) states that the sulci of the surface give the general effect but not the actual arrangement. However, closer examination of the drawing reveals that, like the rest of the figures of the page, the brain of the ox is represented, and it is possible to define the coronal, transverse, marginal, entomarginal, ectomarginal, supra-sylvian and lateral sulci or fissures of the brain of that animal.

fig 4. Outline sketch suggestive of the base of the brain.

fig 5. The base of the brain and the rete mirabile.

The rete mirabile, a plexus of vessels at the base of the brain, is found in ruminants and is prominent in calves. It played an important role in the Galenical physiology since it is the apparatus which was supposed to distil the animal spirit or psychic pneuma from the vital spirit contained in the arteries. The animal spirits are distributed throughout the nervous system as the motive force of "sensibility", both motor and sensory, and the nerves were therefore held to be hollow for this purpose. In the figure the frontal, temporal and occipital poles of the cerebrum, as well as the cerebellum, are distinctly shown, but there are no details of structure.

fig 6. Figure of unknown significance.

This curious figure may possibly represent the vermis of the cerebellum. In common with most mediaeval writers, Leonardo elsewhere regards the choroid plexus as the vermis which was supposed to move within the ventricular system acting as a valve to permit or interrupt the flow of thought and sense impressions within the system. This idea was derived through a misunderstanding from Galen and elaborated by the Arabs. However, anatomists of the period were beginning to recognize that the vermis of the cerebellum more closely resembled a segmented worm and thus altered their interpretation of Galen's opinion.

fig 7. Wax injection of the cerebral ventricles, viewed laterally.

The fourth, third and lateral ventricles are lettered a, b, c, respectively. The site of the injection, as in fig. 1, has been the third ventricle from the base. In the accompanying note Leonardo localizes the sense of touch to the fourth ventricle which he holds to be in close communication with the brachial plexus as well as with the spinal medulla, cf. 131, 145,155.

Since we have clearly seen that the ventricle a [IVth ventricle] *is at the end of the medulla where all the nerves which provide the sense of touch come together, we can then conclude that the sense of touch passes*

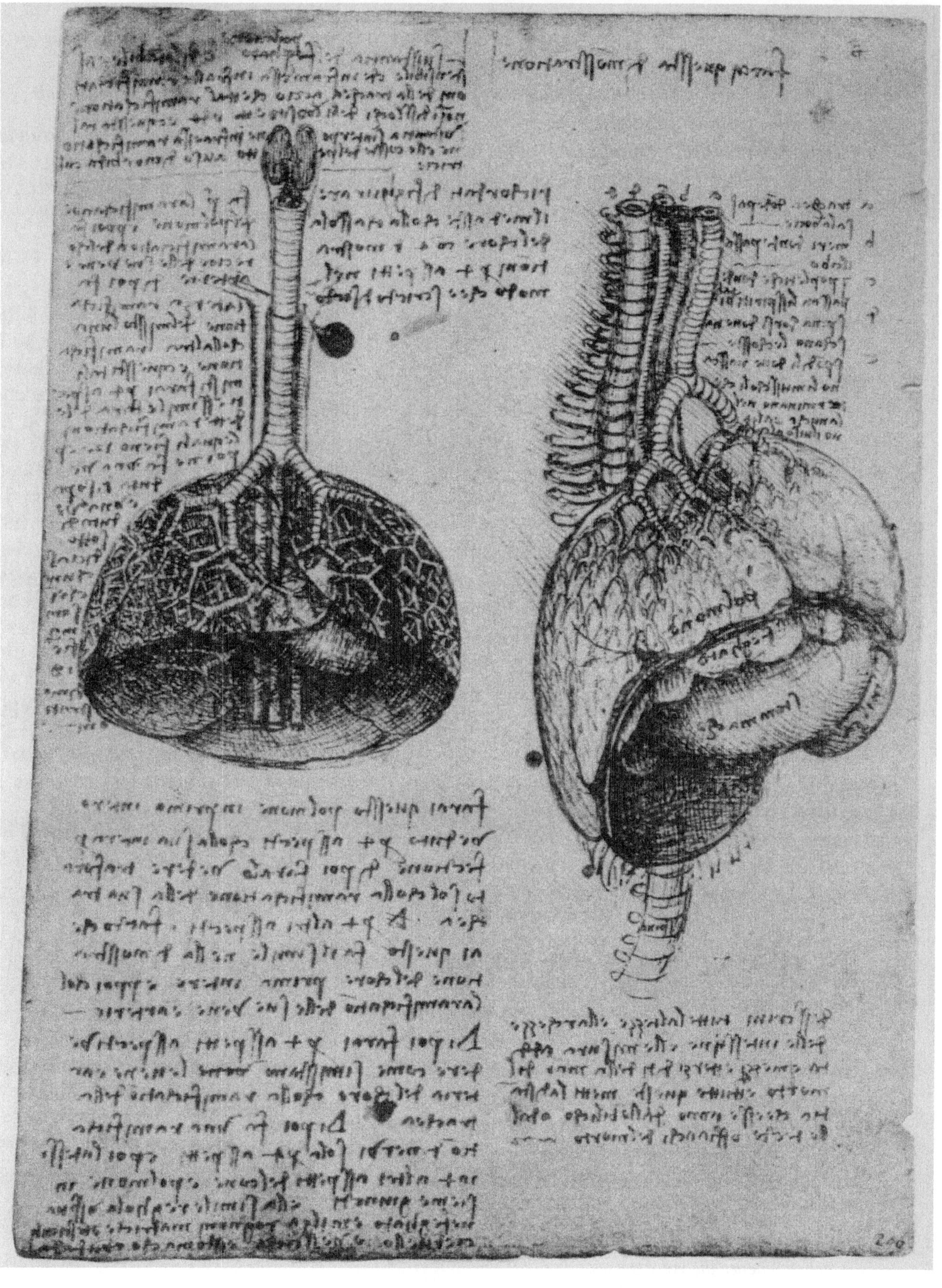

Figs I, 2. Respiratory system

to this ventricle, in view of the fact that in all processes Nature operates in the shortest time and way possible and so would the sense, in the shortest time.

fig 8. Diagram illustrating localization of the sensus communis.

The sketch roughly indicates the position of the third ventricle in the center of the base of the brain. To this ventricle converge a series of lines representing the optic nerves anteriorly, and the acoustic and trigeminal laterally, so establishing this ventricle as the site of the *sensus communis.*

Respiratory system

fig I. The trachea, bronchi and lungs (p. 131).

The primary purpose of the figure is to show the structure of the lung. The position of the heart, the presence of cardiac and intermediate lobes all point to the animal source of the specimen, probably the pig. The three structures observed at the diaphragmatic surface are presumably from left to right, the inferior (posterior) vena cava, the oesophagus and the aorta. On the substance of the parenchyma of the lung, Leonardo writes:

The substance of the lung is dilatable and extensible. It lies between the ramifications of the trachea [i.e., bronchi] *in order that those ramifications may not be displaced from their position, and this substance is interposed between these ramifications and the ribs of the chest to act as a soft covering.*

Since Leonardo assumed that the total cross-sectional area of the terminal bronchi was equal to the cross-sectional area of the trachea (cf. 177), he considered the tidal and complemental air but not the residual air. Thus the parenchyma plays a passive role in respiration as related above. However, elsewhere the residual air is recognized. Proposed methods of illustration follow in the notes:

Remember to represent the mediastinum with the capsule of the heart in 4 demonstrations from 4 aspects in the manner which is described below.

First make the ramification of the lung and then make the ramification of the heart, that is, of its veins and arteries. Afterwards make the third ramification of the combination of one ramification with the other. You will make these combinations from 4 aspects and you will do the same for the said ramification [as in the figure], *so that there will be 12. Then make a view of each from above and one from below that there will be in all 18 demonstrations.*

You will first draw this lung intact, seen in 4 aspects, in its entire perfection. Then you will represent it as seen permeated by the ramification of its trachea only from 4 aspects. Having done this, do the same in the demonstration of the heart: first intact, and then with the ramifications of its veins and arteries.

Afterwards you will do it from 4 aspects to show how the veins and arteries of the heart intermingle with the ramification of the trachea. Then make a ramification of the nerves alone from 4 aspects, and then interweave them in 4 other views of the heart and lung combined together. Observe the same rule with the liver, spleen kidneys, womb, testicles [ie., gonads], *brain, bladder and stomach.*

fig 2. The lungs, diaphragm and subdiaphragmatic viscera in relationship to the spinal column.

The following structures are named: lung, liver, stomach, spleen, diaphragm, spine, from above downwards. Animal features are again in evidence as in the lobulation of the lung and liver. Above the figure is written You *will make this demonstration.* The key to the lettered structures is given as follows:

a. trachea whence the voice passes.

b. oesophagus whence the food passes.

c. *apoplectic arteries* [carotid] *whence the vital spirits pass.*

d. dorsal spine whence the ribs arise.

e. spondyles [vertebrae] *whence the muscles arise which end in the nape of the neck (nucha) and elevate the face towards the sky.*

The *arteriae apoplecticae,* or as Leonardo calls them *ipopletiche,* is the old term for the carotid arteries as employed by Mundinus and so named as the cause of apoplexy. The carotid arteries, of Greek origin, meaning sleep-inducing, were sometimes translated as *arteriae somni,* or *arteriae soporales.*

Always interested in the relative proportions of the human body, Leonardo proposes to give the sizes of the viscera in terms of the length of a finger.

Describe all the heights and widths of the entrails and measure them by fingers, and by halves and thirds of a finger of the dead mans hand. In all these, put down the distance which they have from the umbilicus, or the nipples of the flanks of the deceased.

The figures on this page will be enumerated from right to left in the intended sequence. In general the illustrations are typical of the period when Leonardo was attempting to fit the findings of animal dissection both to traditional theory and to the body of man.

fig I. The great vessels of the heart and lung (p. 134).

The purpose of the figure is to illustrate the supposed pathways for the passage of air to the heart. In Galenical physiology the basic principle of life, the pneuma, is drawn into the lungs with air. It then passes by way of the vein-like artery, arteria venalis, or our pulmonary vein to the left ventricle where, together with the blood which sweats through the interventricular septum, it forms the vital spirits for distribution by way of the arterial system. From the heart, impurities or so-called "sooty vapors" are carried back to the lung by way of the artery-like vein, vena arterialis, or our pulmonary artery, to be exhaled to the outer air. In order to fit the theory to anatomical structure, Leonardo shows the heart, considered to be a two-chambered organ, providing a pulmonary artery above and a pulmonary vein below on either side to the hilus of the lung. On the left side these vessels are lettered m and n, respectively. Not only is his anatomy in error, but his knowledge of Galenical theory is at fault since Galen and his mediaeval followers have the pulmonary artery correctly passing from the right ventricle and the pulmonary vein to the left ventricle. Above the heart we observe a common brachiocephalic trunk arising from the arch of the aorta, which reminds us how great was Leonardo's dependence upon animal anatomy for his knowledge of the distribution of the vessels. The vena cava, hepatic vein, and other structures are easily identified. However, two vessels are shown passing from the spleen. One of these is undoubtedly the splenic vein regarded as the portal vein, and the other represents perhaps the splenic and hepatic arteries in continuity. At any rate, these vessels are shown very diagrammatically.

Below the figure is a note, much of which is lost, but in which the physiological theory discussed above is presented, although later Leonardo discards the notion that air can pass directly to the lung. Above the figure is a brief remark, *Dust causes damage,* doubtless with reference to the lung.

The air sent back from the lung to the heart cannot enter the heart if it has no opening. Therefore it is necessary that there be two passages. When the lung sends forth the air through the trachea, at the same time it must also send air through one of these passages into the cavity of the heart, and through a second passage the air must escape from the heart and return, together with the other air which leaves through the aforesaid trachea, the passage of the lung. Necessity causes the air to be distributed through the spongy entrails of the lung [and], *on being pressed out, every vesicle to be closed in that region. … When joined together [presumably the passages to the heart], they are much narrower than the trachea [and], thus it happens that when one and the same quantity of air is forced at the same time through a narrower passage than it enters, it moves more speedily the narrower the passage, and, consequently, the more … the speedier it is.*

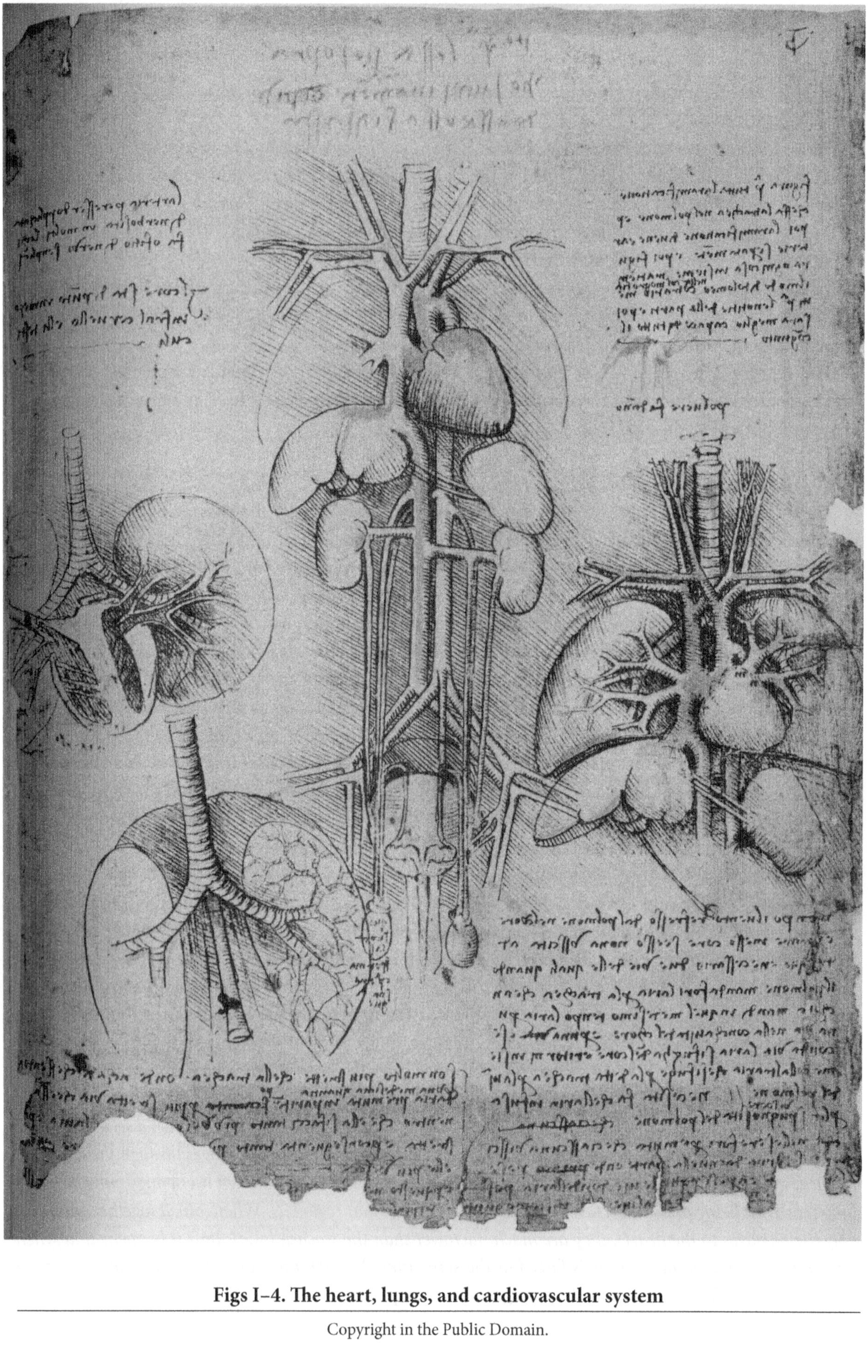

Figs I–4. The heart, lungs, and cardiovascular system

fig 2. General schema of the cardiovascular system seen from behind.

The arrangement of the vessels in the upper part f the figure is essentially the same as that of fig. 1, except that the structures are viewed from behind'Be low, the inferior vena cava, descending aorta and their branches are shown. It will be noted that the right kidney lies at a higher level than the left, as in animals The bladder, seminal vesicle, ductus deferens, epididymis, testis, ejaculatory duct and urethra are all evident, but the prostate, relatively inconspicuous in animals, is lacking. Written on the testis is the remark *Here the sperm is concocted and it was first blood* which again reflects Leonardo's acceptance of Galenical theory and change from his earlier quasi-Aristotelian opinions. Arteries were distinguished by their possession of two tunics, and veins only one. The second coat is regarded as supplying a suspensory apparatus for the cardiovascular system.

Owing to its being double [coated], the artery by its sinewyness (nervosita) performs in many places the office of simple sinews.

It is observed further that, *The heart is exactly in the middle between the brain and the testicles.*

fig 3. The heart and the pulmonary vessels.

The figure is complementary to fig. 1. The right and left ventricular cavities are shown separated by the interventricular septum containing the mythical pores through which the blood sweats in the creation of the vital spirits. From each cavity a pulmonary artery and a pulmonary vein pass to and from the lung as required by Leonardo's incorrect interpretation of Galenical theory. In the right ventricular cavity three moderator bands, Leonardo's unique discovery, are illustrated.

fig 4. The trachea and ramifications of the bronchi.

Above and to the right Leonardo reminds himself to draw a figure such as this.

First draw the entire ramification which the trachea makes in the lung and then the ramification of the veins and arteries separately. Next draw everything together, but follow the method of Ptolemy in his geography in reverse. Then you will better understand the whole put together.

In his proposed "order of the book" on anatomy Leonardo states that it is his intention to adopt the plan used in Ptolemy's cosmography, from which Leonardo quotes almost verbatim. The Ptolemy Cosmography was first printed in 1462 and thereafter there were numerous editions, the later ones containing the maps to which Leonardo refers.

At the top of the page is a note, probably written at a much earlier date, on a plan of illustration, *First place the bones, next put upon them successively* [the structures] *further removed from the bones.*

In this, among the latest of Leonardo's anatomical studies, we find far less reliance upon written traditional authority and greater dependence upon direct observation. This is expressed in a marginal note on the superiority of the illustration, and especially composite illustration, over the written word in biological investigation.

With what words, O Writer, will you describe with like perfection the entire configuration which the drawing here does? Lacking knowledge, this you describe confusedly and leave little conception of the true shape of things which you, in self-deception, make believe that you can fully satisfy your auditors when you must speak of the configuration of some bodily structure bounded by surfaces. But I counsel you not to encumber yourself with words unless you are speaking to the blind. If, however, you wish to demonstrate in words to the ears and not to the eyes of men, speak of substantial or natural things and do not meddle with things appertaining to the eyes by making them enter through the ears, for you will be far surpassed by the work of the painter.

With what words will you describe this heart so as not to fill a book? The longer you write on the details, the more you will confuse the mind of the auditor. You will always be in need of commentators or

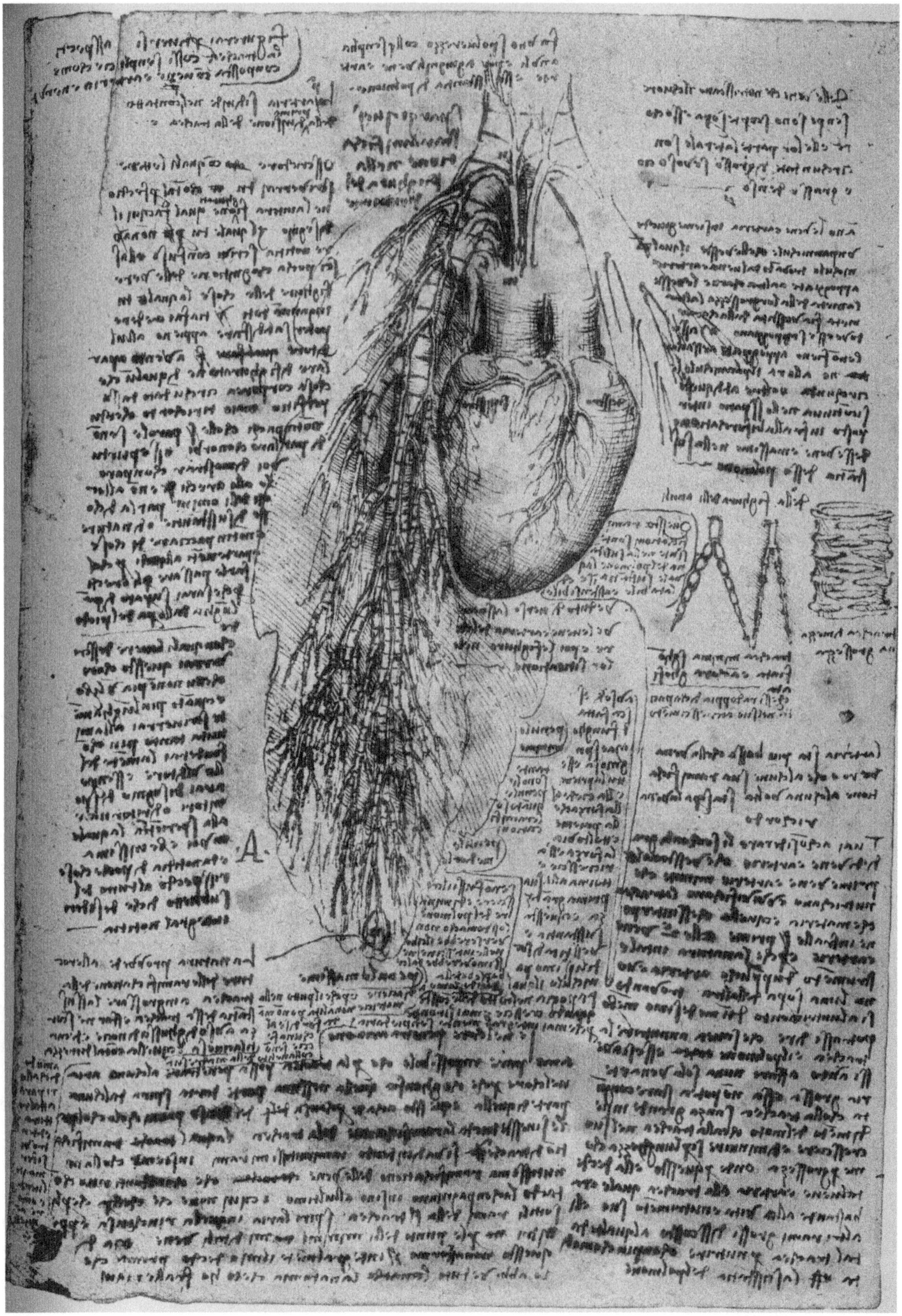

Fig I. The heart, trachea, and bronchial tree. Posterior view.

be required to return to experience, which in your case is very brief, and gives knowledge of but few things concerning the whole subject of which you desire an entire knowledge.

fig I. The heart, trachea and bronchial tree: posterior aspect (p. 136).

The notes pertaining to the figure are scattered irregularly and are here rearranged in some degree of logical sequence. The figure is based upon the findings in the ox. The posterior aspect of the heart is shown as noted by the words, *Seen from behind*, and *right* and *left* placed upon the respective ventricles. The great and lesser cardiac veins and the inferior interventricular and circumflex branches of the right coronary artery are shown ramifying on its surface. Leonardo makes a number of notes on the coronary vessels.

ON THE VESSELS WHICH NOURISH THE HEART.

They always lie naked upon the heart and their lateral portions are surrounded by suet-like fat, that is, dense fat.

Here he follows the traditional classifications of fat into hard and soft. He reminds himself that, *There is the vein and the artery of the hearty and then draw them in position.*

The atria are not shown. Arising from the base of the heart are presumably the pulmonary artery on the left and the superior (anterior) vena cava on the right. Bronchfel arteries, n m, spring from the pulmonary to pass to the bifurcation of the trachea, and branches follow the ramifications of the bronchi. To distinguish the bronchial arteries from branches of the pulmonary vessels, they are called vessels of the first order. *The first* [i.e., bronchial] *artery divides at its point of contact with the first division of the trachea. ...*

A dual blood supply to the lung by way of the bronchial as well as pulmonary vessels was a source of puzzlement. Leonardo correctly concludes that the bronchial vessels supply the parenchyma. On reading his note it should be remembered that the term trachea is applied to the entire bronchial tree.

A REMINDER.

You have to consider the second order [i.e., pulmonary] *of veins and arteries which cover the first* [i.e., bronchial] *veins and arteries which nourish and vivify the trachea, what material is it that interposes itself between the first and second* [order of] *veins and arteries, and why in such an instrument did Nature duplicate artery and vein, one upon the other, finding themselves for the nourishment of one and the same member. You could say that the trachea and the lung had to be nourished and if you had to do this with a single large vein-like artery (venarteria* [=pulmonary vein]*), this* [vessel] *could not remain attached to the trachea without great hindrance to the motion which occurs with the expansion and contraction of the trachea in length as well as in width. Consequently, for this reason she* [i.e., Nature] *gave such* [bronchial] *veins and arteries to the trachea as were needed for its life and nourishment, and separated a little from the trachea the other large* [pulmonary] *branches to nourish the substance of the lung with greater convenience.*

Further details on the arrangement of the pulmonary vessels within the substance of the lung are described.

The [pulmonary] *veins and arteries, which are united, have a membrane which clothes them. If this membrane finds such a vein and artery applied to some other fleshy it clothes half their width and the other half will be clothed by the flesh to which they are applied. But if they are not applied to this flesh, then the membrane surrounds them or in addition to this is continued into the space interposed between the bifurcation of these vessels, and especially in the substance of the lung.*

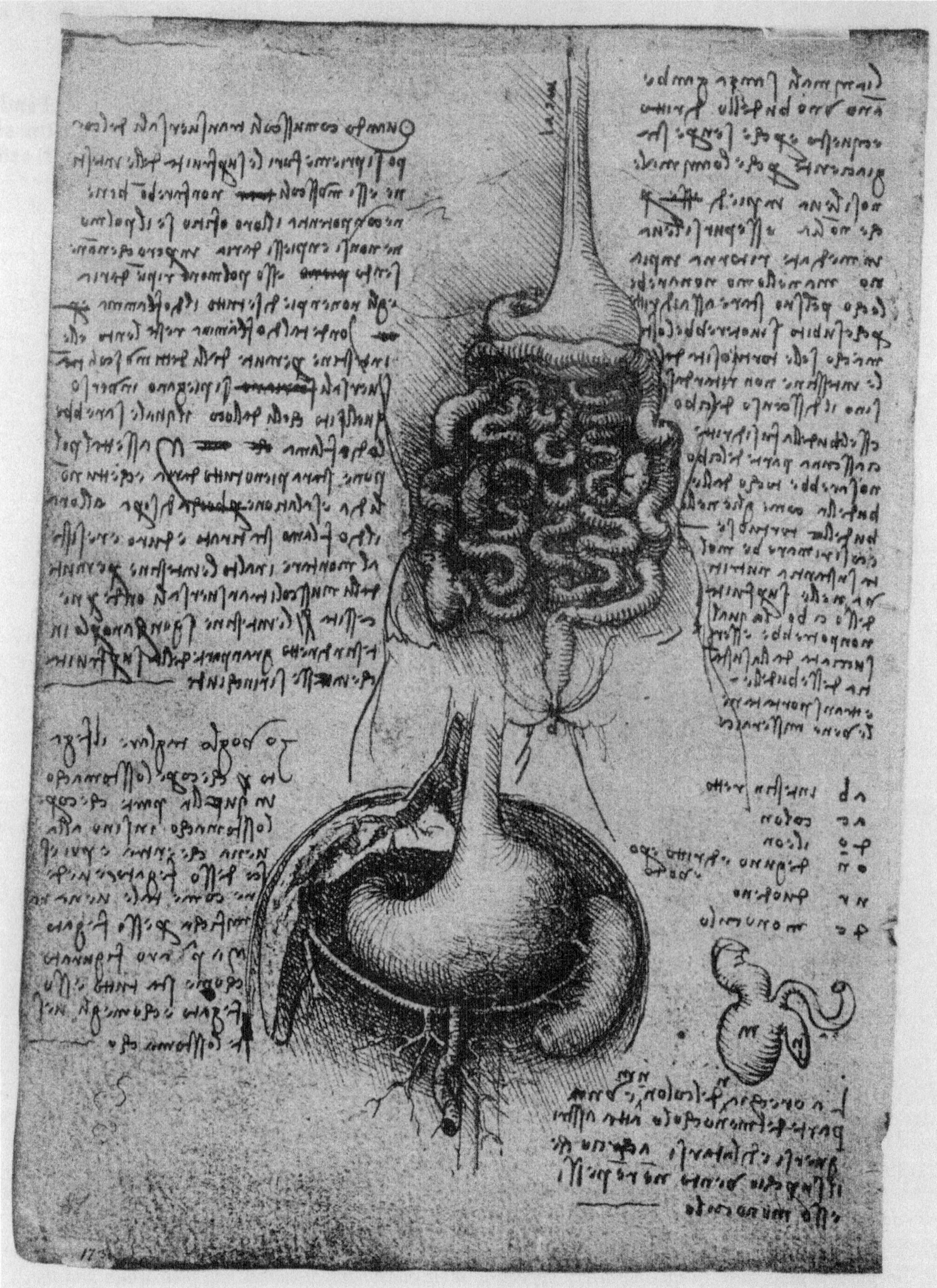

Figs I–3. Alimentary system

The [pulmonary] *artery lies somewhat below the veiny although some of its ramifications sometimes lie above the vein.*

By the above statement Leonardo means that the artery is more closely related to its bronchus. We learn elsewhere that this arrangement is needed since the artery conveying heat requires to be cooled by the incoming air more than the vein.

The bronchial tree and parenchyma of the lung are described:

These [bronchial] *ramifications are interwoven with the substance of the lung. This substance is in itself dilatable and extensible like the tinder made from a fungus. But it is spongy and if you press it, it yields to the force which compresses it, and if the force is removed, it increases again to its original size. This substance is clothed by a very thin membrane* [pleura] *which is opposed to the rib space. When it* [i.e., lung] *enlarges, it never ruptures because it is never entirely filled with air.*

Along the right margin of the king the pennate appearance of the first, second and third orders of branchings of the bronchus are noted from above downwards in picturesque terms as *The smallest feathers; The middle-sized feathers; The largest feathers; and the statement that There are as many feathers as there are ramifications.*

At the lower pole of the lung is an encircled area labelled N, representing some pathological process, possibly a tubercle which is described in these terms:

Nature prevents rupture of the ramifications of the trachea by thickening the substance of the trachea and making a crusty like the shell of a nut. It is cartilaginous, and this with its hardness, like a callus, repairs the rupture and in the interior, powder and an aqueous humor remain.

ALIMENTARY SYSTEM

The drawings on this page are part of the series continued on 192, and appear by style and content to be based on the dissection of the centenarian, cf. 156.

fig I. The alimentary tract (p. 139).

The oesophagus (meri) is so indicated. Other organs identified are: a by the straight intestine [rectum]; *a c, colon; d o, ileum; o n, on right, jejunum* [so-called] *because it is empty; n r, duodenum; d c, caecum (monoculus).*

The jejunum, as Leonardo remarks, was so called because it is often found empty. The monoculus or one-eyed gut was the old term for caecum but sometimes means appendix. Leonardo compares the alimentary tract of reptiles with that of man and concludes that the human intestines, because of the upright position of man, are highly coiled to delay the descent of their contents.

Animals without legs have a straight bowel, and this is because they always remain horizontal and because an animal which has no feet cannot raise itself upright and, even if it did, it immediately returns to the horizontal. But in man this would not be the case since he stands quite vertically, for the stomach would immediately empty itself if the tortuosities of the intestines did not retard the descent of the food. And if the bowel were straight, each part of the food would not come in contact with the bowel as occurs in a tortuous bowel. And much of the nutritive substance would remain in the superfluities, which would not be sucked up by the substance of the bowels and transported in the portal (miseraice) veins.

fig 2. The subdiaphragmatic organs: liver, stomach and spleen.

The hepatic and portal or miseriaic veins are especially well shown because of their importance to then current theory. Galen held that the chyle or intestinal juice was sucked up by the portal vein to be transported to the liver where it was transformed into blood to renew the continual metabolic loss. The figure is to be supplemented by others.

I wish to cut the liver which covers the stomach in that part which covers the stomach as far as the [portal] *vein which enters and then emerges from the liver* [as the hepatic vein] *and to see how this vein ramifies in the liver. But first I will illustrate how the intact liver lies and how it clothes the stomach.*

These ideas are carried out in part in 130. Peristalsis and evacuation are due, according to Leonardo, to the compressive action of the diaphragm and anterior abdominal wall on the stomach and intestines in the movements of respiration, cf. 178, 187. This theory is referred to in the accompanying note.

As the superfluities are forced out of the intestines by means of the transverse muscles of the body, these muscles would not fulfill their office well or with power if the lung were not filled with air. Since, if the lung were not filled with air it would not occupy in its entirety the diaphragm. Hence the diaphragm would remain relaxed and the intestines, compressed by the said transverse muscles, would bend outwards the region which gives way to them. This would be the diaphragm. But if the lung remains entirely full of air which you do not allow to escape above by expiration, then the diaphragm remains taut and hard, and resists the upward ascent of the intestines compressed by the transverse muscles. Thus of necessity the intestines rid themselves of a great part of the superfluities which are contained within them by way of the rectum.

fig 3. The caecum and vermiform appendix.

The auricle [appendix] *n, of the colon n m, is a part of the monoculus* [caecum] *and is capable of contracting and dilating so that excessive wind does not rupture the monoculus.*

Owing to the assumption that the anatomy of certain animals, especially the pig, was identical to that of man, there was great confusion among mediaeval anatomists as to the distinction between the appendix and the caecum. The above illustration is one of the earliest representations of the human appendix known. The earliest published figure of this organ appears in the *Anatomica mundini*, Marburg, 1541, of Johann Dryander.

GENERAL ANATOMY AND GENITO-URINARY SYSTEM

This, the most famous of the Leonardine anatomical illustrations, belongs to the period when Leonardo was coming more decidedly under the influence of Galenical teachings (p.141). It will be noted that the outlines of the figure have been pricked for transfer, giving rise to the incomplete copy on 203.

The illustration is a unique attempt to represent in graphic form both anatomical detail and certain of the principles of the Galenical physiological system. In this respect it fore-shadows the method adopted by Vesalius in the first three of his *Tabulae anatomicae* of 1538. The representational aspects are, however, to receive fuller treatment as evidenced by the note at the top of the page.

Also make this demonstration as seen from the side so that knowledge may be given how far one part lies behind the other. Then make one from behind that knowledge may be given of the veins possessed by the spine and by the heart, and of the greater vessels.

These figures illustrating the general physiology and anatomy of the female were perhaps to constitute an introduction to the embryological section of his proposed work. This is suggested by an accompanying note which points to figures of somewhat later date such as 210, 213–14, of the foetus in utero.

Your series shall be with the beginning of the formation of the child in the womb, stating which part of it is formed first, and so successively putting in its parts according to the periods of pregnancy until birth and how it is nourished, learning partly from the eggs laid by hens.

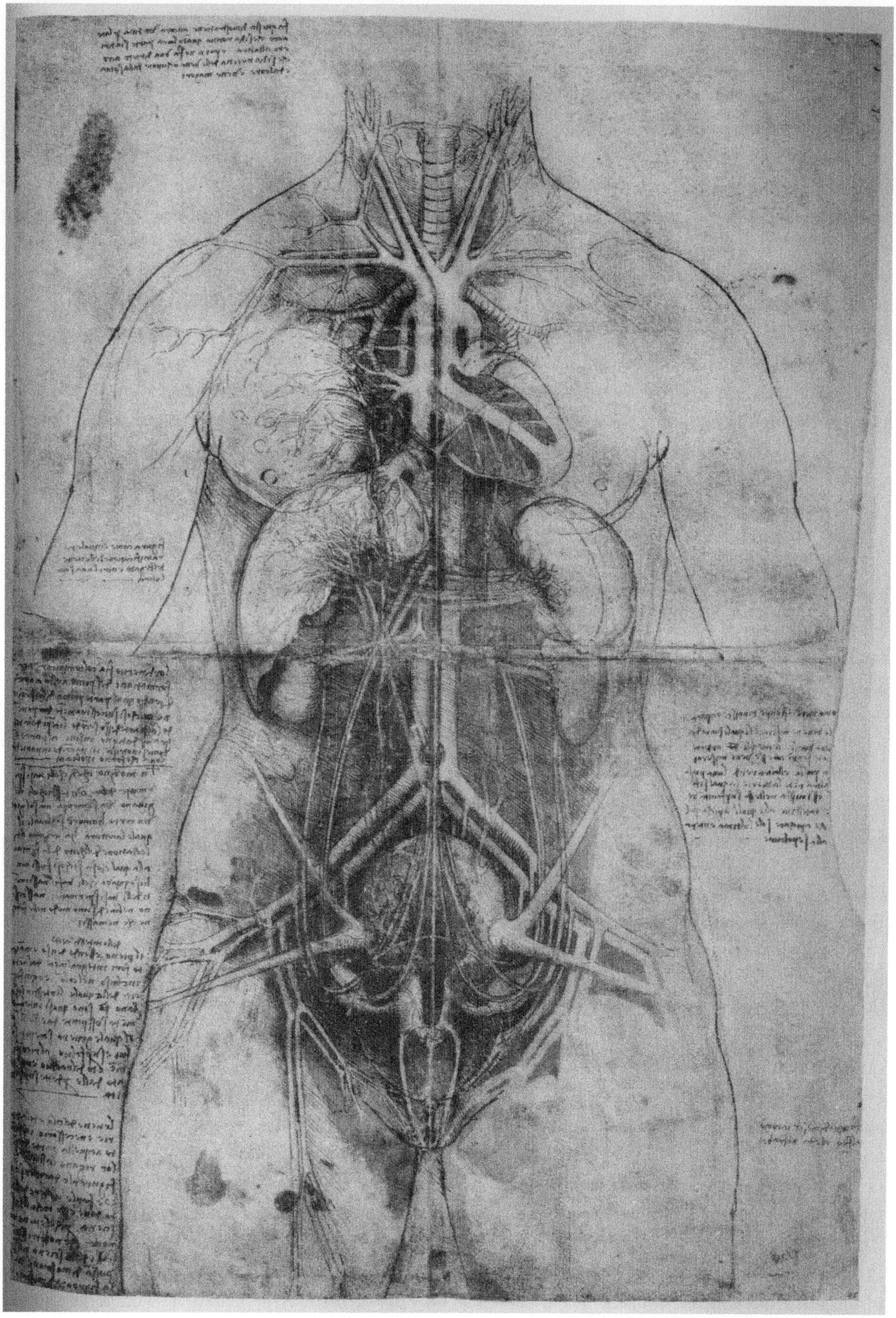

Graphic details of Leonardo's *General Anatomy*

Several features of the illustration should not be overlooked. In the first place it should be recognized that the anatomical details are drawn for the most part from dissections made on animals. This will become apparent as the figure is discussed from above downwards in association with Leonardo's marginal memoranda. The trachea and bronchi remind us that Leonardo is thinking of the pneuma or world-spirit drawn in with the inspired air to be carried to the left ventricle for the formation of the vital spirit. The heart is characteristically represented as a two-chambered and solely ventricular organ, containing, as in the ox, moderator bands in both ventricles, and the interventricular septum shown prominently since through its supposed pores blood sweats to the left side for the completion of the vital spirits. The atria exist as auricular appendages only to participate in a complicated way in the formation of the natural heat as described.

The vena cava opens directly into the right ventricle and is associated with the ebb and flow movement of the blood containing the nutritive natural spirits. It receives the azygos vein thought to nourish the thoracic walls, but the arrangement of this and other branches reflect animal anatomy. The blood is drawn by the hepatic veins from the liver, the blood-making organ, which has received the chyle by way of the portal system for elaboration into blood and natural spirits. The relations of these systems is to be elucidated in further detail. *Represent how and what ramification of the vessels of the liver enters one beneath the other* [i.e., relations of hepatic artery to portal vein].

The gall bladder and the spleen are shown since they form the yellow and black bile respectively, as well as remove the so-called excrements or waste products of metabolism. The yellow bile is filtered out by the kidneys, thus coloring the urine. The kidneys occupy the relative positions found in animals. Their ureters pass to the bladder which is indicated as a circle lying anterior to the uterus. The black bile or melancholia is discharged in part through a hypothetical vein to the stomach to whet the appetite, but the most part is eliminated by way of haemorrhoidal veins into the rectum upon which Leonardo remarks: *The fullness of the rectum, being dense, is expelled entirely by the wind contained in the colon. All the faeces of which the intestines empty themselves, are almost entirely driven out by this wind. This causes a noise when it is in excess following the filling up of the vacuum left by the aforementioned superfluities.*

Like the vena cava, the branchings of the aorta are of the ungulate type. Not only does a typical brachiocephalic trunk spring from the aortic arch, but the pattern of arrangement of the external iliac vessels is also derived probably from the ox. The major vessels are to be represented from behind. *The vena chilis* [cava] *and arteries: it is necessary with respect to that part where they follow the spine to represent them from the reverse, that* is, *make them visible from the side where they touch the spine because the smaller veins which nourish the bones of the spine cannot be shown in the figure demonstrated.*

The representation of the uterus is a curious admixture of traditional notions and accurate observation. It is a globular or pisiform structure of exaggerated size possibly to indicate the organ in pregnancy. From the fundus extend on either side two structures which may be interpreted as the uterine tubes and round ligaments but certainly not recognized as such. It is more than probable that these structures derive from some confused prototype and are the so-called cornua of earlier authorities. The ovarian or spermatic arteries and veins may be traced to the ovaries or "testicles". These vessels carry blood and vital spirit to the organ which is converted into semen. The semen leaves the ovary by way of a short passage also called the "spermatic or seminal vessel" to enter the uterus in the region of the cervix. Elsewhere (201) Leonardo shows this passage entering at a higher level in approximately the position of the suspensory ligament of the ovary. Leonardo now discards the Aristotelian view on generation as reflected by Mundinus that the seed is from the male alone, the female acting only as the soil, and adopts the teaching of the Arabic writers that both sexes contribute m equal part. *It is you, Mundinus, who states that the "spermatic vessels" or testicles* [ovaries] *do not secrete real semen but only a certain saliva-like humor which Nature has ordained for the delectation women in coition, in which case, if it were so, it would not be necessary that origin of the spermatic vessels derive in the same way in the female as in the male.*

On the right side, a vein in part corresponding to the superior epigastric extends from the uterus to the breast. In the Galenical physiology this vessel carries the retained menses to be converted into milk. It is variously shown as a branch of a uterine, hypogastric or umbilical vessel.

A further note beginning with the statement, *Man dies and always regenerates in part,* has been so destroyed that the few remaining words make little sense. The body of the note seems to be concerned with the function of the meseriaic or portal vein. These few words, which do not merit translation, suggest that Leonardo was thinking in part of the cause of death of the centenarian (cf. 128) which he ascribed to hepatic insufficiency.

A final note reminds him of *The females of Messer lacomo Alfredo and "Lleda ne' Fabri".*

Embryology

fig I. The foetus in utero.

This large drawing of the foetus in utero is the first of the series as indicated by the asterisk. Two features of the illustration require comment. First, Leonardo had no knowledge of the coverings of the human foetus and therefore illustrates their attachment by a stylized cotyledonous placenta of ungulates shown in detail in figs. 2–5, and more realistically in 211. Second, the ovary is connected to the uterus by a so-called spermatic duct implanted immediately above the cervix but in other drawings corresponding to the suspensory ligament of the ovary, cf. 201 and 202. The accompanying note is unusual in its denial of the presence of the foetal heart beat, but subscribes to a common mediaeval notion on the transmission of the soul to transform the animal body into man.

The heart of this child does not beat nor does it breathe because it continually lies in water. If it breathed it would drown and breathing is not necessary because vivified and nourished by the life and food of the mother. This food nourishes this creature not otherwise than it does with other members of the mother, that is, the hands, feet and other members. One and the same soul governs these two bodies, and the desires, fears and pains are common to this creature as are all other animal [nervous] *members.. From this it occurs that the thing desired by the mother is often found impressed upon those members of the infant which the mother herself holds at the time of the desire, and a sudden fright kills both mother and child. Therefore, one concludes that one and the same soul governs the bodies and one and the same nourishes both.*

On the connection between the maternal and foetal circulation, a question which was to take some centuries to answer, Leonardo is at this stage uncertain.

See how the great vessels of the mother pass into the uterus, then to the secundines and then to the umbilical cord.

figs 2–5. Details of the ungulate placenta.

As previously mentioned, Leonardo knew little or nothing of the discoidal placenta of man, cf. 173. Here he illustrates the details of a cotyledonary arrangement as in the ungulates. The first of the smaller illustrations is quaintly called, *The mother of the cotyledons, that is, female cotyledons.* The second and fourth figures of the group show, *The male cotyledons,* and in the larger or third figure we are shown, *How the three membranes of the uterus tie themselves together by means of the cotyledons.*

Leonardo was greatly interested in what happened to the cotyledons at parturitions and raises the question whether the maternal or foetal cotyledon remains attached to the uterus. *The cotyledons have male and female* [parts]. *You will now note whether the male or female remains attached to the uterus of*

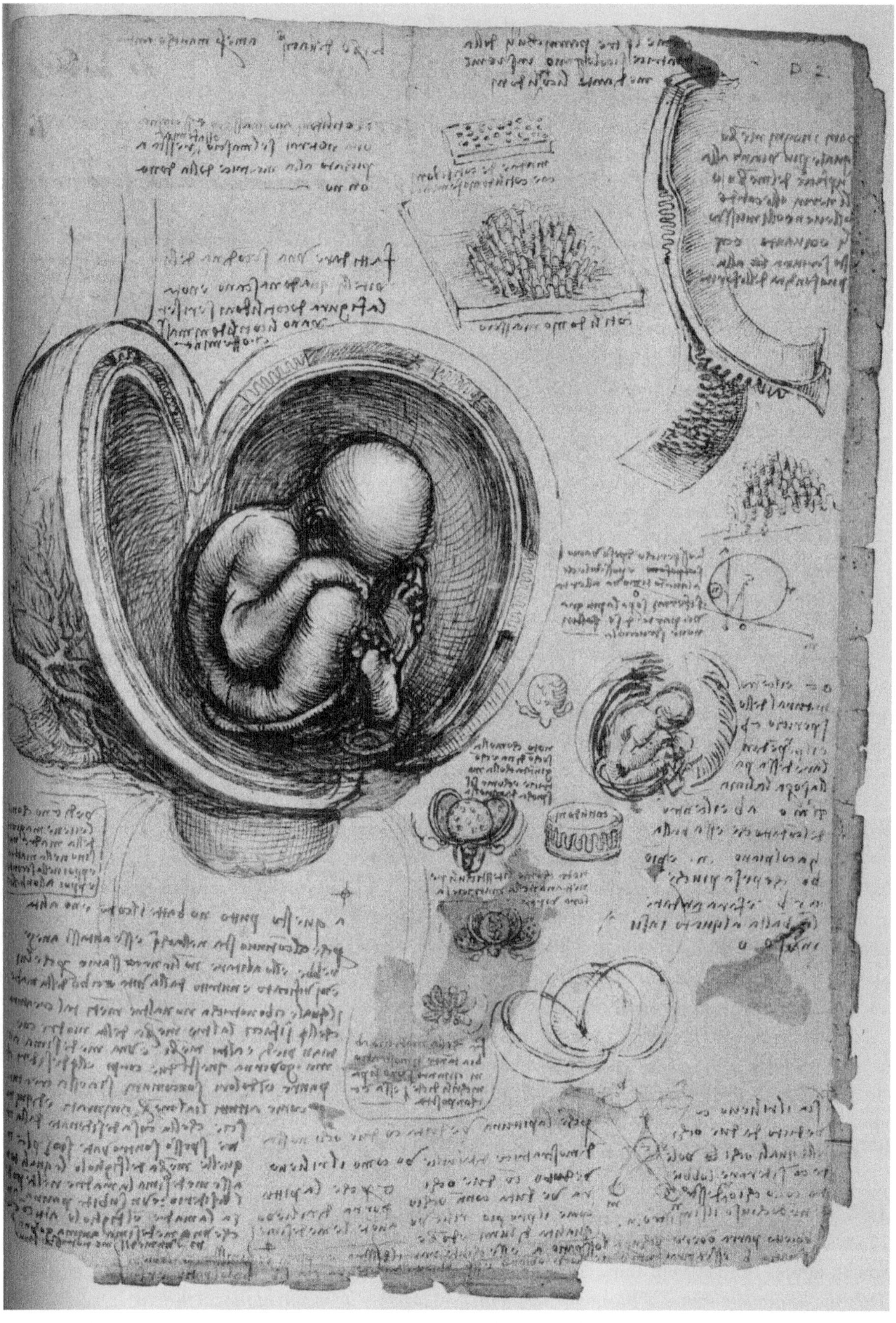

Figs I–14. Embriology, placenta, foetus, and others

the woman or not. An answer is sought from the conceptus of a calf, *Obtain the secundine of calves when they are born and note the shape of the cotyledons and if they keep the male or female cotyledons.* The question is finally resolved on 211.

fig 6. An unrelated diagram and note on the behavior of an eccentrically weighted sphere.

fig 7. Minute sketch of uterus, ovaries, and indications of cotyledons.

fig 8. Preliminary sketch of foetus in utero to show successive coverings.

fig 9. Uterus laid open to expose the conceptus.

The so-called "male and female" cotyledons are shown. On either side are the ovaries and the presumed "spermatic duct" extending to the interior of the uterus, cf. 202. *Note how the testicles* [ovaries] *pass their faculty into the uterus.* In answer to the question raised under figs. 2–5, Leonardo states, *I note how the secundines are united to the uterus and how they separate from it* [on parturition].

fig 10. Diagram of the interdigitating cotyledons.

On the figure is written the word, *cotyledons.*

figs 11–13. Diagrams of the uterus and foetal membranes laid open.

These preliminary sketches are to show the membranes by laying each open successively. In the first, fig. 11, the uterine wall and chorion have been split to expose the amnion with the foetus shining through. Leonardo's intention is expressed thus: *Make it so that the uterus has as many demonstrations as there are membranes of which it is composed.*

fig 14. Diagram on binocular vision.

Why a picture seen with one eye will not demonstrate such relief as the relief [customarily] *seen with both eyes. This is because the picture seen with one eye will have the degree of relief, as a relief proper having the same amount of light and shade. Let the relief c, be seen with both eyes* [m and n]. *If you were to observe the object with the right eye m, keeping the left eye n, closed, the object would appear to the eye in, or would occupy, the space a. If you were to close the right eye and open the left, the object would occupy the space b. And if you were to open completely both eyes, the object would no longer occupy a and b, but the space e r.*

Other memoranda: *Place in every member what is closer to the surface of the member, either the nerves, the cords, the vessels or the muscles and how far. This book will serve for* [the appreciation of] *the depth of wounds.*

The book "On water" to Messer Marco Antonio.

For Leonardo's book on water, cf. 113. This mayor may not be a reference to Marcantonio della Torre, the anatomist whom Leonardo presumably met at Pavia. However, the name Marcantonio was a very common one.

Chapter 8

Andreas Vesalius: *De Humani Corporis Fabrica* (1543)

HISTORICAL HIGHLIGHTS

- Andreas Vesalius (1514–1564)
- Born in Brussels, Belgium
- Attended University of Louvain, 1530
- Continued medical studies at Paris under Guinter, Sylvius and Ferne
- Earned Bachelor of Medicine degree (1537) at Louvain
- Received Doctor of Medicine *magna cum laude* degree at Padua (1537)
- Produced one book of incredible importance, *De Humani Corporis Fabrica* (1543)
- The *Fabrica* showed in precise manner the new anatomy of the human body
- Distanced himself from Galen's anatomy
- Illustrations were unique and giving a great deal of information. Jan Calcar offered his drawing ability to the project

THE WRITINGS OF ANDREAS VESALIUS

PREFACE TO THE ANATOMY OF THE HUMAN BODY

Addressed to The Most Great and Invincible Emperor The Divine Charles V[1]

Those engaged in the arts and sciences, Most Gracious Emperor Charles, find many serious obstacles to the exact study and successful application of them. In the first place, no slight inconvenience results from too great separation between branches of study which serve for the perfection of one art. But much worse is the mischievous distribution among different practitioners of the practical applications of the art. This has been carried so far that those who have set before themselves the

1 Charles V (1500–1558), ruler over Austria, the German Empire, the Low Countries, Spain, and the Spanish domains beyond the seas, was perhaps the most conscientious and serious, as well as the most powerful, monarch of his day.

attainment of an art embrace one part of it to the neglect of the rest, although they are intimately bound up with it and can by no means be separated from it. Such never achieve any notable result; they never attain their goal or succeed in basing their art upon a proper foundation.

I shall pass over all the other arts in silence and confine myself to a few remarks on that which presides over the health of mankind. This, of all the arts which the mind of man has discovered, is by far the most beneficial, necessary, abstruse, and laborious. But in bygone times, that is to say after the Gothic deluge[2] and after the reign of Mansor at Bochara in Persia,[3] under whom, as we know, the Arabs still lived as was right on terms of familiarity with the Greeks, medicine began to be sore distempered. Its primary instrument, the employment of the hand in healing, was so neglected that it was relegated to vulgar fellows with no instruction whatsoever in the branches of knowledge that subserve the art of medicine.

In ancient times there were three medical sects, to wit, the Dogmatic, the Empirical, and the Methodical, but the exponents of each of these embraced the whole of the art as the means to preserve health and to war against disease. To this end they referred all that they individually thought necessary in their particular sects, and employed the service of a threefold aid to health: first, a theory of diet; secondly, the whole use of drugs; and thirdly, manual operation. This last, above the rest, nicely proves the saying that medicine is the addition of that which is defective and the removal of that which is in excess; as often as we resort to the art of medicine for the treatment of disease we have occasion to employ it; and time and experience have taught, by the benefits it has conferred, that it is the greatest aid to human health.

This triple manner of treatment was equally familiar to the doctors of each sect; and those who applied manual operation according to the nature of the affection expended no less care in training their hands than in establishing a theory of diet, or in learning to recognize and compound drugs. This, not to mention his other books, is clearly shown by those most perfect of the compositions of Hippocrates: "On the Function of the Doctor," "On Fractures of Bones," "On Dislocations of Joints and Similar Ailments." Nay, more, Galen, after Hippocrates the prince of medicine, in addition to the fact that he boasts from time to time that the care of the gladiators of Pergamum was entrusted to his sole charge, and that when age was now becoming a burden he was reluctant for the monkeys he had for dissection to be skinned by the help of slaves, frequently impresses on us his joy in manual dexterity and how zealously he, in common with the other doctors of Asia, employed it. Indeed, there is no one of the ancients who does not seem as solicitous to hand down to posterity the method of cure which is effected by the hand as those methods which depend on diet and drugs.

But it was especially after the ruin spread by the Goths, when all the sciences, which before had flourished gloriously and were practiced as was fitting, went to ruin, that more fashionable doctors, first in Italy, in imitation of the old Romans, despising the work of the hand, began to delegate to slaves the manual attentions which they judged needful for their patients, and themselves merely to stand over them like master builders. Then, when all the rest also who practiced the true art of healing gradually declined the unpleasant duties of their profession, without, however, abating any of their claim to money or honor, they quickly fell away from the standard of the doctors of old. Methods of cooking, and all the preparation of food for the sick, they left to nurses; compounding of drugs they left to the apothecaries;

2 That is, after the barbarian invasions that accompanied the fall of the Roman Empire in the West.

3 Mansor, or Al-Mansur (about 712–775), caliph of the victorious Moslem Empire, when its power was rapidly approaching its height. He founded the splendid new capital at Bagdad, increased commerce with the Greeks at Constantinople and urged the translation of Greek philosophy and science into Arabic. For several centuries thereafter Arab medicine was the best in the European world.

manual operation to barbers. Thus in course of time the art of healing has been so wretchedly rent asunder that certain doctors, advertising themselves under the name of physicians, have arrogated to themselves alone the prescription of drugs and diet for obscure diseases, and have relegated the rest of medicine to those whom they call surgeons and scarcely regard as slaves, disgracefully banishing from themselves the chief and most ancient branch of the medical art, and that which principally (if indeed there be any other) bases itself upon the investigation of nature. …

But it was not at all my purpose to set one instrument of medicine above the rest, since the triple art of healing, as it is called, cannot at all be disunited and wrenched asunder, but belongs in its entirety to the same practitioner; and for the due attainment of this triple art, all the parts of medicine have been established and prepared on an equal footing, so that the individual parts are brought into use with a success proportioned to the degree in which one combines the cumulative force of all. How rarely indeed a disease occurs which does not at once require the triple manner of treatment; that is to say, a proper diet must be prescribed, some service must be rendered by medicine, and some by the hand.[4] Therefore the tyros in this art must by every means be exhorted to follow the Greeks in despising the whisperings of those physicians (save the mark!), and, as the fundamental nature and rational basis of the art prescribes, to apply their hands also to the treatment, lest they should rend the body of medicine and make of it a force destructive of the common life of man.

And they must be urged to this with all the greater earnestness because men today who have had an irreproachable training in the art are seen to abstain from the use of the hand as from the plague, and for this very reason, lest they should be slandered by the masters of the profession as barbers before the ignorant mob, and should henceforth lack equal gain and honor with those less than half doctors, losing their standing both with the uneducated commonalty and with princes. For it is indeed above all other things the wide prevalence of this hateful error that prevents us even in our age from taking up the healing art as a whole, makes us confine ourselves merely to the treatment of internal complaints, and, if I may utter the blunt truth once for all, causes us, to the great detriment of mankind, to study to be healers only in a very limited degree.

For when, in the first place, the whole compounding of drugs was handed over to the apothecaries, then the doctors promptly lost the knowledge of simple medicines which is absolutely essential to them; and they became responsible for the fact that the druggists' shops were filled with barbarous terms and false remedies, and also that so many elegant compositions of the ancients were lost to us, several of which have not yet come to light; and, finally, they prepared an endless task for the learned men, not only of our own age, but for those who preceded it by some years, who devoted themselves with indefatigable zeal to research in simple medicines; so much so that they may be regarded as having gone far to restore the knowledge of them to its former brilliance.

But this perverse distribution of the instruments of healing among a variety of craftsmen inflicted a much more odious shipwreck and a far more cruel blow upon the chief branch of natural philosophy [anatomy], to which, since it comprises the natural history of man and should rightly be regarded as the firm foundation of the whole art of medicine and its essential preliminary, Hippocrates and Plato attached so much importance that they did not hesitate to put it first among the parts of medicine. For though originally it was the prime object of the doctors' care, and though they strained every nerve to acquire it, it finally began to perish miserably when the doctors themselves, by resigning manual operations to others, ruined anatomy. For when the doctors supposed that only the care of internal complaints concerned them, considering a mere knowledge of the viscera as more than enough for

4 That is, by surgery.

them, they neglected the structure of the bones and muscles, as well as of the nerves, veins, and arteries which run through bones and muscles, as of no importance for them. And further, when the whole conduct of manual operations was entrusted to barbers, not only did doctors lose the true knowledge of the viscera, but the practice of dissection soon died out, doubtless for the reason that the doctors did not attempt to operate, while those to whom the manual skill was resigned were too ignorant to read the writings of the teachers of anatomy.

It is thus utterly impossible for this class of men to preserve for us a difficult art which they have acquired only mechanically. And equally inevitably this deplorable dismemberment of the art of healing has introduced into our schools the detestable procedure now in vogue, that one man should carry out the dissection of the human body, and another give the description of the parts. These latter are perched up aloft in a pulpit like jackdaws, and with a notable air of disdain they drone out information about facts they have never approached at first hand, but which they merely commit to memory from the books of others, or of which they have descriptions before their eyes; the former are so ignorant of languages that they are unable to explain their dissections to the onlookers and botch what ought to be exhibited in accordance with the instruction of the physician, who never applies his hand to the dissection, and contemptuously steers the ship out of the manual, as the saying goes. Thus everything is wrongly taught, days are wasted in absurd questions, and in the confusion less is offered to the onlooker than a butcher in his stall could teach a doctor. I omit all mention of those schools in which there is scarcely even a thought of opening a human body to exhibit its structure. So far had ancient medicine fallen some years ago from its pristine glory. …

But this effort [to restore anatomy] could by no manner of means have succeeded if, when I was studying medicine at Paris, I had not myself applied my hand to this business, but had acquiesced in the casual and superficial display to me and my fellow students by certain barbers of a few organs at one or two public dissections. For in such a perfunctory manner was anatomy then treated in the place where we have lived to see medicine happily reborn that I myself, having trained myself without guidance in the dissection of brute creatures, at the third dissection at which it was my fortune ever to be present (this, as was the custom there, was concerned exclusively or principally with the viscera), led on by the encouragement of my fellow students and teachers, performed in public a more thorough dissection than was wont to be done. Later I attempted a second dissection, my purpose being to exhibit the muscles of the hand together with a more accurate dissection of the viscera. For except for eight muscles of the abdomen, disgracefully mangled and in the wrong order, no one (I speak the simple truth) ever demonstrated to me any single muscle, or any single bone, much less the network of nerves, veins, and arteries.

Subsequently at Louvain, where I had to return on account of the disturbance of war, because during eighteen years the doctors there had not even dreamed of anatomy, and in order that I might help the students of that academy, and that I myself might acquire greater skill in a matter both obscure and in my judgment of prime importance for the whole of medicine, I did somewhat more accurately than at Paris expound the whole structure of the human body in the course of dissecting, with the result that the younger teachers of that academy now appear to spend great and very serious study in acquiring a knowledge of the parts of man, clearly understanding what invaluable material for philosophizing is presented to them from this knowledge. Furthermore at Padua, in the most famous gymnasium of the whole world,[5] I was charged with the teaching of surgical medicine five years by the illustrious Senate of Venice, which is far the most liberal in the endowment of the highest branches of learning. And since

5 It is interesting to note how many of the great original scientists of the sixteenth and seventeenth centuries studied or taught at Padua, then the university city for Venice.

the carrying out of anatomical inquiry is of importance for surgical medicine, I devoted much effort to the investigation of the structure of man, and so directed my inquiries, and, exploding the ridiculous fashion of the schools, so taught the subject that we could not find in my procedure anything that fell short of the tradition of the ancients.

However, the supineness of the medical profession has seen to it only too well that the writings of Eudemus, Herophilus, Marinus Andreas, Lycus, and other princes of anatomy should not be preserved to us, since not even a fragment of any page has survived of all those famous writers whom Galen mentions, to the number of more than twenty, in his second commentary to the book of Hippocrates on "The Nature of Man" Nay, even of his own anatomical writings scarcely the half has been saved from destruction. But those who followed Galen, among whom I place Oribasius, Theophilus, the Arabs, and all our own writers whom I have read to date, all of them (and they must pardon me for saying this), if they handed on anything worth reading, borrowed it from him. And, believe me, the careful reader will discover that there is nothing they were further from attempting than the dissection of bodies. They placed an absolute trust in I know not what quality of the writing of their chief, and in the neglect of dissection by the rest, and shamefully reduced Galen to convenient summaries, never departing from him by so much as the breadth of a nail, that is, supposing they succeed in arriving at his meaning. Nay, they place it in the forefront of their books that their own writings are pieced together from the teachings of Galen, and that all that is theirs is his. And so completely have all surrendered to his authority that no doctor has been found to declare that in the anatomical books of Galen even the slightest error has ever been found, much less could now be found; though all the time (apart from the fact that Galen frequently corrects himself, and in later books, after acquiring more experience, removes oversights that he had committed in earlier books, and sometimes teaches contradictory views) it is quite clear to us, from the revival of the art of dissection, from a painstaking perusal of the works of Galen, and from a restoration of them in several places, of which we have no reason to be ashamed, that Galen himself never dissected a human body lately dead. Nay, more, deceived by his monkeys (although it is admitted that human bodies dried, and prepared as it were for an inspection of the bones, did come under his observation), he frequently wrongly controverts the ancient doctors who had trained themselves by dissecting human corpses.

And again, how many false observations you will find him to have made even on his monkeys. I shall say nothing about the astonishing fact that in the manifold and infinite divergences of the organs of the human body from those of the monkey Galen hardly noticed anything except in the fingers and the bend of the knee—which he would certainly have passed over with the rest, if they had not been obvious to him without dissection. But at the moment I do not propose to criticize the false statements of Galen, easily the foremost among the teachers of anatomy; and much less would I wish to be regarded now in the beginning as disloyal to the author of all good things and lacking in respect for his authority. For I am not unaware how the medical profession (in this so different from the followers of Aristotle) are wont to be upset when in more than two hundred instances, in the conduct of the single course of anatomy I now exhibit in the schools, they see that Galen has failed to give a true description of the interrelation, use, and function of the parts of man—how they scowl at times, and examine every inch of the dissection in their determination to defend him. Yet they too, drawn by the love of truth, gradually abandon that attitude and, growing less emphatic, begin to put faith in their own not ineffectual sight and powers of reason rather than in the writings of Galen. These true paradoxes, won not by slavish reliance on the efforts of others, nor supported merely by masses of authorities, they eagerly communicate in their correspondence to their friends; they exhort them so earnestly and so friendly-wise to examine for themselves, and to come at last to a true knowledge of anatomy, that there is ground for hope that anatomy will ere long be cultivated in all our academies as it was of old in Alexandria.

And that the muses might the more smile upon this hope, I have, so far as in me lay, and in addition to my other publications on this subject—which certain plagiarists, thinking me far away from Germany, have put out there as their own—made a completely fresh arrangement in seven books of my information about the parts of the human body in the order in which I am wont to lay the same before that learned assembly in this city, as well as at Bologna and at Pisa. Thus those present at the dissections will have a record of what was there demonstrated, and will be able to expound anatomy to others with less trouble. And also the books will be by no means useless to those who have no opportunity for personal examination, for they relate with sufficient fullness the number, position, shape, substance, connection with other parts, use and function of each part of the human body, together with many similar facts which we are wont to unravel during dissection concerning the nature of the parts, and also the method of dissection applicable to dead and living animals. Moreover, the books contain representations of all the parts inserted in the text of the discourse, in such a way that they place before the eyes of the student of nature's works, as it were, a dissected corpse.

Thus in the first book I have described the nature of all bones and cartilages, which, since the other parts are supported by them, and must be described in accordance with them, are the first to be known by students of anatomy. The second book treats of the ligaments by which bones and cartilages are linked one with another, and then the muscles that affect the movements that depend upon our will. The third comprises the close network of veins which carry to the muscles and bones and the other parts the ordinary blood by which they are nourished, and of arteries which control the mixture of innate heat and vital spirit. The fourth treats of the branches not only of the nerves which convey the animal spirit to the muscles, but of all the other nerves as well. The fifth explains the structure of the organs that subserve nutrition effected through food and drink; and furthermore, on account of the proximity of their position, it contains also the instruments designed by the Most High Creator for the propagation of the species. The sixth is devoted to the heart, the *fomes* of the vital faculty, and the parts that subserve it. The seventh describes the harmony between the structure of the brain and the organs of sense, without, however, repeating from the fourth book the description of the network of nerves arising from the brain. …

But here there comes into my mind the judgment of certain men who vehemently condemn the practice of setting before the eyes of students, as we do with the parts of plants, delineations, be they never so accurate, of the parts of the human body. These, they say, ought to be learned not by pictures but by careful dissection and examination of the things themselves. As if, forsooth, my object in adding to the text of my discourse images of the parts, which are most faithful, and which I wish could be free from the risk of being spoiled by the printers, was that students should rely upon them and refrain from dissecting bodies; whereas my practice has rather been to encourage students of medicine in every way I could to perform dissections with their own hands. Assuredly, if the practice of the ancients had lasted down to our day, namely, to train boys at home in carrying out dissections, just as in making their letters and in reading, I would gladly consent to our dispensing not only with pictures but with all commentaries. For the ancients only began to write about dissection when they decided that honor demanded that they should communicate the art not only to their children but to strangers whom they respected for their virtue. For, as soon as boys were no longer trained in dissection, the inevitable consequence at once followed that they learned anatomy less well, since the training had been abolished with which they had been wont to begin in youth. So much so that when the art had deserted the family of the Asclepiads,[6] and had been now for many centuries on the decline, books were needed to preserve a complete view of

6 An association of the alleged descendants of Asclepius, the Greek god of medicine and healing; later, a school for the training of physicians.

it. Yet how greatly pictures aid the understanding of these things, and how much more accurately they put the things before the eyes than even the clearest language, nobody can have failed to experience in geometry and the other mathematical disciplines.

But, however that may be, I have done my best to this single end, namely, in an equally recondite and laborious matter, to aid as many as possible, and truly and completely to describe the structure of the human body—which is built up not of some ten or twelve parts (as seems to those who give it a passing glance) but of some thousands of different parts—and to bring to students of medicine a substantial contribution toward the understanding of those books of Galen treating of this branch of learning, which of all his writings most require the assistance of a teacher.

Moreover, I am aware how little authority my efforts will carry by reason of my youth (I am still in my twenty-eighth year); and how little, on account of the frequency with which I draw attention to the falsity of Galen's pronouncements, I shall be sheltered from the attacks of those who have not—as I have done in the schools of Italy—applied themselves earnestly to anatomy, and who, being now old men devoured by envy at the true discoveries of youths, will be ashamed, together with all the other sectaries of Galen, that they have been hitherto so purblind, failing to notice what I now set forth, yet arrogating to themselves a mighty reputation in the art—[I know, I say, how little authority my efforts will carry] unless they come forth auspiciously into the light, commended by the great patronage of some divine power. And, inasmuch as it cannot be more safely sheltered or more splendidly adorned than by the imperishable name of the Divine Charles, the Most Great and Invincible Emperor, I beseech Your Majesty to allow this useful work of mine, which on many accounts and for many reasons is dangerous to itself, to circulate for a short time under Your Majesty's auspices, glory, and patronage, until through experience of the facts, through judgment which matures with time, and through learning, I may make the fruit of my toil worthy of the Most High and Best Prince, or may offer another gift worthy of acceptance on another subj chosen from our art.

Padua, *August 1, a.d. 1542.*

WHAT MAY BE LEARNED BY DISSECTION OF THE DEAD AND WHAT OF THE LIVING

Just as the dissection of the dead teaches well the number, position and shape of each part, and most accurately the nature and composition of its material substance, thus also the dissection of a living animal clearly demonstrates at once the function itself, at another time it shows very clearly the reasons for the existence of the parts. Therefore, even though students deservedly first come to be skilled in the study of dead animals, afterward when about to investigate the action and use of the parts of the body they must become acquainted with the living animal. …

Examination of the Uses of the Veins and Arteries

Also when inquiring into the use of the veins the work is scarcely one for the dissection of the living, since we shall become sufficiently acquainted in the case of the dead with the fact that these veins carry the blood through the whole body and that any part is not nourished in which a prominent vein has been severed in wounds.

Likewise concerning the arteries we scarcely require a dissection of the living although it will be allowable for anyone to lay bare the artery running into the groin and to obstruct it with a band and to observe that the part of the artery cut off by the band pulsates no longer.

And thus it is observed by the easy experiment of opening an artery at any time in living animals that blood is contained in the arteries naturally.

In order that on the other hand we may be more certain that the material contained in the arteries is not the producer of the pulsation, for in truth this force depends for its strength upon the heart. Besides, because we see that an artery bound by a cord no longer beats under the cord, it will be permitted to undertake an extensive dissection of the artery of the groin or of the thigh, and to take a small tube made of a reed of such a thickness as is the capacity of the artery and to insert it by cutting in such a way that the upper part of the tube reaches higher into the cavity of the artery than the upper part of the dissection, and in the same manner also that the lower portion of the tube is introduced downward farther than the lower part of the dissection, and thus the ligature of the artery which constricts its caliber above the canulla is passed by a circuit.

To be sure, when this is done the blood and likewise the vital spirit run through the artery even as far as the foot; in fact the whole portion of the artery replaced by the canulla beats no longer. Moreover, when the ligature has been cut, that part of the artery which is beyond the canulla shows no less pulsation than the portion above.

We shall see next how much force is actually carried to the brain from the heart by the arteries. Now in this demonstration thou shalt wonder greatly at a vivisection of Galen in which he advises that all things be cut off which are common to the brain and heart, always excepting the arteries which seek the head through the transverse processes of the cervical vertebrae and carry also besides a substantial portion of the vital spirit into the primary sinuses of the dural mater and also in like manner into the brain. So much so that it is not surprising that the brain performs its functions under these conditions for a long time, which Galen observed could easily be done, for the animal breathes for a long time during this dissection, and sometimes moves about. If indeed it runs, and therefore requires much breath, it falls not long afterwards, although the brain will still afterwards receive the essense of the animal spirit from those arteries which I have closely observed seek the skull through the transverse processes of the cervical vertebrae. …

To Johannes Oporinus

PROFESSOR OF GREEK AT BASEL AND VERY DEAR FRIEND

GREETINGS. Through the agency of the Milanese merchants, the Danoni, you will shortly receive, with this letter, the plates engraved for my books DE HUMANI CORPORIS FABRICA and its EPITOME. I trust that they will reach Basel intact and safely since, lest they be defaced in any way or suffer any other damage during their cartage, I carefully packed them with the help of the engraver and Nicolaus Stopius, trustworthy manager here for the firm of Bomberg, a youth well versed in the humanities. Between the series of plates we have placed separately their proofs as well as the letter-press for the individual figures, on each of which I have written where it is to go so that their arrangement and disposition might present no difficulty to you and your workmen and hence prevent the plates being printed out of order. You will readily observe from the proof where the type of characters must be changed, since by means of lines I have separated that part of the letter-press which comprises the account of the organs, divided in the

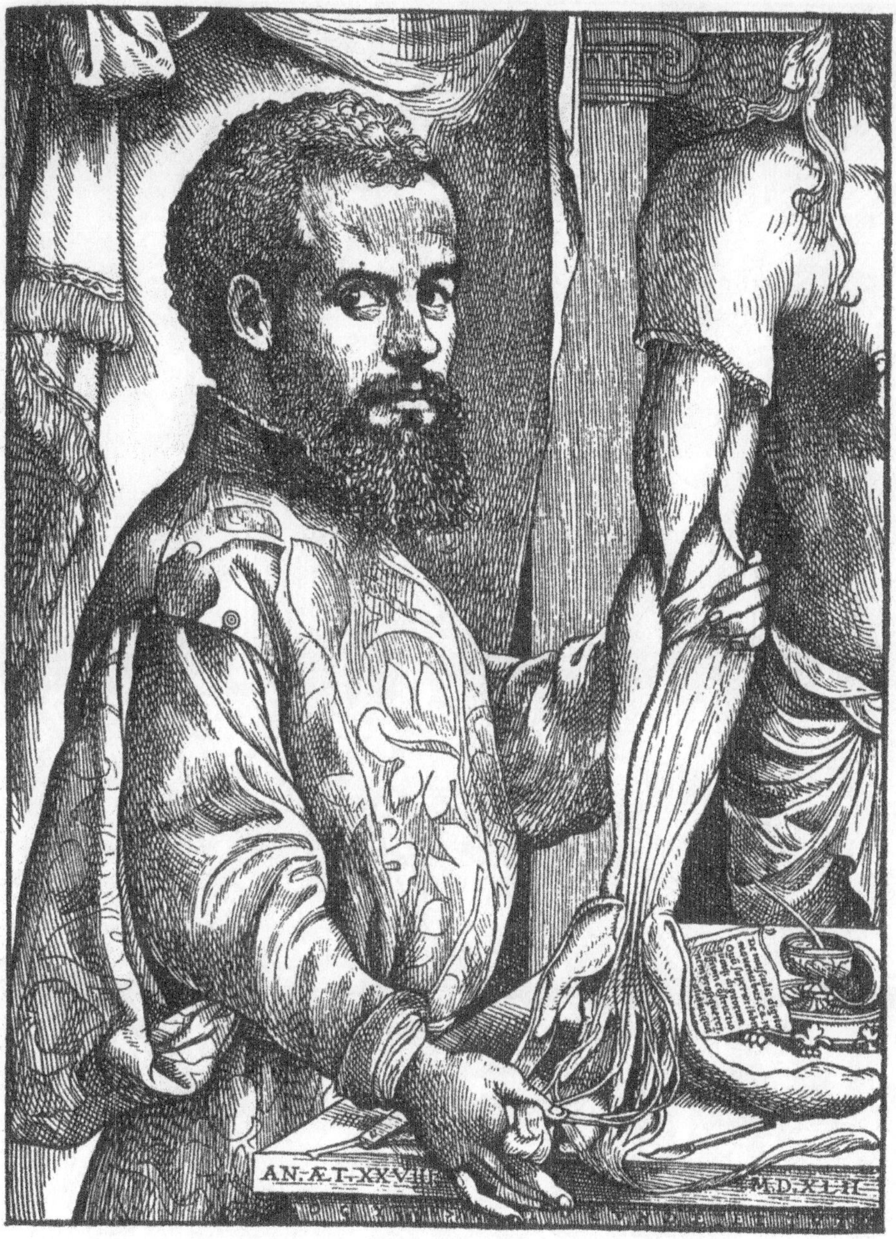

PLATE 1. Woodcut portrait of Andreas Vesalius

continuous descriptive text into separate chapters, from that which aids in the explanation of the characters found engraved on the plates. For this reason the latter is called the Index of the figures and their characters. In the continuous course of the text, nowhere interrupted by references to figures, you will employ the small type which printers call "superlinear" to indicate those annotations which I have added to the inner margin, not so much through industry as through labor and tedium, in order that they might serve as a commentary for the reader and indicate in whatever plate the part under discussion may be seen; on the other hand, the annotations seen on the outer margin present to some extent a summary of the discussion. To avoid prolixity, wherever an indicated figure is attached to the chapter

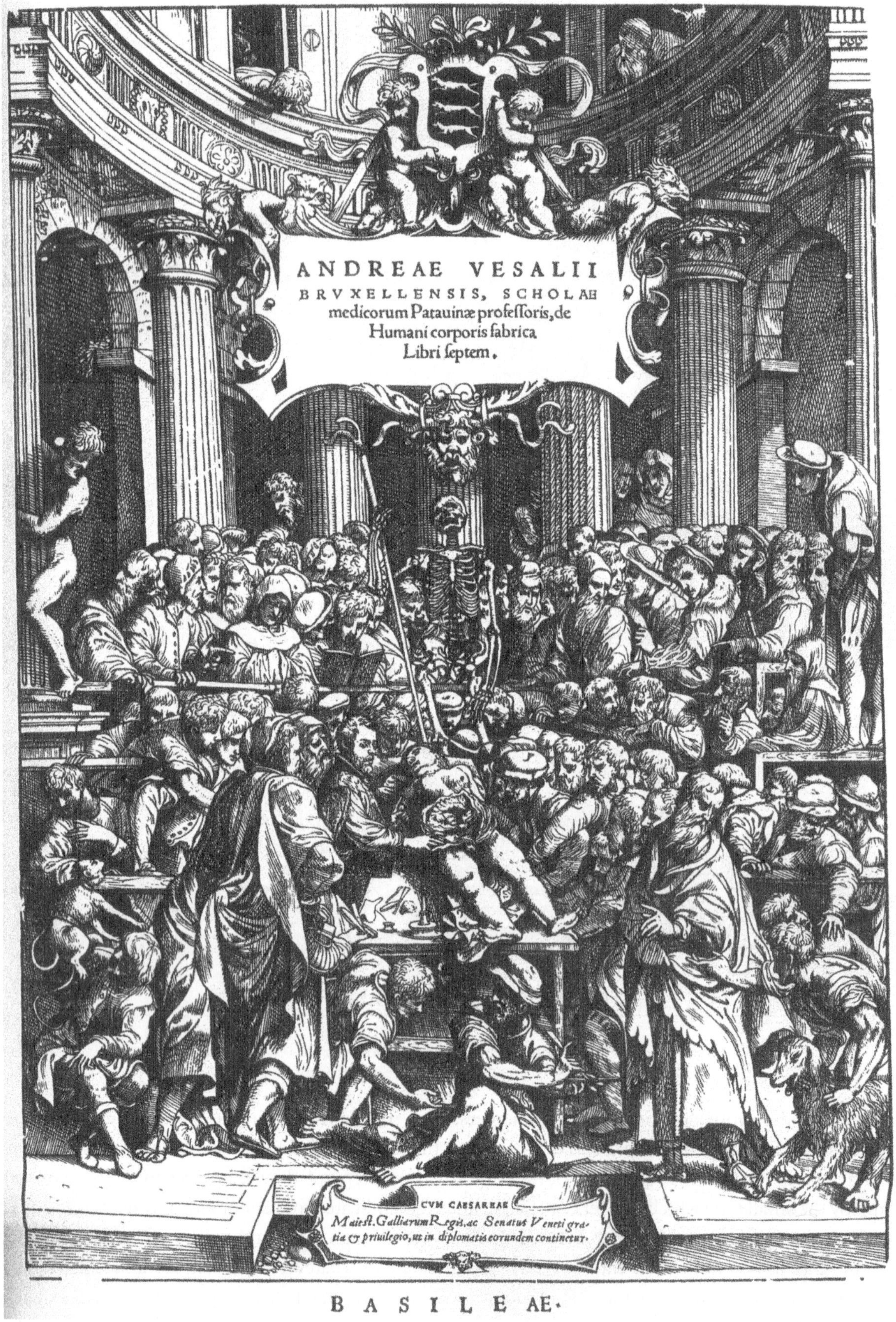

Andreas Vesalius, Plate 2 from *De Humani Corporis Fabrica.* Copyright in the Public Domain.

containing the annotation I have observed the practice of providing no chapter number in the inner margin, although I have included it if the figure is placed in another chapter. Again, if the figure is found in the "book" where the annotation occurs, I do not subjoin the number of the "book" to the figure. You will End clearly explained in the titles of the "books" and in the indices of the characters why I have decided that the plates ought to be gathered in this or that place. For signs with which to designate the parts in any delineation, we have carved on the plates characters of the sort constantly employed in printing shops; first we used upper-case Latin letters and then, lowercase; thereafter, lower-case Greek and then some upper-case which are not identical with the Latin ones; but since all of these did not suffice, we used numerals even though other indicative signs occur in ordinary types. In the description of these indices it should be observed that an indicating character having only a single reference is placed in the margin of the book. But if it does not have a single indication and is described as well by another character, I have added a period to it in the margin so that it, as well as the others in the series, would be clear to the reader. Elsewhere I wrote to you at length of this procedure and why I believed that the index of characters should not be confused with the account of the parts. But now I urge and exhort you most earnestly to execute everything as handsomely and swiftly as possible so as to satisfy in my undertaking the expectations which all conceive of your printing shop, now for the first time, under the happy auspices of the Muses, completely devoted to the greater convenience of student. Special care should be employed on the impression of the plates which are not to be printed like ordinary textbooks with simple line engravings; nowhere should the import of the picture be neglected, unless perhaps where the delineation is [verbally] complemented. And although here your judgment is such that I have promised myself nothing other than your industry and care, I desire above all that in the printing you copy as closely as possible the proof struck off by the engraver as a specimen, which you will find enclosed in its place together with the wood blocks; for thus no character, although concealed in the shading, will lie hidden from the careful and observant reader. Likewise take care of what I consider most artistic and so pleasing in these pictures, that the thickness of the lines which produce gradation in the shadows is tastefully rendered. But this is not the reason that I write to you since everything depends on the smoothness and solidity of the paper, and above all, on the carefulness of your efforts. And may each plate issued from your printing shop be of the same quality as the several copies of the proofs which we now send. I shall strive to journey to you soon, and I shall remain in Basel, if not for the whole period of printing, at least for some time. I shall bring with me a copy of the decree of the Venetian Senate warning everyone not to print the plates without my consent My mother will send you from Brussels an imperial license inasmuch as you generally have one in all the books which you print for the first time. It was obtained for me some time ago, and thus far we have not been able to get it renewed and validated for a longer period of years. The Bishop of Montpellier, ambassador to Venice, will obtain for me the license of the French king. I have no concern on this score so long as I am not compelled to fill a page with copies of official decrees. For what the decrees of Princes are worth among booksellers and publishers, now very thickly sown in every corner, is well known from the fate of my *Anatomical Tables* first printed three years ago in Venice and thereafter, although decorated with pompous titles, issued miserably depraved throughout. For in an edition from Augsburg my letter to Narcissus Vertunus, first physician to the Emperor and to the King of Naples, and a rare example of the physicians of our age, was replaced by a preface written by some German babbler who, unworthily decrying Avicenna and the rest of the Arabic writers, enumerates me among the concise Galenists, and (to deceive the purchaser) falsely asserts that I have compressed into six tables what Galen diffusely expressed in more than thirty books. Then adding that he has translated the Latin into German, he affirms that he employed the Greek and Arabic words, although actually not only has he entirely suppressed them, but he omitted all which he was unable to translate and whatever gave value to the *Tables* in the first place; furthermore, the Venetian plates were wretchedly reproduced. But he of Cologne who put his hand to the same plates is by far more crude and unskilled than the Augsburg engraver; and although some one in Cologne wrote in praise of the printer, that not only was he able to observe the construction of man better from my plates than from the dissection of the human fabric, but also that they had made from my most elegant figures much more pleasing ones, although, as it happens, they corrupted the pictures and added a delineation of the nerves imitated with little success from a rough sketch which I had drawn, with an index added, for one or two friends who sought it from me during the progress of the work. At Paris they have printed the first three very elegantly, but the others, I imagine because of engraving difficulties, they have omitted, although if they were considered for the sake of students, the first [three] might best have been dispensed with. Moreover, that one of Strasburg whom Fuchs reviled with so great an outcry because of certain forgeries, and whom I am able to name on other grounds as a plagiarist, deserves the very worst from students, because the plates, which could never be large enough for students, he contracted so abominably, colored so shamefully, surrounded them beyond all reason with the Augsburg text and published as his own. Still another seems envious of the latter's glory, and having compiled from all sides without discrimination, from the books and pictures of others, is preparing to publish books of the sort issued at Marburg and Frankfurt. I gladly tolerate, indeed, greatly admire the divine and most felicitous talents of the Italians, in contradistinction to my judgment of German physicians, because the latter seek the services of certain sordid printers who, for the sake of any mean profit which can be squeezed out, dare to issue any type of writing which the physicians abridge, alter or simply copy and publish as apparently new and in their own name, while the decrees of Princes remain silent. I write these things that you may understand how little I believe that you will do that sort of printing, but rather I feel compelled to state that gladly I will transmit the plates to any diligent printer whomsoever, and in whatever way I can, offer the use of my literary efforts. Likewise, I shall attempt in every way in my power to hinder any inept person from reproducing the plates, made with so much labor for the general use of students, so that regardless of whatever turgid title is prefixed to them, they may not come into human hands as if they had been issued carelessly by me. And in particular, this is the reason why I have prepared the plates at my own expense, and now once again I shall urge you to preserve them faultlessly and elegantly by your efforts.

Farewell. Venice, September 5th. Your Andreas Vesalius.

Plate 11 of *De Humani Corporis Fabrica*

11:1–9 [I:xv]. The first figure presents part of the occipital bone heed from the other bones and observable 011 the external aspect of the base of the skull.

The inclusion of the occipital bone in the series on the cervical vertebrae was not only to reveal the shape of the opposing articular surfaces of the atlanto-occipital joint but also to show that the occipital condyles of man differed markedly in shape from the description of Galen which had been taken from quadrupeds.

The second figure contains the first cervical or vertebra of the neck represented on its antero-superior aspect.

The third figure exposes to view the postero-superior aspect of the first cervical vertebra.

The fourth figure exhibits the first cervical vertebra delineated from the postero-inferior aspect.

The fifth figure displays the anterior aspect of the second cervical vertebra.

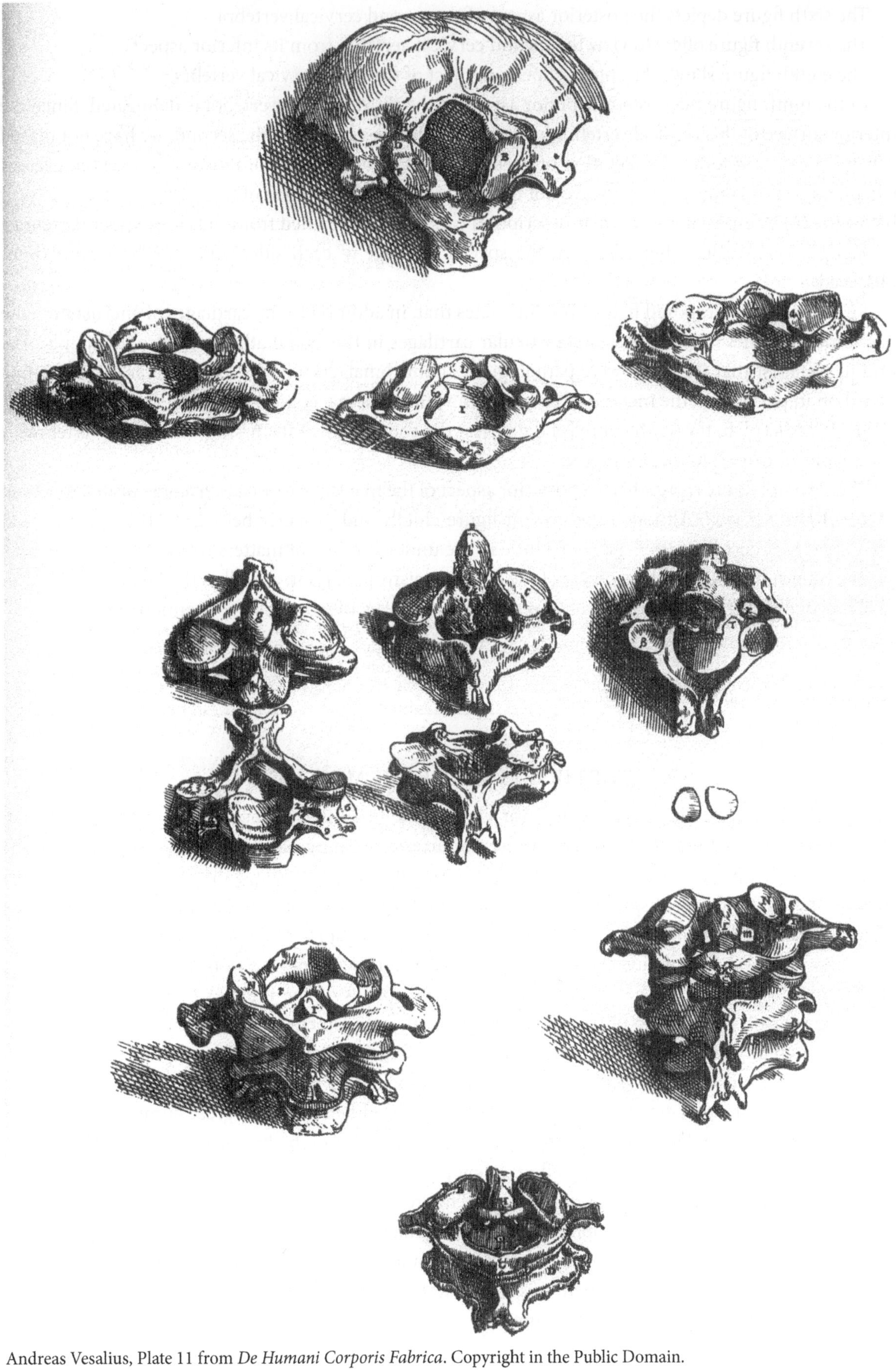

Andreas Vesalius, Plate 11 from *De Humani Corporis Fabrica*. Copyright in the Public Domain.

The sixth figure depicts the posterior aspect of the second cervical vertebra.

The seventh figure offers to view the second cervical vertebra from its inferior aspect.

The eighth figure shows the antero-superior aspect of the third cervical vertebra.

In the ninth figure the postero-superior aspect of the third cervical vertebra is delineated. Since the interior surface of this cervical vertebra resembles the inferior surface of the second, we have not placed it here so as to avoid the presentation of perhaps an excessive number of illustrations for the present Chapter. For the same reason, we have not depicted individually the rest of the cervical vertebrae lying below the third, especially since their description can be readily gained from the three upper vertebrae.

11:10 [I:xv]. We have here depicted the special cartilage of each side, which we have sometimes observed.

Regarding this interposed figure, Vesalius states that, in addition to the cartilages of encrustation, he has sometimes met with irregular interarticular cartilages in the lateral atlanto-epistrophic joints. The findings suggest that the joints were pathological, chondromalacia, or that the articular cartilages had flaked off in part due to the method of preparation which was maceration in boiling water.

II:11–12 [I:xv]. In the tenth figure [of the series] the connection of the first three cervical vertebrae is seen depicted from the anterior aspect.

The eleventh figure represents the posterior aspect of the first three cervical vertebrae united together.

11:13 [I:xv; II:xxx]. Although the present figure chiefly and properly belongs to the second book, I have placed it here because it aids not a little in the understanding of matters treated at this time. …

The transverse and apical ligaments of the atlanto-epistrophic joint, as well as the ligamenta flava, an easily recognized. The illustration will be reproduced once again in book II, as mentioned.

Plate 24 of *De Humani Corporis Fabrica*

THE FIRST PLATE OF THE MUSCLES

24 [II]. The first plate illustrates the anterior view of the body from which I have cut away the skin *together* with the fat, and all the sinews, veins and arteries existing on the surface. No portion of the membrane which we call fleshy [deep fascia] has been left, even in those regions in which this *becomes* muscle-like. This we have displayed in the third plate, there dissected in many regions, so that in that plate, as well as in the second and the ninth, the fleshy membranes are not so obscure. These plates *display a* total view of the scheme of muscles such as only painters and sculptors are wont to consider. …

The first, together with the second, third and ninth plates of the muscles series, was apparently designed not only to reveal to physicians the superficial arrangement of the muscles but also, as indicated by Vesalius' own introductory statement, for the special use of artists and sculptors. Indeed, it has been in the latter use that these illustrations, especially plates 25 and 26, have been employed almost continuously for the past 400 years and may be found in modified form in a great number of textbooks on anatomy for art students today. Likewise, from plate 25 an écorché has been constructed of which occasional examples may be encountered in art supply shops.

One of the characteristic features of all Vesalian figures is the attempt to represent the dissected body in dynamic fashion with greater emphasis on the living than the dead. In the dissections at a deeper level this has given rise to a rather bizarre and ragged appearance of the figures, but it serves to emphasize the fact that in the sixteenth century there was no separation between morphology and function. On the significance of the backgrounds to the figures the reader should consult the introduction.

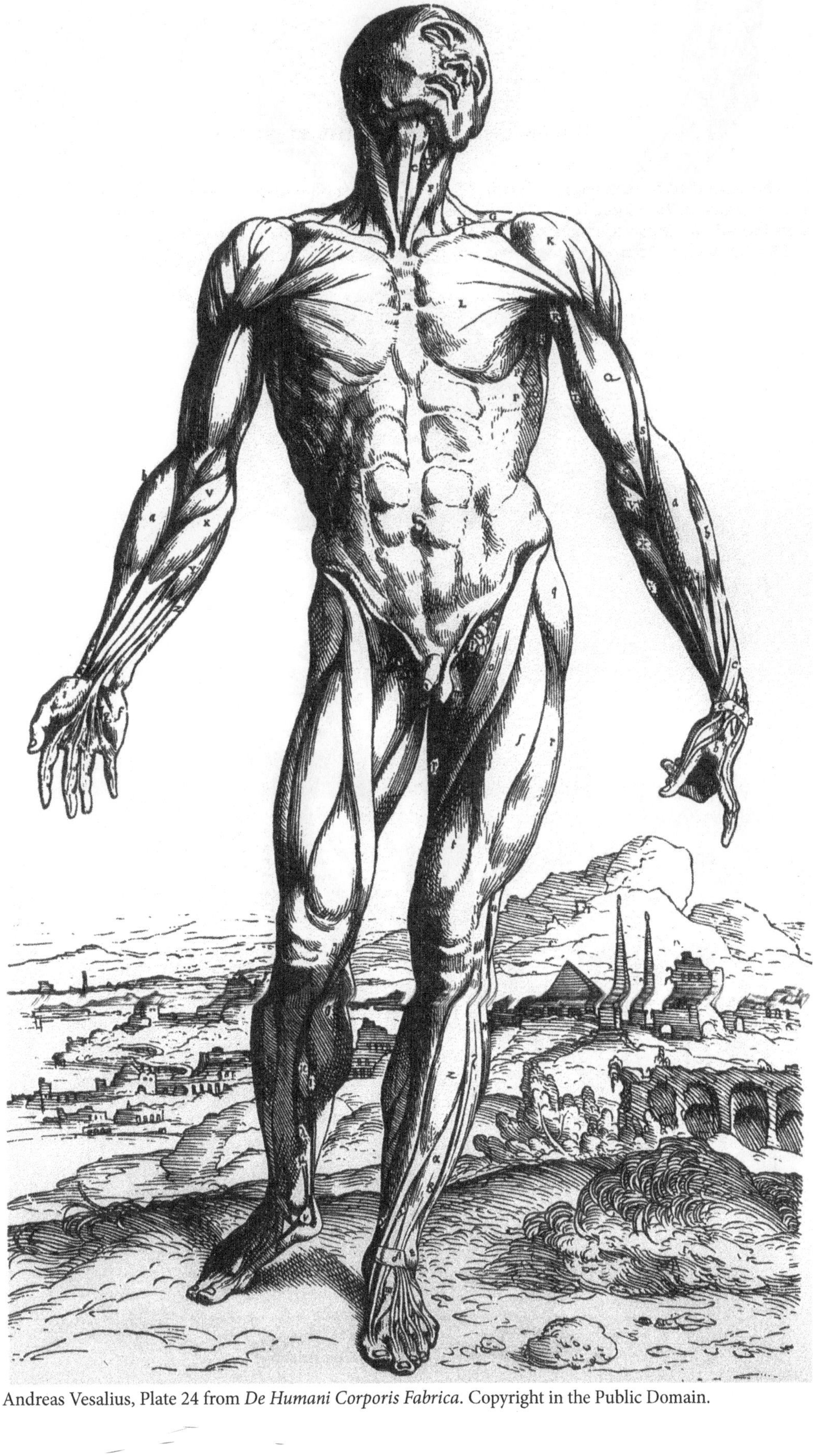

Andreas Vesalius, Plate 24 from *De Humani Corporis Fabrica*. Copyright in the Public Domain.

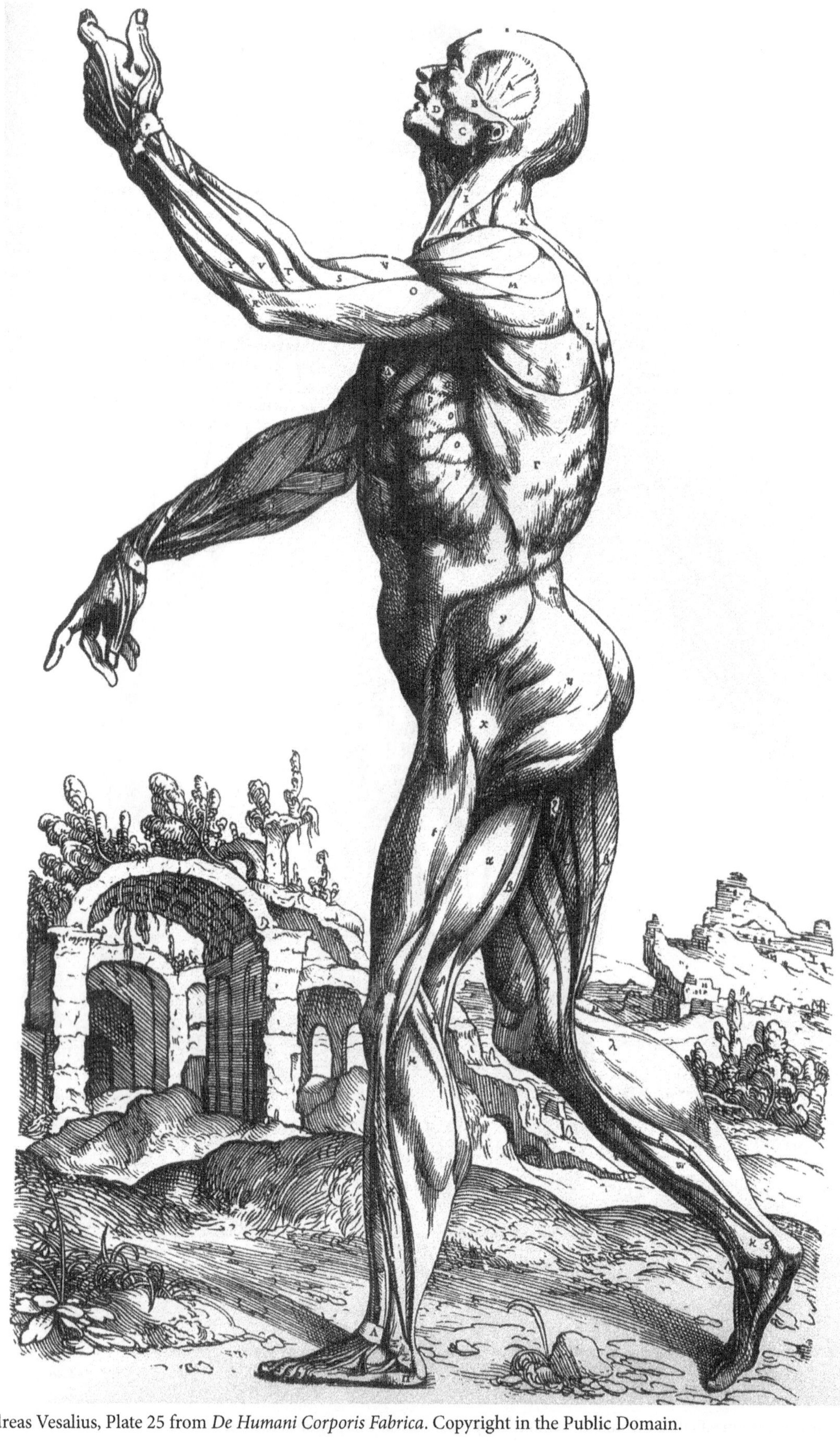

Andreas Vesalius, Plate 25 from *De Humani Corporis Fabrica*. Copyright in the Public Domain.

Plate 25 of *De Humani Corporis Fabrica*

THE SECOND PLATE OF THE MUSCLES

25 [II]. The second plate corresponds entirely to the first since it concerns the dissection, which has been turned to the side to display the same muscles as the former, together with the bony regions, prominent on the surface and somewhat excarnate. Therefore almost the entire surface, as well as the head since it is osseous in only a little less than its entirety, is consequently indicated by very few letters.

Plate 28 of *De Humani Corporis Fabrica*

THE FIFTH PLATE OF THE MUSCLES

28 [II]. Just as the fourth plate shows many muscles dissected and lifted away, which were seen intact in the third plate, so the fifth in the sequence of dissection has many removed which were fully uncovered in the fourth. This plate also exposes many which will be shown reflected in the sixth. Meanwhile it should not be neglected that we have advised the reader immediately at the beginning of this book that the plates expressing the anterior surface of the body mutually correspond in order with the dissections which display the posterior surface; that is to say, just as if this were to follow the tenth plate, for the present [plate] nowhere makes apparent muscles which are shown reflected in the tenth plate.

The extension of the rectus abdominis muscle to the level of the first rib, an arrangement found only in lower forms, appears at first sight to be a glaring blunder on the part of Vesalius. However, it should be recognized that Vesalius not infrequently incorporated many of his observations on comparative anatomy in his illustrations of the human figure. This may have been done to economize on space but is perhaps more truly a reflection of his teleological outlook since Vesalius characteristically introduces into his text theoretical arguments as to what position a structure found in animals would occupy if it occurred in man, thus revealing the errors of Galen. The telescoping of human with other mamalian findings in the illustrations is very confusing unless careful attention is given to the text, and superficial judgments of the illustrations alone have often resulted in Vesalius being unjustly accused of committing errors of the Galenical sort. In this particular instance Vesalius specifically states that the upper part of the muscle is a tendinous extension found in apes and dogs. The massiveness of the scalenus anterior muscle is to demonstrate the findings in dogs and is better seen in the next plate.

The continuation of the dissection consists of the excision of the sternomastoid displacement of the digastric, removal of the mylohyoid and sternohyoid muscles and separation of the sternothyroids to reveal the trachea. The right clavicle has been hinged laterally on the acromioclavicular joint. The left pectoralis minor has been removed. The left internal oblique is now seen hanging from the side of the subject, and the right has been excised. In the upper extremities the right deltoid and right flexor carpi ulnaris are detached from their origins, but only their tendons are apparent on the left. The muscles turned down in the right thigh are rectus femoris and gracilis and in the right leg, extensor digitorum longus. Extensor hallucis longus has been left intact.

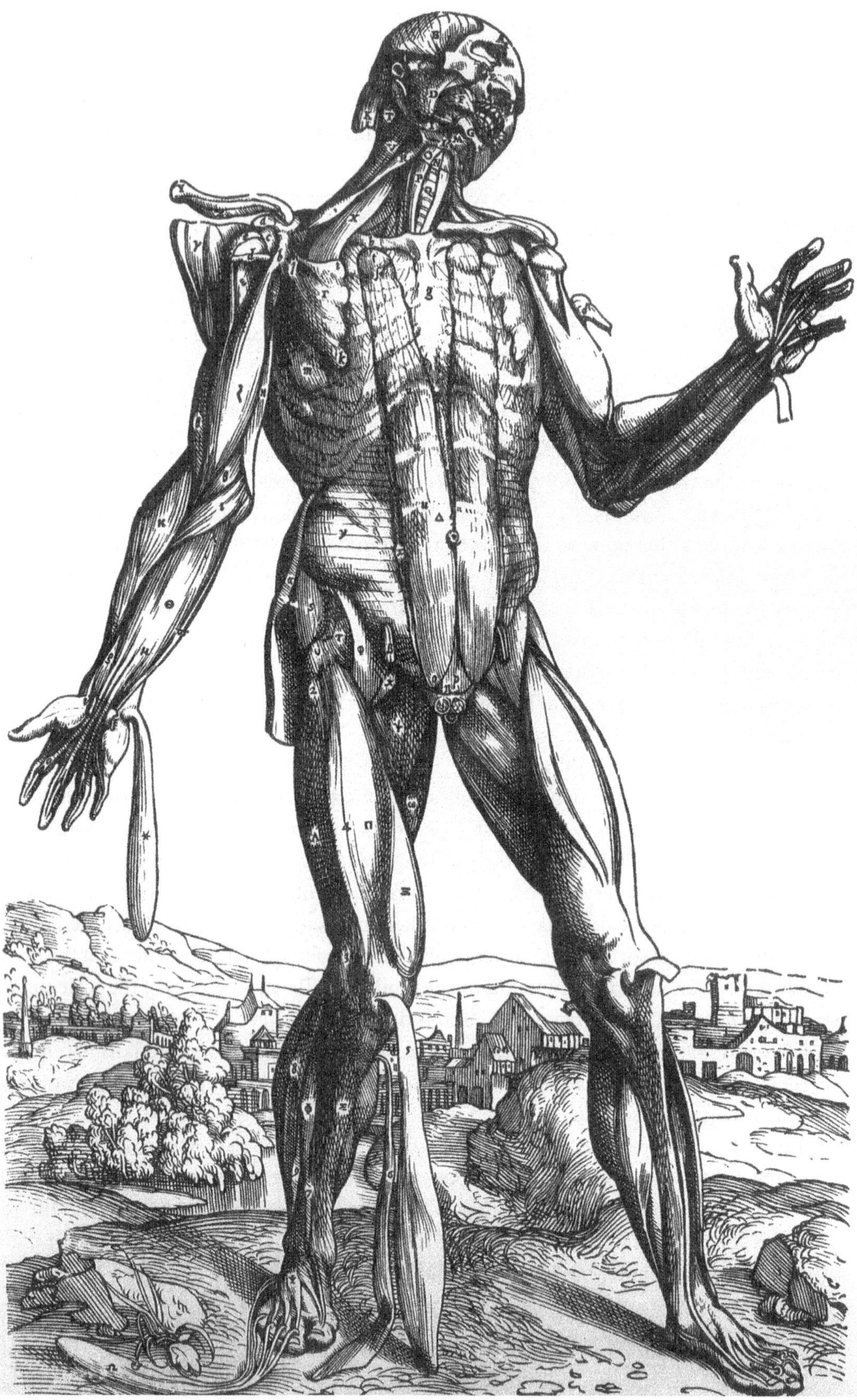

Andreas Vesalius, Plate 28 from *De Humani Corporis Fabrica*. Copyright in the Public Domain.

Plate 42 of *De Humani Corporis Fabrica*

42:1 [II:xxxviii]. In the present figure we have roughly outlined the sides, and nature and arrangement of the fibers of the muscle which we here describe. …

A marginal figure to show the outline of the scalene muscles, so named from their resemblance to a scalene triangle. Vesalius regarded the three scalenes as one muscle.

42:2 [II:xxvi]. A schematic figure to illustrate the outline of the trapezius muscle in which DE represents the scapular spine, above; and below, the shape of the trapezius as described by Galen in his work On the Administration of Dissection, book 4.

42:3 [II:xxxviii]. The present figure represents to some extent the boundaries of the muscle, here discussed.

Another marginal figure to show the outline of the quadratus lumborum muscle and how it receives its name.

42:4 [II:i]. A small figure inset in the text to illustrate the function of certain ligaments such as the transverse ligament of the ankle in preventing tendons from rising out of their beds during contraction.

42:5 [I:xl, 2nd ed.]. We illustrate in this figure the instrument with which the harder bones are perforated with little difficulty.

Vesalius initiated the technique of articulating the skeleton which has not changed materially up to the present. For this purpose he appended to the second edition of the Fabrica this illustration of a crude drill to facilitate the introduction of the wire supports.

42:6 [VII:xix], In this figure you will observe a pig tied to the board which we usually provide for the administration of vivisections and which we represented together with the rest of our anatomical instruments in the last Chapter of the first book, so that the manner in which it is employed in our schools will to some extent be apparent.

This figure properly belongs to the chapter of the seventh book in which Vesalius repeats after the lapse of more than a thousand years the experiments in physiology described by Galen. However, it is convenient to view it here in order to appreciate the manner in which his vivisection board illustrated below was employed.

42:7 [II:vii; I:xli, 2nd ed.]. In the present figure we have placed a board such as we employ in vivisections, resting on a table. On this board we have arranged almost everything which could be used in the administration of dissections or in an entire Anatomy.

41:10 [II:xxi]. The eighth figure differs from the seventh in this respect, that here we have resected the four straight muscles [posterior cricoarytenoids] which connect the third cartilage [arytenoid] to the second [cricoid], thus revealing the second cartilage more clearly.

The illustration closely resembles the previous figure except that the removal of the posterior cricoarytenoid muscles reveals the lamina of the cricoid.

41:11 [II:ixxi]. The ninth figure differs from the eighth since in addition to the muscles already mentioned, we have lifted away the four oblique muscles [lateral cricoarytenoid] joining the third cartilage [arytenoid] to the second [cricoid], as well as the two muscles [oblique arytenoids] placed at the base of the third cartilage, preserving together with the three cartilages only those muscles [thyroarytenoids] which bind the third cartilage to the first [thyroid].

The muscular process of the arytenoid cartilage is now clearly exposed, which would lead one to believe "An administration," a term derived from Galen, was the step-by-step technical procedure employed in dissection, whereas "an Anatomy" was the term used to describe a course of anatomical instruction which included the preparation of teaching specimens often other than the parts of man

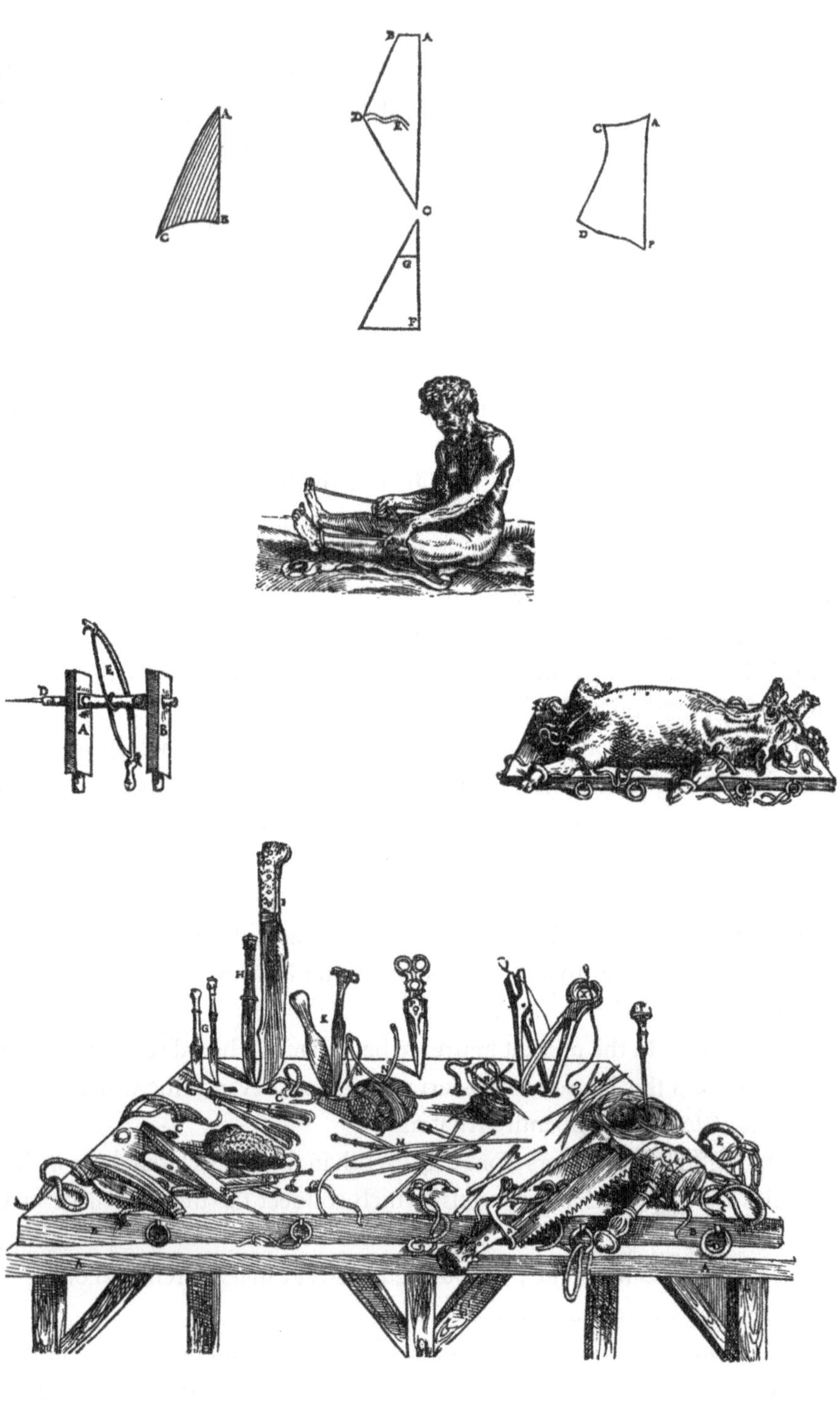

Andreas Vesalius, Plate 42 from *De Humani Corporis Fabrica*. Copyright in the Public Domain.

that the structure which Vesalius contends is a deep portion of the thyroarytenoid muscle is, in fact, the cricovocal membrane.

41:12 [II:xxi]. The tenth figure offers for observation the anterior aspect of the larynx itself in which the first cartilage [thyroid] has now been removed and only the muscles joining the third cartilage [arytenoid] to the first together with the second [cricoid] and third cartilages themselves appear.

The removal of the thyroid cartilage reveals what Vesalius believed to be a deep portion of the thyroary tenoid muscles but which, for reasons stated above, an probably the cricovocal membranes incompletely dis sected so that the ventricular folds are left attached Above and posteriorly are the apices of the arytenoid cartilages and below the anterior ring of the cricoid.

41:13 [II:xxi]. The eleventh figure, as in the two which follow, we have delineated in order to display the "reed" or fissure of the larynx. Therefore the larynx is here illustrated freed from the rest of the stem of the rough artery [trachea] and the common [extrinsic] larynge muscles. In addition, its operculum [epiglottis] is ...

Plate 44 of *De Humani Corporis Fabrica*

44 [III:vi]. A delineation of the entire vena cava freed from all parts.

In the general scheme of the venous system several unusual features may be observed. Following traditional views, the vena cava is regarded as a single continuous vessel. This was due in part to reliance upon the anatomy of the domestic animals, and especially that of the ape, and in part to the conception that the heart was a two-chambered organ. The portion of the vessel seen connecting the superior to the inferior vena cava is therefore the left atrium of modern anatomists, hence the aperture observed in this region represents the right atrioventricular orifice, and the vein marked E is the coronary sinus. Posteriorly at F is the vena azygos greatly exaggerated in size and concerning the therapeutic importance of which Vesalius wrote his Venesection Letter. The arrangement of the veins at the root of the neck is certainly not human and suggests the brachiocephalic vessels of lower animals. Oddly enough, Vesalius usually shows the external jugular as larger than the internal jugular veins, once again indicating that he had not rid himself of the Galenical influence. Too much attention should not be given to the representation of the venous sinuses of the cranial cavity since he was very confused and uncertain as to their disposition. Note the nonhuman position of the renal veins, the right being higher than the left, as derived from the opinions of Aristotle and Galen.

The arrangement of the venous system was of first importance to the sixteenth-century physician since it formed the basis for phlebotomy, the sheet anchor of the therapeutics of the day. It will be observed that in consequence the venous system is portrayed in great detail whereas the arterial system is glossed over and only the major vessels shown.

Plate 71 of *De Humani Corporis Fabrica*

71:1 [VII: fig. 12]. In this figure the head is represented from the left side, the right being somewhat elevated. Here we have evulsed the cerebellum from the cavity of the skull while only that portion of the brain remains which was still preserved in the eighth and ninth figures [70:1, 70:3]. However, this portion of the brain does not lie in position but has been elevated and reflected to some extent posteriorly from the base of the skull so that the processes [olfactory] of the brain, in form not unlike nerves and

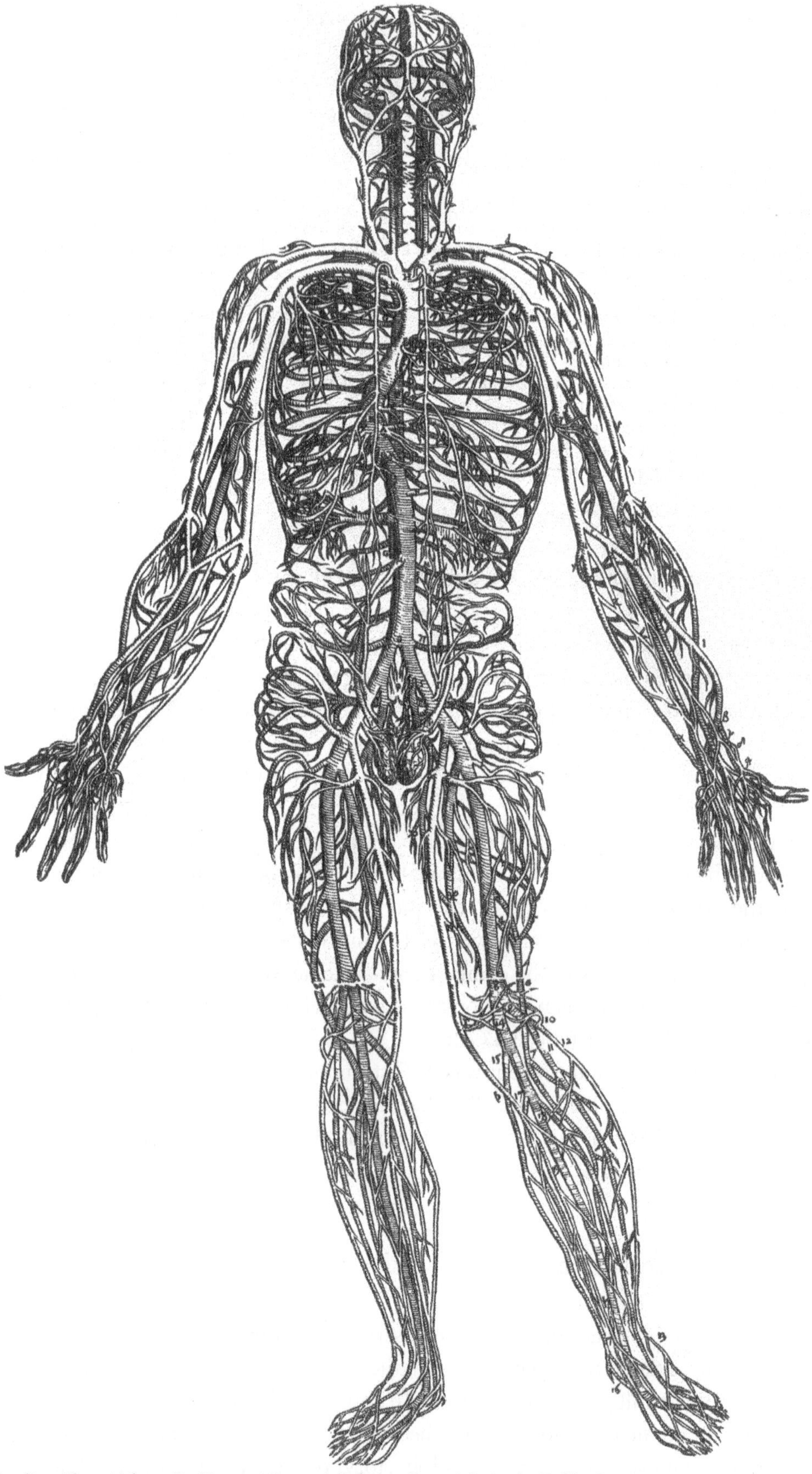

Andreas Vesalius, Plate 44 from *De Humani Corporis Fabrica*. Copyright in the Public Domain.

which subserve smell, may come into view. The left process has been lifted up with the brain from its position while the right still remains connected to the dural membrane of the brain where it covers the eighth bone of the head [ethmoid].

Following Galen, the olfactory are not classified with the cranial nerves but, owing to appearances in animals, regarded as hollow processes or extensions of the lateral ventricles. The remaining structures here seen are readily identified.

71:2 [VII: fig. 13]. This figure rests entirely upon its occiput, and all the brain substance which still remains hangs reflected downwards into the posterior parts so that the olfactory organs, the connection of the visual nerves and the largest branches of the sleep-inducing [carotid] artery might conic into sight.

The optic chiasma, O, M, N; the infundibulum, S; the internal carotid P, dividing into the anterior and middle cerebral arteries R and Q, but not correctly identified; and the olfactory tracts L, are exposed. I is a cerebral vein connecting with the sphenoparietal sinus; H and K are the anterior and middle meningeal vessels. Other lettering refers to the brain, attachment of the falx cerebri and the ethmoid.

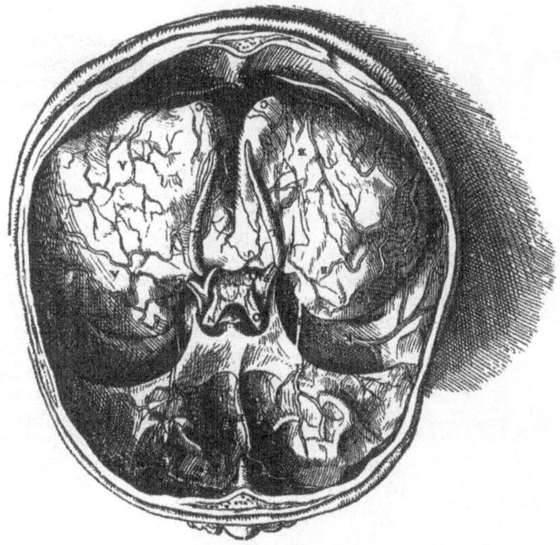

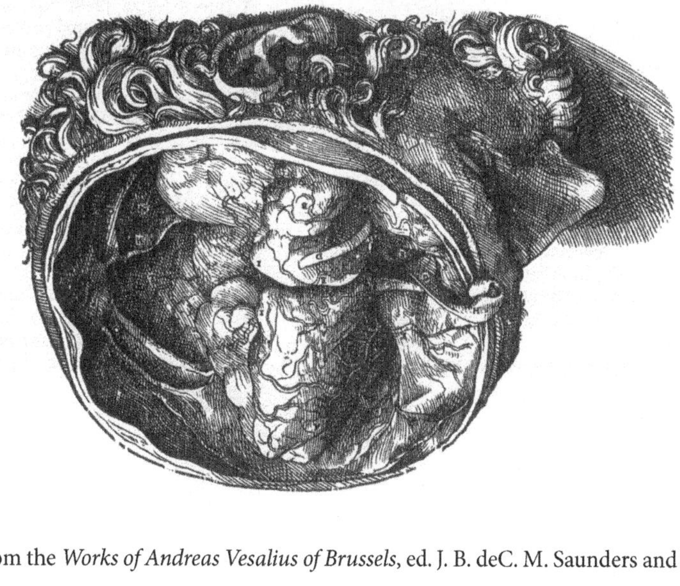

Andreas Vesalius, Plate 71 from The Illustrations From the *Works of Andreas Vesalius of Brussels*, ed. J. B. deC. M. Saunders and Charles D. O'Malley, pp. 197.

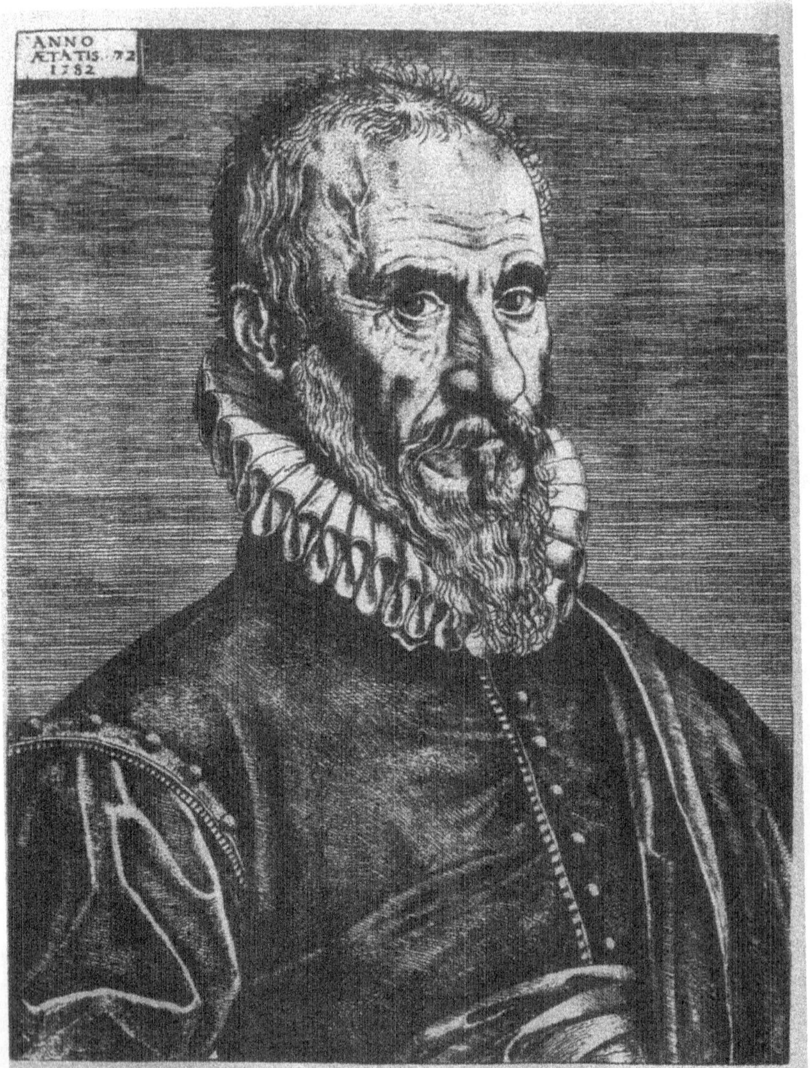

AMBROISE PARÉ

ÆT. 72

Engraved by Stephanus Delaulne 1582

Source: www.sil.si.edu/digitalcollections/hst/scientific-identity/CF/by_name_display_results.cfm?scientist=Par%C3%A9,%20 Ambroise.

Chapter 9

Ambroise Paré: *On Gunshot Wounds* (1545); *The Apologie and Treatise of Ambroise Paré Containing the Voyages Made Into Divers Places with Many of His Writings Upon Surgery* (1585)

HISTORICAL HIGHLIGHTS

- Ambroise Paré (1510–1590)
- Born at Laval, Mayenne, France
- Became apprentice to a barber-surgeon
- Acted as house surgical student at Hôtel-Dieu, Paris
- Was master barber-surgeon and entered military service under Maréchal Montejan
- Became royal surgeon for Kings Henry II, Francis II, Charles IX and Henry III
- Finished books of *On Gunshot Wounds* (1545) and *The Apologie and Treatise of Ambroise Paré Containing the Voyages Made Into Divers Places with Many of His Writings Upon Surgery* (1585)
- Introduced ligature of arteries instead of cauterization during amputation
- Contributed to design of limb and ocular prostheses
- Pioneered battlefield medicine
- Introduced the "Crow's beak" instrument for arterial ligature
- He said, "*Je le pansai.*" "*Dieu le guérit.*" ("I bandaged him". "God healed him".)

THE WRITINGS OF AMBROISE PARÉ

Introduction

What Chyrurgerie is.

Chyrurgerie is an Art, which teacheth the way by reason, how by the operation of the hand we may cure prevent and mitigate diseases, which accidentally happen unto us. Others have thought good to describe it otherwise, as that; it is that part of Physicke which undertaketh the cure of diseases by the sole industry of the hand; as by cutting, burning, sawing off, uniting fractures, restoring dislocations, and performing other workes, of which we shall hereafter treate. Chyrurgery also is thus defined by the Author of the medicinall Definitions; The quicke motion of an intrepide hand joyned with experience:

or an artificiall action by the hands used in Physicke, for some convenient intent. Yet none must thinke to attaine to any great perfection in this Art, without the helpe of the other two parts of Physicke; I say of Diet and Pharmacie, and the divers application of proper medicines, respecting the condition of the causes, diseases, symptomes, and the like circumstances, which comprehended under the names of things naturall, not naturall, and besides nature (as they commonly call them) wee intend to describe in their proper place. But if any reply, that there be many which doe the workes of Chirurgery, without any knowledge of such like things, who notwithstanding have cured desperate diseases with happy successe; let them take this for an answer,, that such things happen rather by chance, than by the industry of the Art, and that they are not provident that commit themselves to such. Because that for some one happy chance, a thousand dangerous errors happen afterwards, as *Galen* (in divers places of his Method) speakes against the Emperickes. Wherefore seeing wee have set downe Chirurgery to be a diligent operation of the hands, strengthened by the assistance of Diet and Pharmacie, wee will mow shew, what, and of what nature the operations of it aire.

Of Chirurgicall operations.

Five things are proper to the dutie of a Chirurgian; To take away that which is superfluous; to restore to their places, such things as are displaced; to separate those things which are joyned together; to joyne those which are separated; and to supply the defects of nature. Thou shalt fare more easily and happily attaine to the knowledge of these things by long use and much exercise, than by much reading of Bookes, or daily hearing of Teachers. For speech how perspicuous and elegant soever it be, cannot so vively expresse any thing, as that which is subjected to the faithfull eyes and hands.

Wee have examples of taking away that which abounds, in the amputation, or cutting off a finger, if any have sixe on one hand, or any other monstrous member that may grow out: in the lopping off a putrified part inwardly corrupted; in the extraction of a dead child, the secondine, mole or such like bodies out of a womans wombe; in taking downe of all Tumors, as Wens, Warts, Polypus, Cancers, and fleshiy excrescenses of the like nature; in the pulling forth of bullets, of peeces of maile, of darts, arrowes, shells, splinters, amd of all kind of weapons in what part of the body soever thaey be. And hee taketh away that which redounds, which plucks away the haires of the eye-lids which trouble the eye by their turning in towards it: who cuts away the web, possessing all the **Adnata,* and part of the **Cornea:* who letteth forth suppurated matter; who taketh out stones in what part soever of the body they grow; who puis out a rotten or otherwise hurtfull tooth, or cuts a naile that runs into the flesh; who cuts away part of the *uvula,* or haires that grow on the eye-lids; who taketh off a Cataract; who cuts the navill or fore-skinne of a child newly borne, or the skinnie caruncles of womens privities.

*Two tunicles of the eyes.

Examples of placing those things which are out of their naturall site, are manifest in restoring dislocated bones; in replacing of the guts and Kall fallen into the cods, or out of the navill or belly by a wound, or of the falling downe of the wombe, fundament, or great gut, or the eye hanging out of its circle, or proper place.

But wee may take examples of disjoyning those things which are continued from the fingers growing together, either by some chance, as burning, or by the imbeciltie of the forming facultie: by the disjunction of the membrane called *Hymen*, or any other troubling the necke of the wombe, by the dissection of the ligament of the tongue, which hinders children from sucking and speaking, and of that which hinders the *Glans* from being uncovered of the foreskinne; by the devision of a varicous veine, or of a halfe cut nerve or tendon, causing convulsion: by the division of the membrane stopping the auditory passage, the nose, mouth, or fundament, or the stubborne sticking together of the haires of the eye-lids. Referre to this place all the workes done by Causticks, the Saw, Trepan, Lancet, Cupping glasses, Incision Knife, Leaches, either for evacuation, derivation or revulsion sake.

The Chirurgion drawes together things separated, which healeth wounds by stitching them, by bolstering, binding, giving rest to, and fit placing the part: which repaires fractures; restores luxated parts; who by binding the vessell, staieth the violent effusion of bloud: who cicatriseth cloven lips, commonly called hare-lips; who reduces to equalitie the cavities of Ulcers, and Fistula's.

But hee repaires those things which are defective, either from the infancy, or afterwards by accident, as much as Art and Nature will suffer, who sets on an eare, an eye, a nose, one or more teeth; who fils the hollownesse of the palat eaten by the Poxe, with a thinne plate of gold or silver, or such like; who supplies the defect of the tongue in part cut off, by some new addition; who fastens to a hand, an arme or legge with fit ligaments workemanlike: who fits a doublet bumbasted, or made with iron plates to make the body straight; who fills a shooe too big with corke, or fastens a stocking or socke to a lame mans girdle to helpe his gate. We will treate more fully of all these in our following Worke. But in performing those things with the hands, we cannot but cause paine: (for who can without paine cut off an arme, or legge, devide and teare asunder the necke of the bladder, restore bones put out of their places, open ulcers, bind up wounds, and apply cauteries, and doe such like?) notwithstanding the matter often comes to that passe, that unlesse wee use a judicious hand, wee must either die, or leade the remnant of our lives in perpetuall misery. Who therefore can justly abhorre a Chirurgion for this, or accuse him of crueltie? or desire they may be served, as in ancient times the Romanes served *Archagalus,* who at the first made him free of the Citie, but presently after, because he did somwhat too cruelly burne, cut and performe the other workes of a good Chirurgion, they drew him from his house into the Campus Martius and there stoned him to death, as wee have read it recorded by *Sextus Cheroneus Plutarches* Neece by his daughter. Truly it was an inhumane kind of ingratitude, so cruelly to murder a man intent to the workes of so necessary an Art. But the Senate could not approve the act, wherefore to expiate the crime as well as then they could, they made his Statue in gold, placed it in *AEsculapius* his Temple, and dedicated it to his perpetuall memorie. For my part I very well like that saying of *Celsus;* A Chirurgeon must have a strong, stable, and intrepide hand, and a minde resolute and mercilesse; so that to heale him he taketh in hand, he be not moved to make more haste than the thing requires; or to cut lesse than is needfull; but which doth Si things as if he were nothing affected with their cries; not giving heed to the judgement of the vaine common people, who speake ill of Chirurgions because of their ignorance.

Of Aneurismas

Of an *Aneurisma,* that is, the dilatation, or springing of an Artery, veine, or Sinnew.

AN *Aneurisma* is a soft tumor yeelding to the touch, made by the bloud and spirit powred forth under the flesh and Muscles, by the dilatation or relaxation of an Artery. Yet the author of the definitions seemes to call any dilatation of any venous vessell by the name of an *Aneurisma. Galen* calls an *Aneurisma* an opening made of the *Anastomosis* of an Artery. Also an *Aneurisma* is made, when an Artery that is wounded closeth too slowly, the substance which is above it being in the meane time agglutinated, filled with flesh and cicatrized, which doth not seldome happen in opening of Arteries unskilfully performed and negligently cured; therefore *Aneurismaes* are absolutely made by the *Anastomosis,* springing, breaking, *Erosion,* and wounding of the Arteries. These happen in all parts of the body, but more frequently in the throat, especially in women after a painfull travaile. For when as they more strongly strive to hold their breath, for the more powerfull expulsion of the birth, it happens that the Artery is dilated and broken, whence followes an effusion of bloud and spirits under the skin. The signes are, a swelling, one while great, another small, with a pulsation and a colour not varying from the native constitution of the skinne. It is a soft tumor, and so yeelding to the impression of the fingers that if it peradventure be small, it wholy vanisheth, the Arterious bloud and spirits flying backe into the body of the Artery, but presendy assoone as you take your fingers away, they returne againe with like celerity. Some *Aneurismaes* doe not onely when they are pressed, but also of themselves make a sensible hissing, if you lay your eare neare to them, by reason of the motion of the vitall spirit rushing with great violence through the straitnes ot the passage.

Wherefore in *Aneurismaes* in which there is a great rupture of the Artery, such a noyse is not heard, because the spirit is carryed through a larger passage. Great *Aneurismaes* under the Arme pits, in the Groines and in other parts wherein there are large vessells, admit no cure, because so great an eruption of blood and spirit often followes uppon such an incision, that death prevents both art and Cure. Which I observed a few yeares agoe in a certaine preist of Saint *Andrewes* of the Arches, M. *John Maillet* dwelling with the chiefe President *Christopher de Thou.* Who having an *Aneurisma* at the setting on of the shoulder about the bignes of a Wall-nut, I charged him, hee should not let it be opened, for if he did, it would bring him into manifest danger of his life, and that it would be more safe for him, to breake the violence thereof with double clothes steeped in the juyce of Night-shade and Houseleeke, with new and whayey cheese mixt therewith: Or with *Unguentum de Bolo* or *Emplastrum contra rupturam* and such other refrigerating and astringent medicines, if hee would lay upon it a thin plate of Lead, and would use shorter breeches that his doublet might serve to hold it too, to which hee might fasten his breeches instead of a swathe, and in the meane time he should eschew all things which attenuate and inflame the blood, but especially he should keepe himselfe from all great straining of his voyce. Although he had used this Diet for a yeare, yet he could not so handle the matter but that the tumor increased, which he observing goes to a Barber, who supposing the tumor to be of the kinde of vulgar inpostumes, applies to it in the Evening a Causticke causing an Eschar so to open it. In the Morning such an abundance of blood flowed forth from the tumor being opened, that he therewith astonished, implores all possible ayde, and bidds that I should be called to stay this his great bleeding, and he repented that he had not followed my directions. Wherefore I am called, but when I was scarce over the threshould, he gave up his ghost with his blood. Wherefore I diligently admonish the young Chirurgion that hee do not rashly open *Aneurismas* unlesse they be small in an ignoble part, and not indued with large vessells, but rather let him performe the cure after this manner. Cut the skinne which lyes over it untill the Artery appeare, and then separate it with your knife from the particles about it, then thrust a blunt and crooked needle with a thred in it under it, binde it, then cut it off and so expect the falling off, of the thred of it selfe whiles nature covers the orifices of the cut Artery with new flesh, then the residue of the cure may be performed after the manner of simple wounds. The *Aneurismaes* which happen in the internall parts are uncurable. Such as frequently happen to those who have often had the unction and sweat for the cure of the French disease, because the blood, being so attenuated and heated therewith that it cannot be contayned in the receptacles of the Artery, it distends it to that largenesse as to hold a mans fist; Which I have observed in the dead body of a certaine Taylor, who by an *Aneurisma* of the Arterious veine suddenly whilest hee was playing at Tennis fell downe dead, the vessell being broken: his body being opened I found a great quantity of blood powred forth into the Capacity of the Chest, but the body of the

Artery was dilated to that largenesse I formerly mentioned, and the inner Coate thereof was bony. For which cause within a while after I shewed it to the great admiration of the beholders in the Physitions Schole whilest I publiquely dissected a body there; the whilst he lived said he felt a beating and a great heate over all his body by the force of the pulsation of all the Arteryes, by occasion whereof hee often swounded. Doctor *Sylvius* the Kings professor of Physicke at that time forbad him the use of Wine, and wished him to use boyled water for his drinke, and Crudds and new Cheeses for his meate, and to apply them in forme of Cataplasmes upon the grieved and swolne part. At night he used a ptisan of Barley meale and Poppy-seedes, and was purged now and then with a Clyster of refrigerating and emollient things, or with Cassia alone, by which medicines hee said hee found himselfe much better. The cause of such a bony constitution of the Arteries by *Aneurismaes* is, for that the hot and fervid blood first dilates the Coates of an Artery, then breakes them; which when it happens, it then borrowes from the neighbouring bodies a fit matter to restore the loosed continuity thereof.

This matter whilest by little and little it is dried and hardened, it degenerates into a Gristely or else a bony substance, just by the force of the same materiall and efficient causes, by which stones are generated in the reines and bladder. For the more terrestriall portion of the blood is dried and condensed by the power of the unnaturall heat contayned in the part affected with an *Aneurismae*; whereby it comes to passe that the substance added to the dilated and broken Artery is turned into a body of a bony consistence. In which the singular providence of nature, the handmaide of God is shewed, as that which, as it were by making and opposing a new wall or bancke, would hinder and breake the violence of the raging blood swelling with the abundance of the vitall spirits; unlesse any had rather to refer the cause of that hardnesse to the continuall application of refrigerating and astringent medicines. Which have power to condensate and harden, as may not obscurely be gathered by the writings of *Galen*. But beware you be not deceived by the forementioned signes; For sometimes in large *Aneurismaes* you can perceive no pulsation, neither can you force the blood into the Artery by the pressure of your fingers, either because the quantity of such blood is greater than which can be contayned in the ancient receptacles of the Artery, or because it is condensate and concrete into Clods, whereupon wanting the benefit of ventilation from the heart, it presently putrifies; Thence ensue great paine, a Gangren, and mortification of the part, and lastly the death of the Creature.

Of Hernia

Of the Tumors of the Groines and Codds, called *Hernias,* that is, Ruptures.

THE ancient Phisitions have made many kindes of Ruptures, yet indeede there are onely three to be called by that name, that is, the *Intestinalis,* or that of the guts, the *Zirbalis,* or that of the kali, and that which is mixed of them both. The other kindes of Ruptures have come into this order, rather by similitude, than any truth of the thing: for in them the Gut, or Kali doe not forsake their places.

The Greekes have given to all these severall names, both from the seat of the tumor, as also from their matter. For thus they have called an unperfect rupture which descends not beyond the Groines, nor falls downe into the Codds, *Bubonocele*: but the compleate which penetrates into the Codde, if it be by falling downe of the Gut, *Enterocele:* if from the Kali, *Epiplocele;* if from them both together, they name it *Entero-epiplocele:* but if the tumor proceede from a waterish humor, they terme it *Hydrocele;* if from winde, *Physocele*, if from both, *Hydrophysocele;* if a fleshie excrescence shall grow about the testicle, or in the substance thereof, it is named *Sarcocele*. If the veines interwoven, and divaricated diverse wayes shall be swollen in the Codde and Testicles, the tumor obtaines the name of a *Cirsocele.* But if the humors shall be shut up, or sent thither, the name is imposed upon the tumor, from the predominant humor, as we have noted in the beginning of our Tractate of tumors. The causes are many, as all too violent motions, a stroake, a fall from a high place, vomiting, a cough, leaping, riding upon a trotting horse, the sounding of trumpets, or sackbuts, the carrying, or lifting up of a heavy burden, racking, also the too immoderate use of vistide and flatulent meates; for all such things may either relaxe or breake the *Peritonœum,* as that which is a thinne and extended membrane. The signes of a *Bubonocele* are a round tumor in the Groine, which pressed, is easily forced in. The signes of an *Enterocele,* are a hard tumor in the Codde, which forced, returneth backe and departeth with a certaine murmour and paine; but the tumor proceeding of the Kall, is laxe and feeles soft like Wooll, and which is more difficultly forced in, than that which proceeds from the Guts, but yet without murmuring and paine: for the substance of the Guts, seeing it is one, and continued to it selfe, they doe not onely mutually succeede each other, but by a certaine consequence doe, as in a dance draw each other, so to avoide distention, which in their membranous body cannot be without paine, by reason of their change of place from that which is naturall, into that against nature: none of all which can befall the Kali, seeing it is a stupide body, and almost without sence, heavy, dull, and immoveable. The signes that the *Peritonœum* is broken, are the sudden increase of the tumor, and a sharpe and cutting paine; for when the *Peritonœum* is onely relaxed, the tumor grow- eth by little and little, and so consequently with small paine; yet such paine returnes so often, as the tumor is renewed by the falling downe of the Gut, or Kall, which happens not the *Peritonœum* being broken: for the way being once open, and passable to the falling body, the tumor is renued without any distention, and so without any paine to speake of The rest of the signes shall be handled in their places. Sometimes it happens that the Guts, and Kall, do so firmely adhere to the processe of the *Peritonœum,* that they can not be driven back into their proper seate. This stubborne adhesion happens by the intervention of the viscide matter, or by meanes of some excoriation caused by the rude hand of a Chirurgion, in too violently forcing of the Gut, or Kall, into their place. But also, too long stay of the gut in the codde, and the neglect of wearing a Trusse, may give occasion to such adhesion. A perfect and inveterate rupture by the breaking of the processe of the *Peritonœum* in men of full growth, never, or very seldomes admits of cure. But you must note, that by great ruptures of the *Peritonœum,* the Guts may fall into the codde, to the bignesse of a mans head, without much paine and danger of life, because the excrements, as they may easily enter, by reason of the largenesse of the place and rupture, so also they may easily returne.

Of the cure of Ruptures.

Because children are very subject to Ruptures, but those truely not fleshy or varicous, but watry, windy, and especially of the Guts, by reason of continuall and painefull crying and coughing: Therefore in the first place we will treate of their cure. Wherefore the Chirurgion, called to restore the Gut which is fallen downe, shall place the child, either on a table, or in a bed, so that his head shall be low, but his buttocks, and thighes higher; then shall he force with his hands by little and little, and gently, the Gut into its proper place; and shall foment the Groine with the astringent fomentation, described in the falling downe of the wombe. Then let him apply this remedy. *Rx, Prcescript. decoctionis quantum sufficit, farince hordei & fabarum, an.* 3j, *pulver. Aloes, Mastiches, Myrtyll & Sarcoco. an.* 3ss, *Boli Armeni* 3ij. Let them be incorporated and made a cataplasme according to Art. For the same purpose he may apply *Emplastrum contra Rupturam:* but the chiefe of the cure consists in folded clothes, and Trusses, and ligatures artificially made, that the restored gut may be contained in its place, for which purpose he shall keepe the child seated in his cradle for 30. or 40. dayes, as we mentioned before; and keepe him from crying, shouting, and coughing. *Aetius* bids steepe paper 3. dayes in water, and apply it made into a ball to the groine, the gut being first put up; for that remedy by 3. dayes adhesion wil keep it from falling down. But it wil be, as I suppose more effectuall, if the paper be steeped not in common, but in the astringent water, described in the falling downe of the wombe. Truely I have healed many by the helpe of such remedies, and have delivered them from the hands of Gelders, which are greedy of childrens testicles, by reason of the great gaine they receive from thence. They by a crafty cozenage, perswade the Parents, that the falling downe of the Gut into the Codde, is uncurable: which thing notwithstanding, experience convinceth to be false, if so be the cure be performed according to the forementioned manner, when the *Peritoneum* is onely relaxed, and not broken: for the processe thereof by which the Gut doth fall as in a steepe way, in progresse of time and age is straitned and knit together, whilest also in the meane time the guts grow thicker.

A certaine Chirurgion who deserveth credit, hath told me that he hath cured many children as thus: He beates a loadstone into fine powder, and gives it in pappe, and then hee annointes with hony the Groine, by which the gut came out, and then strewed it over with fine filings of iron. He administred this kinde of remedy for ten or twelve dayes: The part, for other things, being bound up with a ligature and trusse as was fitting. The efficacie of this remedy seemeth to consist in this; that the loadestone by a naturall desire of drawing the iron which is strewed upon the Groine, joynes to it the fleshy and fatty particles interposed betweene them, by a certaine violent impetuosity, which on every side pressing and bending the loosenesse of the *Peritoneum,* yea verily adjoyning themselves to it, in processe of rime by a firme adhesion intercept the passage and falling downe of the Gut or Kall; which may seeme no more abhorring from reason, than that we behold the loadstone it selfe through the thicknesse of a table, to draw iron after it any way. The same Chirurgion affirmed, that he frequently and happily used the following medicine. Hee burnt into ashes in an Oven red Snailes, shut up in an earthen pot, and gave the powder of them to little children in pappe, but to those which were bigger, in broath.

But we must despaire of nothing in this disease, for the cure may happily proceede in men of full growth, as of fortie yeare old, who have filled the three demensions of the body, as this following relation testifies.

There was a certaine Priest in the Parish of Saint *Andrewes*, called *John Moret*, whose office it was to sing an Epistle with a loud voice as often as the solemnitie of the day, and the thing required. Wherefore seeing he was troubled with the *Enterocele*, he came to me, requiring helpe, saying, he was troubled with a grievous paine, especially then, when he stretched his voice in the Epistle.

When I had seene the bignesse of the *Enterocele*, I perswaded him to get another to serve in his place; so having gotten leave of M. *Curio*, Clearke and Deacon of Divinity, he committed himselfe unto me: I handled him according unto Art, and commanded him he should never goe without a Trusse; and he followed my directions. When I met him some five or sixe yeares after, I asked him how he did, he answered very well, for he was wholly freed from the disease with which he was formerly troubled; which I could not perswade my selfe of, before that I had found that hee had told mee the truth, by the diligent observation of his genitals. But some sixe moneths after, he dying of a Pleurisie, I came to *Curio's* house where hee died, and desired leave to open his body, that I might observe whether nature had done any tiling at all in the passage through which the gut fell down. I call God to witnesse, that I found a certaine fatty substance about the processe of the *Peritonœum* about the bignesse of a little egge, and it did sticke so hard to that place, that I could scarce pull it away without the rending of the neighbouring parts. And this was the speedy cause of his cure. But it is most worthy of observation, and admiration, that Nature but a little helped by Art, healeth diseases which are thought incurable. The chiefe of the cure consists in this, that we firmerly stay the gut in its place, after the same manner as these two Figures shew.

In the meane time we must not omit diet. We must forbidde the use of all things, which may either relaxe, dilate, or breake the processe of the *Peritonœum*, of which I have already treated sufficiently. Sometimes, but especially in old men, the guts cannot be restored into their place by reason of the quantity of the excrements hardened in them: In this case they must not be too violently forced, but the Patient must be kept in his bed, and lying with his head low, and his knees higher up; let the following Cataplasmes be applied.

Rx, rad. altn. & lil ana. 3ij. seminis lini. & fcenug. an. 3ss, fol malvce, viol. & pariet. an. m. ss. Let them be boiled in faire water, afterwards beaten, and drawne through a searce,[1] adding thereto of new Butter without salt, and oyle of Lillies, as much as shall suffice. Make a Cataplasme in the forme of a liquid pultis. Let it be applied hot to the Codde, and bottome of the belly; by the helpe of this remedy when it had beene applied all night, the guts have not seldome beene seene of themselves, without the hand of a Chirurgion, to have returned into their proper place. The windinesse being resolved, which hindered the going backe of the excrements into another gut, whereby they might be evacuated and expelled. But if the excrements will not goe backe thus, the flatulencies, yet resisting and undiscussed, an emollient and carminative Clyster is to be admitted with a little Chymicall oyle of Turpentine, Dill, Juniper or Fennill. Clysters of Muscadine, oyle of Wallnuts and *Aqua vitœ*, and a small quantitie of any the aforesaid oyles, are good for the same purpose.

It often happens that the guts cannot yet be restored, because the processe of the *Peritonœum* is not wide enough. For when the excrements are fallen downe with the gut into the codde; they grow hard by little and little, and encrease by the accesse of flatulencies caused by resolution, which cause such a tumor as cannot be put up through that hole, by which a little before it fell downe: whereby it happens that by putrifaction of the matter there contained, come inflammations, and a new accesse of paine; and lastly, a vomitting and evacuation of the excrements by the mouth being hindered from the other passage of the fundament. They vulgarly call this affect *Miserere mei.* That you may helpe this symptome, you must rather assay extreame remedies, than suffer the Patient to die by so filthy and loathsome a death. And we must cure it by Chirurgery after this manner following. We will binde the Patient lying on his backe, upon a Table or Bench; then presently make an incision in the upper part of the codde, not touching the substance of the guts; then we must have a silver Cane or Pipe, of the thicknesse of a Goose quill, round, and gibbous in one part thereof, but somewhat hollowed in the other, as is shewed by this following Figure.

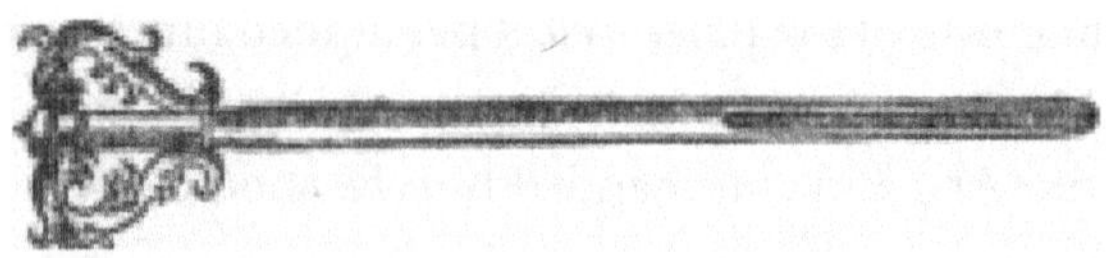

The Figure of the Pipe or Cane

We must put it into the place of the incision, and put it under the production of the *Peritonœum* being cut together with the codde, all the length of the production; that so with a sharpe knife we may divide the processe of the *Peritonœum*, according to that cavity separated from the guts there contained, by the benefit of the Cane in a right line not hurting the guts. When you have made an indifferent incision, the guts must gently be put up into the belly with your fingers, and then so much of the cut *Peritoneum* must be sowed up, as shall seeme sufficient, that by that passage made more straight, nothing may fall into the Codde, after it is cicatrized.

1 i.e. a sieve or strainer.

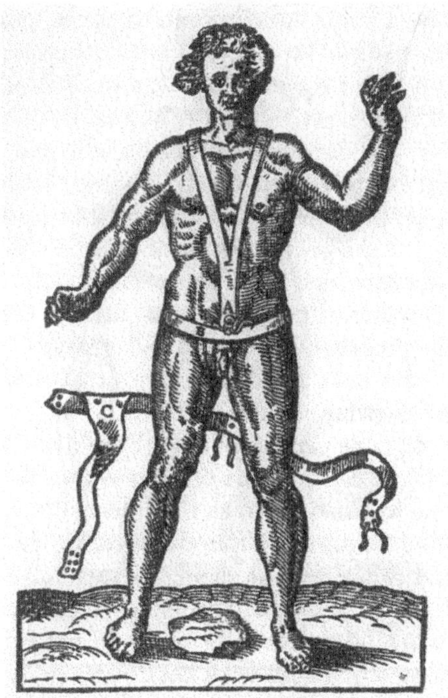

The Figure of a man broken on one side, wearing a Trusse, whose bolster must have three Tuberosities, two on the upper, and one on the lower part; and there must be a hollownesse betweene them in the middest, that they may not too straitly presse the sharebone, and so cause paine. The manner of such a Trusse, I found out not long agoe, and it seemed better and safer than the rest for to hinder the falling downe of the Gut and Kall.

A. Shewes the shoulder band which is tied before and behinde to the girdle of the Trusse.
B. The Trusse.
C. The Cavitie left in the midst of the Tuberosities.

But if there be such abundance of excrements hardned, either by the stay or heate of inflammation, that that incision is not sufficient to force the excrements into theit place, the incision must be made longer, your Cane being thrust up towards the belly: so that it may be sufficient for the free regresse of the guts into the belly. Then sow it up as is fit, and the way will be shut up against the falling downe of the guts or kall; the processe of the *Peritonœum* being made more straight, by reason of the suture; for the rest, the wound shall be cured according to Art. But before you undertake this worke, consider diligently whether the strength of the Patient be sufficient, neither attempt any thing before you have foretold, and declared the danger to the Patients friends.

Of the golden Ligature, or the *Punctus Aureus,* as they call it.

If the Rupture will not be cured by all these meanes, by reason of the great solution of the continuity of the relaxt, or broken *Peritonœum,* and the Patient by the consent of his friends there present, is ready to undergoe the danger in hope of recovery; the cure shall be attempted by that which they call the *Punctus Aureus*, or Golden tie.

For which purpose a Chirurgion which hath a skilfull and sure hand, is to be imploied. He shall make an incision about the share bone, into which he shall thrust a Probe like to the Cane, a little before

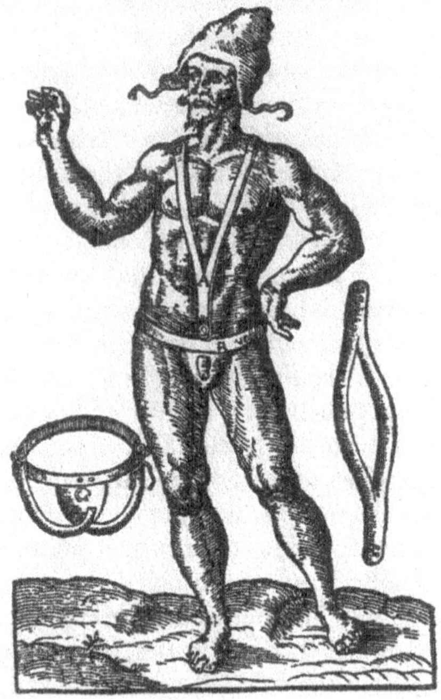

Another Figure of a man having a Rupture on both sides, skewing by what manes, what kinde of Trusse, and what shoulder-band he must be bound on each groine.

A. Sheweth the shoulder-band divided in the middest for the putting through the head.
B. The Trusse, with two bolsters, betweene which is a hole for putting through the yard. The forms of both bolsters ought to be the same with the former.

described; and thrust it long wayes under the processe of the *Peritonœum*, and by lifting it up, separate it from the adjoining fibrous, and nervous bodies, to which it adheres; then presently draw aside the spermatique vessels, with the *Cremaster,* or hanging muscle of the testicle; which being done, he shall draw aside the processe it selfe, alone by it selfe: And he shall take as much thereof, as is too lax, with small and gentle mullets, perforated in the middest, and shall with a needle, having five or sixe threeds, thrust it through as neere as hee can to the spermaticke vessels, and cremaster muscles. But the needle also must be drawne againe into the middest of the remnant of the processe, taking up with it the lipps of the wound; then the threed must be tied on a strait knot, and so much thereof must be left after the section, as may be sufficient to hang out of the wound. This threed will of it selfe be dissolved by little and little by putrefaction: neither must it be drawne out before that nature shall regenerate and restore flesh into the place of the ligature, otherwise all our labour shall be spent in vaine.

And lastly, let the wound be clensed, filled with flesh, and cicatrized, whose callous hardnesse may withstand the falling of the gut, or kall.

There are some Chirurgians who would performe this golden Ligature after another manner. They cut the skinne above the share-bone where the falling downe commonly is, even to the processe of the *Peritonœum*, and they wrap once or twice about it, being uncovered, a small golden wyre, and onely straiten the passage as much as may suffice, to amend the loosenesse of this processe, leaving the spermatique vessels at liberty. Then they twist the ends of the wyre twice or thrice with small mullets, and cut off the remnant thereof; that which remaines after the cutting, they turne in, least with the sharpnesse it should prick the flesh growing upon it. Then leaving the golden wyre there, they cure the wound like to other simple wounds, and they keepe the Patient some fifteene or twenty day in his bed, with his knees some thing higher, and his head some thing lower.

Many are healed by this meanes; others have fallen againe into the disease by reason of the ill twisting of the wire.

There is also another manner of this golden tie, which I judge more quicke and safe, even for that there is no externall body left in that part after the cure. Wherefore they wrappe a leaden wyre in steade of the golden, which comes but once about the processe of the *Peritonœum*, then they twine it as much as neede requires, that is, not too loosely, least it should leave way for the falling downe of the body, neither too straitly, least a Gangrene should come by hindring the passage of the spirits and nourishment. The ends thereof are suffered to hang out; when in processe of time, this contraction of the *Peritonœum* seemes callous, then the wyre is untwisted and gently drawne out. And the rest of the cure performed according to Art. But let not the Chirurgion thrust himselfe upon his worke rashly, without the advice of the Physition, for it diverse times comes to passe, that the testicles are not as yet fallen downe into the Codde by the too great sluggishnesse of nature, in some of a pretty growth, but remaines long in the groines, causing a tumor with paine, which thing may make a good Chirurgion beleeve that it is an *Enterocele.* Therefore whilst he labours by repelling medicines and trusses to force backe this tumor, he encreaseth the paine, and hinders the falling downe of the testicles into the codde. I observed this not long agoe in a Boy, which an unskilfull Chirurgion had long, and grievously troubled, as if he had had a rupture: for when I had observed that there was but one stone in the Codde, and knew the Boy was never gelt, I bid them cast away the plasters, and trusses, and wisht his Parents that they should suffer him to run and leape, that so the idleing stone might be drawne into the Codde, which thing by little and little, and without paine, had the event, as I foretold. That the reason of this effect may be understood, we must know a man differs from a woman, onely in efficacie of heat; but it is the nature of strong heat to drive forth, as of cold to keepe in. Hence it is that the stones in men hang forth in the codde, but in women they He hid in the lower belly. Therefore it happens that in some males more cold by nature, the testicles are shut up some certaine time, untill at length they are forest downe into the codde by youthfull heat. But that we may returne to our former treatise of the codde, although that way of curing ruptures wants not paine and danger, yet it is safer than that which is performed by gelding, which by the cruelty thereof exposes the Patient to manifest danger of death. For the Gelders whilst they feare least when die cure is finshed, the relaxation may remaine, pull with violence the processe of the *Peritonœum* from the parts to which it adheres, and together with it a nerve of the sixth conjugation which runnes to the stones; they offer the same violence to the spermaticke vessels; by which things ensue great paine, convulsion, effiuxe of bloud, inflammation, putrefaction, and lastly death, as I have observed in many whom I have dissected, having died a few dayes after their gelding. Although some escape these dangers, yet they are deprived of the facility of generation for all their life after, for performance whereof nature hath bestowed the testicles, as parts principally necessary for the conservation of mankinde. Through which occasion *Galen* hath not feared to preferre them before the heart; because the heart is the beginning of life, but the testicles of a better life; for it is farre more noble to live well, than simply and absolutely to live; therefore Eunuches degenerate into a womanish nature, for they remaine without beards, their voice is weake, their courage failes them, and they turne cowards; and seeing they are unfit for all humane actions, their life cannot but be miserable. Wherefore I will never subscribe to the cutting out of the stones, unlesse a *Sarcocele* or Gangrene invade them. But that the way of performing the *Punctus aureus* may be better knowne, I have thought good here to set the instruments, by which this operation is performed, before your view.

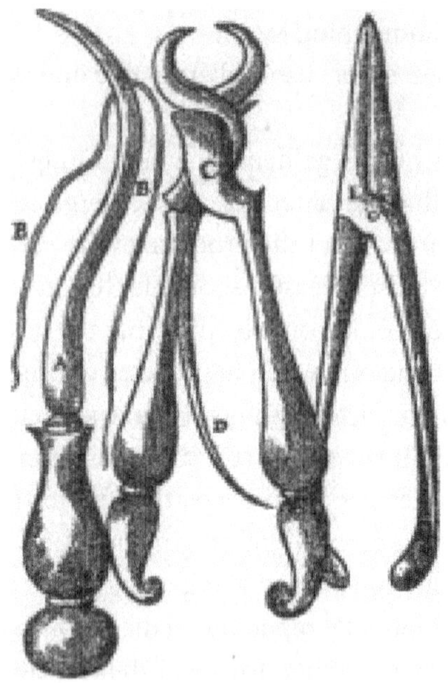

A. Shewes a croked needle, having an eye not farrefrom the point, through which you may put the golden wyre.
B. B. The golden wyre put through the eye of the needle.
C. The mullets or Pincers, to cut away the wast or superfluous ends of the wyre.
D. The springe of the mullets.
E. The mullets to twist the ends of the wyre together.

Another more easie and safe way to restore the Gut and Kall.

Theodoricke and *Guido* have invented another way of performing this operation. They put backe into their places the Gut and Kall being fallen downe, the Patient being so placed, that his thighs are high and his head is somewhat low; then they draw aside the lower portion of the production of the *Peritonaeum,* and also the spermaticke vessels, and cremaster muscle to the *Ischium*; then by applying a causticke fitted to the age and disease, they burne the other part of the processe, directly perpendicular to the share- bone, where the Gut did fall downe. Then they pull off the eschar thus made with a knife even to the quicke, then they apply another causticke in the same place, which may go even to the bone, then procure the falling of this Eschar made on the foresaid processe. And afterwards they heale the ulcer which remaines, which presendy contracting somewhat, a thicke *Callus* so keeps up the Guts and Kall, that it bindes them from falling down into the Cod. This way of restoring the Gut and Kall, though it be safer and more facile; yet the Chirurgion must not attempt it, if the Guts or Kall sticke so fast, agglutinated to the processe of the *Peritonœum*, that they cannot be severed, nor put backe into their places (for from the guts so burnt and violated, greater mischiefe would ensue) if by the broken and too much dilated processe, the bodies thereby restrained, make an exceeding great tumor by their falling downe; if the testicle yet lying in the groine as in a *Bubonocele,* a kinde of *Enterocele,* being not yet descended into the *Scrotum* or Codde; if the Patients be not come to such age as they can keepe themselves from stirring, or hold their excrements whiles the operation is performed.

Of the cure of other kinds of Ruptures.

Epiplocele is the falling downe of the Kali into the Groine, or Codde, it hath the same causes as an *Enterocele*. The signes have beene explained. It is not so dangerous, nor infers a consequence of so many evill symptomes, as the *Enterocele* doth, yet the cure is the same with the other.

Hydrocele is a waterish tumor in the Codde, which is gathered by little and litde betweene the membranes encompassing the testicles, especially the *Dartos* and *Erythroides*; it may be called a particular dropsie, for it proceeds from the same causes, but chiefely from the defect of native heate. The signes are a tumor encreasing slowly without much paine, heavy, and almost of a glassie clearenesse, which you may perceive by holding a candle on the other side, by pressing the Codde above, the water flowes downe, and by pressing it below, it rises upwards, unlesse per-adventure in too great a quantity it fills up the whole capacity of the Codde, yet it can never be forced or put up into the belly as the Kall or Guts may, for oft times it is contained in a Cyste, or bagge; it is distinguished from a *Sarcocele*, by the smoothnesse and equality thereof. The cure must first be tried with resolving, drying, and discussing medicines, repeated often before, and in the Chapter of the Dropsie; this which followes I have often tried with good successe.

Rx, Ung. comitissœ,& desiccat rub. an. 3ij. malaxentur simul; and make a medicine for your case. The water by this kinde of remedy is digested and resolved, or rather dried up, especially if it be not in too great quantity. But if the swelling, by reason of the great quantity of water will not yeeld to those remedies, there is neede of Chirurgery; the Cod and membranes wherein the water is contained, must be thrust through with a Seton, that is, with a large three- square pointed needle, thred with a skeane of silke; you must thrust your needle presently through the holes of the mullets made for that purpose, not touching the substance of the Testicles. The skean of thred must be left there, or removed twise or thrise a day, that the humor may drop downe, and be evacuated by little and little. But if the paine be more vehement by reason of the Seton, and inflammation come upon it, it must be taken away, and neglecting the proper cure of the disease, we must resist the symptomes.

Some Practitioners use not a Seton, but with a Razor, or incision knife, they open the lower part of the Cod, making an incision some halfe fingers breadth long, penetrating even to the contained water; alwayes leaving untouched the substance of the Testicles and vessels, and they keepe the wound open, untill all the water seemes evacuated; truly by this onely way the cure of a watery rupture whose matter is contained in a Cyste, is safe, and to be expected; as wee have said in our Treatise of Tumors in generall.

The *Pneumatocele*, is a flatulent tumor in the Codde, generated by the imbecility of heate residing in the part.

It is knowne by the roundnesse, lenity, renitencie[2] and shining. It is cured by prescribing a convenient diet, by the application of medicines which resolve and discusse flatulencies, as the seeds of Annis, Fennell, Faenugreeke, *Agnus Castus,* Rue, *Origanum*, other things set downe by *Avicen* in his Treatise of Ruptures. I have often used with good successe for this purpose, *Emplastrum Vigonis cum mercurio;* and *Emplastrum Diacalcitheos,* dissolved in some good wine, as Muscadine, with oyle of Bayes.

A *Sarcocele* is a tumor against nature, which is generated about the stones by a schyrrhus flesh. Grosse and viscide humors breed such kind of flesh, which the part could not overcome and assimulate to it selfe; whence this overabundance of flesh proceeds, like as Warts doe. *Varices,* or swollen veines often associate this tumor; and it increases with paine. It is knowne by the hardnesse, asperitie, inequality, and roughnesse. It cannot be cured but by amputation or cutting it away; but you must diligently observe,

2 i.e. resistance.

that the flesh be not growne too high, and have already seazed upon the Groine, for so nothing can be attempted without the danger of life.

But if any may thinke, that he in such a case may somewhat ease the patient by the cutting away of some portion of this same soft flesh, he is deceived. For a *Fungus* will grow, if the least portion thereof be but left, being an evill farre worse than the former; but if the tumor be either small or indifferent, the Chirurgion taking the whole tumor, that is, the testicle, tumefied through the whole substance, with the processe encompassing it, and adhering thereto on every side, and make an incision in the Codde, even to the tumor; then separate all the tumid body, that is, the testicle from the Codde; then let him thrust a needle with a strong threed in it, through the middest of the processe above the region of the swolne testicle; and then presently let him thrust it the second time through the same part of the processe; then shall both the ends of the threed be tied on a knot, the other middle portion of the *Peritonœum* being comprehended in the same knot. This being done, he must cut away the whole processe with the testicle comprehended therein. But the ends of the threed, with which the upper part of the processe was bound, must be suffered to hang some length out of the wound, or incision of the Codde. Then a repercussive medicine shall be applied to the wound, and the neighbouring parts with a convenient ligature. And the cure must be performed as we have formerly mentioned.

The *Cirsocele* is a tumor of veines dilated, and woven with a various and mutuall implication about the testicle and codde, and swelling with a grosse and melancholy bloud. The causes are the same as those of the *Varices*. But the signes are manifest.

To heale this tumor, you must make an incision in the codde, the bredth of two fingers to the *Varix*. Then you must put under the varicous veine, a needle having a double threed in it, as high as you can, that you may binde the rootes thereof: then let the needle be againe put after the same manner about the lower part of the same veine, leaving the space of two fingers between the Ligatures. But before you binde the thread of this lowest Ligature, the *Varix* must bee opened in the middest, almost after the same manner as you open a veine in the arme to let bloud: That so this grosse blood causing a tumor in the Cod, may be evacuated as is usually done in the Cure of the *varices*. The wound that remaines shall be cured by the rules of Art after the manner of other wounds: Leaving the threads in it, which will presently fall away of themselves. To conclude then, it being growne callous especially in the upper part thereof, where die veine was bound, it must be Cicatrized, for so afterwards the bloud cannot be strained, or run that way.

Hernia Humoralis is a tumor generated by the confused mixture of many humors in the Cod or betweene the tunicles which involue the testicles, often also in the proper substance of the testicles. It hath like causes, signes and cure as other tumors. While the cure is in hand, rest, trusses, and fit rowlers to sustaine and beare up the testicles are to be used.

OF WOUNDS IN GENERALL

What a Wound is, what the kindes and differences thereof are, and from whence they may be drawne, or derived.

WOUND is a solution of Continuity, caused by a stroake, fall, or bite, newly done, bloody, and with putrifaction, and filth. They also call it a new simple ulcer; for the solution of continuity happens to all parts of the body; but according to the diversity of the parts, it hath divers names amongst the Greekes. For in the flesh it is called *Helcos*, in the bone *Catagma*, in the nerve *Spasma*, in the ligament *Thlasma*, in the vesselles *Apospasma*, in the Muscles *Regma:* and that solution of continuity, which happens in the vessells, their mouths being open, is termed *Anastomosis,* that which happens by erosion, *Anaurosis*; that which is generated by sweating out and transcolation, *Diapedesis.* That these may bee the more easily understood, I have thought good to describe them in the table on p. 118.

Of the causes of Wounds.

All things which may outwardly assayle the body with force and violence, may be counted the causes of wounds; which are called greene, and properly bloody. These things are either animate, or inanimate. The animate, as the bitings, and prickings of beasts. The Inanimate, as the stroake of an arrow, sword, clubb, gunne, stone, a dagger, and all such like things.

From the variety of such like causes, they have divers shall be powred out into any capacity or belly) that so the part freed from the superfluous quantity of blood may be lesse subject to inflammation. Therefore the lippes of the wounds shall be put together, and shall bee kept so joyned by suture and ligatures: Not truly of all, but onely of those which both by their nature, and magnitude, as also by the condition of the parts in which they are, are worthy and capable of both the remedies. For a simple and small solution of continuity, stands only in neede of the Ligature which we call incarnative, especially, if it be in the Armes or Legges; but that which divides the Muscles transversly, stands in need of both Suture and Ligature; that so the Lippes which are somewhat farre distant from each other, and as it were drawne towards their beginnings, and ends, may bee conjoyned.

If any portion of a fleshy substance by reason of some great cut shall hang downe, it must necessarily be adjoyned and kept in the place by suture. The more notable and large Wounds of all the parts, stand in need of Suture, which doe not easily admit a Ligature, by reason of the figure and site of the part in which they are, as the Eares, Nose, Hairy-scalpe, Eie-liddes, Lippes, Belly and Throat.

There are three sorts of Ligatures, by the joynt consent of all the Ancients. They commonly call the first, a Gluti-native or Incarnative; the second Expulsive, the third Retentive. The Glutinative or Incarnative is fit for simple, greene, and yet bloody wounds. This consists of two ends, and must so be drawne, that beginning on the contrary part of the wound, wee may so goe upwards, partly crossing it, and going downewards againe, we may closely joyne together the lippes of the Wound. But let the Ligature be neither too strait, least it may cause inflammation or paine; nor too loose, least it be of no use, and may not well containe it.

The Expulsive Ligature is fit for sanious and fistulous úlcers, to presse out the filth contained in them. This is performed with one Rowler, having one simple head; the beginning of binding must bee taken from the bottome of the *Sinus*, or bosome thereof; and there it must be bound more straightly, and so by little and little going higher, you must remit something of that rigour, even to the mouth of the Ulcer. That so (as we have said) the sanious matter may be pressed forth.

The Retentive Ligature is fit for such parts as cannot suffer straight binding, such are the Throat, Belly, as also all parts oppressed with paine; For the part vexed with paine, abhorreth binding. The use thereof, is to hold to ocall Medicines. It is performed with a Rowler, which consists some whiles of one, some whiles of more heads. All these Rowlers ought to be of linnen, and such as is neither too new, nor too old; neither too coarse, nor too fine. Their breadth must be proportionable to the parts to which they shall bee applyed; the indication of their large- nesse being taken from their magnitude, figure and site. As wee shall shew more at large in our Tractates of Fractures and Dislocations.

The Chirurgion shall performe the first scope of curing Wounds, which is of preserving the temper of the Wounded part, by appointing a good order of Diet by the Prescript of a Physition, by using universall and locall Medicines. A slender, cold, and moyst Diet must be observed, untill that time be passed, wherein the patient may be safe and free from accidents which are usually feared. Therefore let him bee fed sparingly, especially if he be plethorick; he shall abstaine from salt and spiced flesh, and also from wine; If he shall be of a Cholerick or Sanguine nature: In steed of wine he shall use the decoction of Barly or Liquerice, or Water and Sugar. He shall keepe himselfe quiet; for rest is (in *Celsus* opinion) the very best Medicine. Hee shall avoyde Venery, Contentions, Brawles, Anger, and other perturbations of the minde. When hee shall seeme to bee past danger, it will bee time to fall by little and little to his accustomed maner of diet and life. Universall remedies are Phlebotomies and purging, which have force to divert and hinder defluxion, wherby the temper of the part might be in danger of change.

For Phlebotomy it is not alwayes necessary, as in small wounds and bodies, which are neither troubled with ill humours, nor plethoricke: But it is onely required in great wounds, where there is feare of defluxion, paine, *Delirium,* Raving and unquietnesse; and lastly in a body that is Plethoricke, and when the joynts, tendons, or nerves are wounded. Gentle purgations must bee appointed, because the humours are moved and inraged by stronger; whence there is danger of defluxion and inflammation: wherefore nothing is to be attempted in this case, without the advice of a Physition.

The Topick and particular Medicines are Agglutinative, which ought to be indued with a drying and astrictive quality, whereby they may hold together the lips of the wound, and drive away defluxion, having alwayes regard to the nature of the part and the greatnesse of the disease. The Simple Medicines are *Olibanum, Aloes, Sarcocolla, Bole-Armenick, Terra sigillata, Sanguis Draconis,* Common and Venice Turpentine, Gumme *Elemnii,* Plantane, Horse-tayle, the greater Comfery, *Farina Volatilis,* and many other things of this kind, which wee shall speake of hereafter in our Antidotary.

The fifth scope of healing wounds, is the Correction of those Symptomes or Accidents which are accustomed to follow wounds, which thing verily makes the Chirurgion have much to doe; For he is often forced to omit the proper cure of the disease, so to resist the accidents and symptomes, as bleeding, paine, inflammation, a feaver, convulsion, palsie, talking idly, or distraction, and the like. Of which wee shall treat briefly and particularly, after we have first spoken of Sutures as much as we shall thinke fitting for this place.

Of Sutures.

When Wounds are made alongst the thighes, Legs, and armes, they may easily want Sutures, because the solution of continuity is easily restored by Ligatures, but when they are made overthwart, they require a Suture, because the flesh and all such like parts, being cut are drawne towards the sound parts; whereby it comes to passe that they part the further each from other; wherefore that they may be joyned and so kept, they must be sowed, and if the wound be deepe, you must take up much flesh with your needle; for if you onely take hold of the upper part, the wound is onely superficially healed: but the matter shut up, and gathered together in the bottome of the wound, will cause abscesses and hollow Ulcers: Wherefore now wee must treate of making of Sutures.

The first, called *Interpunctus,* leaves the distance of a fingers breadth, and therfore is fit for the greene wounds of the fleshy parts, which cannot be cured with a Ligature, and in which no heterogeneous or strange body remaines; It is performed after this manner. You must have a smooth needle with a threed in it, having a three square point, that so it may the better enter the skin, with the head of it some what hollowed, that the threed may lie therein; for so the needle will the better goe through. You must also have a litde pipe with a hole or window in the end, which you must hold and thrust against the lip of the wound, that it bee not moved to the one side or other, whilest you thrust thorough the needle. And that wee may see thorough that window when the needle is thrust thorough, and also draw it together with the threed, and withall hold the lip of the wound in more firmly, that it follow not at the drawing forth of the needle and threed. Having thus pierced the lips of the wound, tie a knot, neere to which cut off the threed; least that if any of it bee left below the knot, it may so stick to the Emplasters that it cannot be plucked and separated from them without paine, when they are taken off. But you must note, the first stitch must be thrust through the midst of the wound, and then the second must be in that space which is betweene the midst and one of the ends; but when you have made your stitches, the lips of the wound must not be too closely joyned, but a little space must be left open betweene them, that the matter may have free passage forth, and the inflammation and paine may be avoyded: otherwise if they shall be closely joyned together without any distance betweene, a tumor after arising when the matter shall come to suppuration, the lips will be so much distended that they may easily be broken by the stifnesse of the threed. But you must neither take hold of too much nor too little flesh with your needle, for too little will not hold, and too much causeth paine and inflammation. And besides leaves an ill favoured scarre. Yet in deepe wounds, such as are those which are made in the thicker Muscles, the needle must be thrust home, that so it may comprehend more of the fleshy substance; least the thred drawne away by the weight of the flesh not taken hold of, may bee broken. But oft times wounds are seene made in such places as it will be needfull, the Chirurgion should have a crooked needle and pipe, otherwise the Suture will not succeede according to his desire. Wherefore I have thought good to set forth both their figures, that you may use either as occasion shall serve.

The second Suture is made just after the same manner as the Skinners sowe their fels or furrs. And the guts must be sowed with this kind of Suture, (if they shall be at any time wounded) that the excrements come not forth by the wound.

The third Suture is made by one or more needles having threed in them, thrust through the wound, the threed being wrapped to and againe at the head and the point of the needle, as boyes use to fasten their needle, for feare of losing it, in their caps, or clothes. This kind of Suture is fit in the curing and healing of Hare-lips.

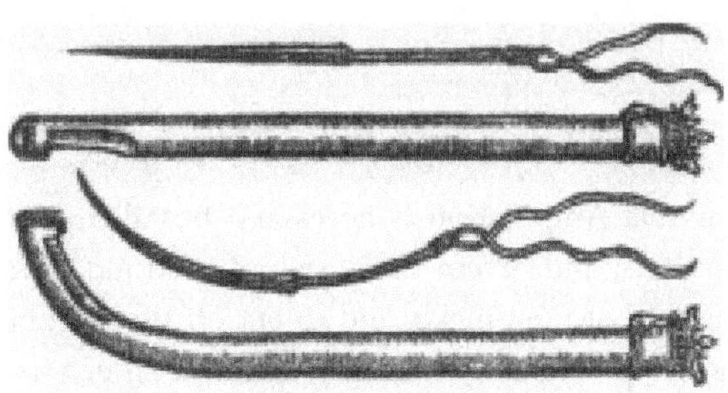

The Figure of Pipes with fenestrels in them, and Needles fit for Sutures.

The fourth kind of Suture is tearmed *Gastroraphia*, invented for the restoring and uniting the great Muscles of the *Epigastrium*, or lower belly, cut with a great wound together with the *Peritonæum* lying under them.

The fifth kind is called the Dry Suture, which we use onely in the wounds of the face.

The signes of a perfect *Necrosis* or Mortification.

YOU shall certainly know that a Gangreene is turned into a Sphacell, or mortification, and that the part is wholly and throughly dead, if it looke of a blacke colour, and bee colder than stone to your touch, the cause of which coldnesse is not occasioned by the frigiditie of the aire; if there bee a great softnesse of the part, so that if you presse it with your finger it rises not againe, but retaines the print of the impression. If the skinne come from the flesh lying under it; if so great and strong a smell exhale (especially in an ulcerated Sphacell) that the standers by cannot endure or suffer it; if a sanious moisture, viscide, greene or blackish flow from thence; if it bee quite destitute of sense and motion, whether it be pulled, beaten, crushed, pricked, burnt, or cut off. Here I must admonish the young Chirurgion, that hee be not deceived concerning the losse or privation of the sense of the part.

For I know very many deceived as thus; the patients pricked on that part would say they felt much paine there. But that feeling is oft deceiptfull, as that which proceeds rather from the strong apprehension of great paine which formerly reigned in the part, than from any facultie of feeling as yet remaining. A most cleare and manifest argument of this false and deceitful sense appeares after the amputation of the member; for a long while after they will complaine of the part which is cut away.

Verily it is a thing wondrous strange and prodigious, and which will scarse be credited, unlesse by such as have seene with their eyes, and heard with their eares the patients who have many moneths after the cutting away of the Legge, grievously complained that they yet felt exceeding great paine of that Leg so cut off. Wherefore have a speciall care least this hinder your intended amputation; a thing pittifull, yet absolutely necessary for to preserve the life of the patient and all the rest of his body, by cutting away of that member which hath all the signes of a Sphacell and perfect mortification; for otherwise the neglected fire will in a moment spread over all the body, and take away all hope of remedy; for thus *Hippocrates* wisheth: That Sections, Ustions, and Terebrations must bee performed as soone as neede requires.

Where Amputation must be made.

It is not sufficient to know that Amputation is necessary; but also you must learne in what place of the dead part, it must bee done, and herein the wisedome and judgement of the Chirurgion is most apparent. Art bids to take hold of the quicke, and to cut off the member in the sound flesh; but the same art wisheth us, to preserve whole that which is sound, as much as in us lies. I will shew thee by a familiar example how thou maist carry thy selfe in these difficulties. Let us suppose, that the foote is mortified even to the anckle; here you must attentively marke in what place you must cut it off. For unlesse you take hold of the quicke flesh in the amputation, or if you leave any putrefaction, you profit nothing by amputation, for it will creepe and spread over the rest of the body. It befits Physicke ordained for the preservation of mankind, to defend from the iron or instrument and all manner of injurie, that which enjoyes life and health. Wherefore you shall cut off as little of that which is sound as you possibly can; yet so that you rather cut away that which is quicke, than leave behind any thing that is perished, according to the advice of *Celsus*. Yet oft times the commodity of the action of the rest of the part, and as it were a certaine ornament thereof, changes this counsell. For if you take these two things into your consideration they will induce you in this propounded case and example, to cut off the Legge some five fingers breadth under the knee. For so the patient may more fitly use the rest of his Legge and with lesse trouble, that is, he may the better goe on a woodden Legge; for otherwise, if according to the common rules of Art, you cut it off close to that which is perished the patient will be forced with trouble to use three Legges instead of two.

For I so knew Captaine *Francis Clerke*, when as his foote was strucken off with an iron bullet shot forth of a man of warre, and afterwards recovered and healed up, hee was much troubled and wearied with the heavy and unprofitable burden of the rest of his Legge, wherefore though whole and sound he caused the rest thereof to bee cut off, some five fingers breadth below his knee; and verily hee useth it with much more ease and facility than before in performance of any motion. Wee must doe otherwise if any such thing happen in the Arme; that is, you must cut off as little of the sound part as you can. For the actions of the Legges much differ from these of the armes, and chiefly in this that the body rests not, neither is carried upon the armes, as it is upon the feete and Legges.

How the section or amputation must be performed.

The first care must be of the patients strength, wherefore let him be nourished with meats of good nutriment, easie digestion, and such as generate many spirits; as with the yolkes of Egges, and bread tosted and dipped in Sacke or Muskedine. Then let him bee placed, as is fit, and drawing the muscles upwards toward the sound parts, let them be tyed with a straite ligature a little above that place of the member which is to be cut off, with a strong and broad fillet like that which women usually bind up their haire withall; This ligature hath a threefold use; the first is, that it hold the muscles drawne up together with the skin, so that retiring backe presently after the performance of the worke, they may cover the ends of the cut bones, and serve them in stead of boulsters or pillowes when they are healed up, and so suffer with lesse paine the compression in susteining the rest of the body; besides also by this meanes the wounds are the sooner healed and cicatrized; for by how much more flesh or skinne is left upon the ends of the bones, by so much they are the sooner healed and cicatrized. The second is, for that it prohibites the fluxe of blood by pressing and shutting up the veines and arteries. The third is, for that it much dulls the sense of the part by stupefying it; the animall spirits by the straite compression being hindred from passing in by the Nerves: Wherefore when you have made your ligature, cut the flesh even to the bone with a sharpe and well cutting incision knife, or with a crooked knife, such as is here expressed.

Now you must note, that there usually lyes betweene the bones, a portion of certaine muscles, which you cannot easily cut with a large incision or dismembring knife; wherefore you must carefully divide it and separate it wholly from the bone, with an instrument made neately like a crooked incision knife. I thought good to advertise thee hereof; for if thou shouldest leave any thing besides the bone to bee divided by the saw, you would put the patient to excessive paine in the performance thereof; for soft things as flesh tendons and membranes, cannot be easily cut with a saw. Therefore when you shall come to the bared bone, all the other parts being wholly cut asunder and divided, you shall nimbly divide it with a little saw about some foote and three inches long, and that as neare to the sound flesh as you can. And then you must smooth the front of the bone which the saw hath made rough.

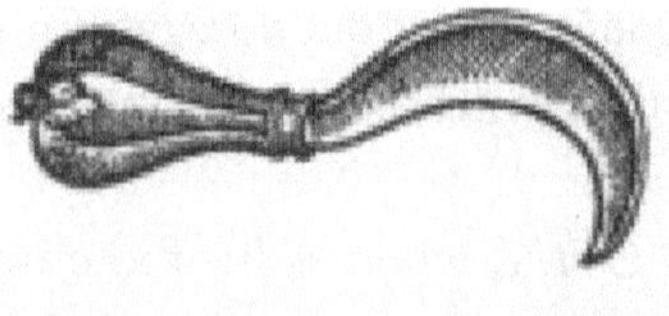

A crooked knife fit for dismembring; or a dismembring knife.

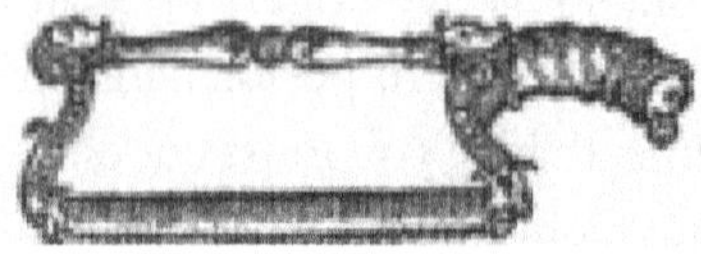

The Figure of such a Saw

How to stanch the bleeding when the member is taken off.

When you have cut off and taken away the member, let it bleed a little according to the strength of the patient, that so the rest of the part may afterwards be lesse obnoxious to inflammation and other symptomes; Then let the Veines and Arteries be bound up as speedily and streightly as you can; that so the course of the flowing blood may bee stopped and wholly stayed. Which may be done by taking hold of the vessells with your Crowes beake, whereof this is the figure.

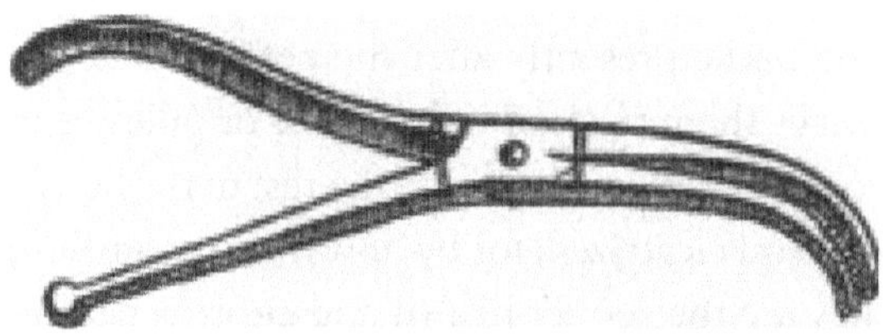

The Crowes beake fit for to draw the vessells forth of the flesh wherein they lye hid, that so they may be tyed or bound fast.

The ends of the vessells lying hid in the flesh, must be taken hold of & drawn with this instrument forth of the muscles whereinto they presently after the amputation withdrew themselves, as all parts are still used to withdraw themselves towards their originalls. In performance of this worke, you neede take no great care, if you together with the vessells comprehend some portion of the neighbouring parts, as of the flesh, for hereof will ensue no harme; but the vessells will so bee consolidated with the more ease, than if they being bloodlesse parts should grow together by themselves. To conclude, when you have so drawne them forth, binde them with a strong double thred.

How after the blood is stanched, you must dresse the wounded member.

When you have tyed the Vessells, loose your Ligature which you made above the place of amputation; then draw together the lippes of the wound with foure stitches made acrosse, having taken good hold of the flesh; for thus you shall draw over the bones that part of the skinne and cut muscles drawne upwards before the amputation, and cover them as close as you can, that so the ayre may the lesse come at them, and that so the wound may bee the more speedily agglutinated. But when wee say, draw together the lippes of the wound with foure stitches, you must not so understand it, as that you must endeavour, to draw them so close as to touch each other, for that is impossible; for the stitches would sooner breake out, and so the part would lye bare. Wherefore it will be sufficient to draw them indifferent close together, that so you may suffer the skinne and flesh thereunder to enjoy its former liberty which it possest before the drawing up, and so in fine by natures assistance, the wound may be the more easily agglutinated.

How you must stoppe the bleeding, if any of the bound up vessels chance to get loose.

The businesse hitherto being performed as we said, if peradventure it happen that any bandage of any of the vessels be unloosed; then must you againe binde the member with that kinde of Ligature which you did before the amputation thereof. Or else, which is better, more easily and lesse painefull, let your servant taking hold of the member with both his hands, pressing his fingers strait, stoppe the passage of the loosed vessell, for so hee may stanch the bleeding. Then let the worke-master take a needle some foure fingers long, square, and having sharpe edges, drawing after it a three or foure doubled strong thred. With this let him binde the vessell after the following manner. Let him thrust his needle on the outside into the flesh, some halfe fingers breadth from the loosed vessell untill he come to the end thereof, then let him put it about it, and bring it backe againe, but so that there be no more than the space of a fingers bredth betweene the going in, and comming forth of the needle. In this space let him put a linnen ragge three or foure times doubled, and thereupon bind somewhat straite the two ends of the thred together. For so he shall hinder the knot from hurting the flesh which lyes under it in the bindings, and also adde strength thereto. For so the bound up orifice of the vessell will in short space be agglutinated to the adjoyning flesh, and that so firmely, that there hath never beene seene, any one drop of blood to have flowed from a vessell so bound up. But if the blood which flowes forth proceede from any small vessell, you must not use this suture and ligature, nor make any such great matter thereof; for it will quickly be stanched by the only application of Astringents presently to be mentioned.

OF FRACTURES

What a Fracture is, and what the differences thereof are.

FRACTURE, in Galens opinion, is the solution of continuitie in a bone, which by the Greeks is called *Catagma*. There are many sorts of hurting or offending the bones: as the drawing them asunder, luxation, or putting them out of joynt; their unnaturall growing together, their cutting or dividing a-sunder; contusion, abscesse, putrefaction, rottennesse, the *periostium* being laid bare, violated or lost; and lastly, that whereof we now treate, a Fracture. Again, the varieties of Fractures are almost infinite. For one is complete and perfect, another imperfect; one runnes long-wise, another transverse, another oblique; one while it is broken into great peeces, another while into little and small scales, which have eyther a blunt, or else a sharpe end, and pricke the adjacent bodies of the muscles, nerves, veines or arteries. It somtimes happens, that the bone is not broken into splinters, that is, long-wayes, but together, and at once into two peeces overthwart, which Fracture is called *Raphanedon*, that is, after the maner of a Raddish.

A Fracture is made *Caryedon*, or like a nut, when as the bone flyes into many small peeces, severed each from other, as when a Nut is broken with a hammer or mallet upon an Anvile: Which fracture is also termed *Alphitidon*, by reason of the resemblance it hath to meale or floure; and such is often seene in fractures made by bullets, shot out of guns and such fiery engines. Contrary to these are those fractures which are called *Schidacidon*, as rent into splinters, or after the manner of a boord or peece of timber, that is, right-downe, and alongst the bone: and these fractures are eyther apparent to the eye, or else not apparent, and therefore called Capillarie, being so small, as that they cannot be perceived by the eye, unlesse you put inke upon them, and then shave them with your Scrapers. Sometimes the bone is only pressed downe by the stroke, sometimes on the contrarie it flyes up, as if it were vaulted. They call it attrition, when the bone is broken into many small fragments, and as it were scales or chips. The fragments of fractured bones are somtimes smooth and polished, other- whiles unequall, and as it were sharpe and rough with little teeth, or prickes. Some fractures touch onely the surface of the bone, fetching off only a scale; othersome change not the site of fractured bones, but only cleaves them length-waies, without the plucking away of any fragment; othersome penetrate even to their marrow.

Furthermore some Fractures are simple and alone by themselves; othersome are accompanied with a troop of other affects and symptomes; as a wound, haemorrhagye, inflammation, gangrene, and the like. Hereunto you may also adde the differences drawne from the parts which the Fractures possesse; as from the head, ribs, limbs, joynts, and other members of the bodie. Adde also these which are taken from the habit of bodies, aged, young, full of ill humors, well tempered; almost all which have their proper and peculiar indications for curing. Now the causes of Fractures, are the too violent assaults or stroaks of all exter- nall things, which may cut, bruise, breake, or shake: in this number of causes may also be reckoned fals from high places, and infinite other things, which would be long and tedious to reckon up.

Of the signes of a Fracture.

We may know by evident signes that a bone is broken: the first whereof, and most certaine, is, when by handling the part which we suspect to be broken, wee feele peeces of the bone severed asunder, and heare a certaine crackling of these peeces under our hands, caused by the attrition of the shattered bones. Another signe is taken from the impotencie of the part, which chiefly bewrayes its selfe, when both the bones, the legge, and brace-bones, the ell and wand[3] are broken. For if onely the brace-bone or wand be broken, the Patient may goe on his legge, and stirre his arme: for the brace-bone serves for the sustaining of the muscles, and not of the bodie, as the legge bone doth. The third signe is drawne from the figure of the part changed besides nature: for it is there hollow, from whence the bone is flowne or gone, but gibbous or bunching out whither it is runne. Great paine in the interim torments the patient by reason of the wronged *periostium*, and that membrane which involves the marrow and the sympathie of the adjacent parts which are compressed or pricked.

Of Prognosticks to be made in Fractures.

Wee must prognosticate in Fractures, whether they are to end in the destruction or welfare of the patient; or whether their cure shall be long or short, easie, or else difficult and dangerous; and lastly, what accidents and symptomes may happen thereupon. Hee shall easily attaine to the knowledge of all these things, who is not onely well seene in the anatomicall description of the bones, but also in the temper, composition and complexion of the whole bodie. Wherefore in the first place, I thinke good to admonish the Surgeon of this, that in winter when all is stiffe with cold, by a little fall, or some such sleight occasion, the bones may be quickly and readily broken. For then the bones, being dryed by the drinesse of the ayre encompassing us, become more brittle; which everie one of the Vulgar usually observe to happen both in waxen and tallow candles: but when the season is moist, the bones are also more moist, and therefore more flexible and yeelding to the violence of the obvious and offending bodie.

3 i.e. the ulna and radius.

Wherefore also you may gather this to the framing of your Prognosticks: That bones by reason of their natural drinesse are not so easily agglutinated and consolidated as flesh; though in Children, according to Galen, by reason of the abundance of their humiditie, the lost substance may bee repaired, according (as they terme it) to the first intention, that is, by restoring of the same kinde of substance or matter. But in others, about the Fractures a certaine hard substance usually concreats, of that nourishment of the broken bone which abounds, which glues together the fragments thereof, being fitly put together. This substance is then termed a *Callus*, and it is so hardened in time, that the bone thereafter in the broken part is seene to be more firme and hard than it is in any other: therefore that usuall saying in Physicke is not without reason; That rest is necessarie lor the uniting of broken bones. For the *Callus* is easily dissolved, if they bee moved before their perfect and solid agglutination. The matter of a *Callus* ought to be indifferent and laudible in quantitie and qualitie, even as blood which flowes for the regeneration of the lost flesh in wounds. It is fit, that there may be sufficient matter for such a *Callus*, that the part have a laudible temper, otherwise there either wil be no *Callus*, or certainly it wil grow more slowly. Fractures are far more easily repaired in yong bodies than in old: for in these there is plentie of the primi- genious and radicall moisture, that is laudably holding and glutinous; and in the other there is store of watrish and excrementitious. By this you may easily conjecture, that you cannot certainely set downe a time necessarie for the generating a *Callus*: for in some it happens later, in some sooner: the cause of which varietie is also to be referred to the constitution of the yeare and region, the temper and diet of the Patient, and maner of Ligation. For, those Patients whose powers are weake, and blood watrish and thin, in these the generation of a *Callus* uses to be more slow: On the contrarie, strong powers hasten to agglutinate the bones, if there be plentie of grosse and viscous matter; whereby it comes to passe, that meats of grosser nutriment are to bee used, and medicines applyed which may helpe forwards the endeavour of nature, as we shall declare hereafter. When the bones are broken neare unto the joynts, the motion afterwards uses to be more difficult, especially if the *Callus*, which is substituted, be somewhat thicke and bunching forth. But if, together with the violence and force of the Fracture, the joynts shall bee broken and bruised, the motion will not only bee lost, but the life brought in danger, by reason of the greatnesse of the inflammation, which usually happens in such affects, and the excesse of paine in a tendinous body. These fractures wherein both the bones of the arme or legge are broken, are more difficult to cure, than those which happen but to one of them. For they are handled & kept in their places with more difficulty, because that which remaines whole, serves the other for a rest or stay to which it may leane. Moreover, there is longer time required to substitute a *Callus* to a great bone, than to a little one. Againe these bones which are more rare and spongie, are sooner glued together by the interposition of a *Callus*, than these which are dense and solid. A *Callus* sooner growes in sanguine, than in cholerick bodies. But broken bones cannot be so happily agglutinated, nor restored in any body, but that alwaies some asperity or unequall protuberancie may bee seene on that part where the *Callus* is generated. Wherfore the Surgeon ought to make artificiall Ligations, that the *Callus* may not stand out too far, nor sinke downe too low. That Fracture is least troublesome which is simple; on the contrarie, that is more troublesome which is made into splinters; but that is most troublesome and worst of all which is in small and sharp fragments, because there is clanger of convulsion by pricking a nerve, or the *periostium*. Sometimes the fragments of a broken bone keep themselves in their due place: they also oft times fly forth thereof, so that one of them gets above another; which when it happens, you may perceive an inequality by the depression of the one part and the bunching forth of the other, as also paine by the pricking: besides also the member is made shorter than it was, and than the sound member on the opposite side is, and more swolne by the contraction of the muscles towards their originall. Wherefore when a bone is broken, if you perceive anie thing so depressed, presently putting your hand on both sides above and below, stretch forth the bone as forcibly as you can; for otherwise, the muscles and nerves, stretched and contracted, will never of their owne accord suffer the bones to be restored to their proper seat and themselves. This extension must bee performed in the first dayes, for afterwards there will happen inflammation: which being present, it is dangerous to draw the nerves and tendons too violently; for hence would ensue an impostume, convulsion, gangrene and mortification. Therefore Hippocrates forbids you to defer such extension untill the third, or fourth day. Fractures are thought dangerous, whose fragments are great, and fly out, especially in these bones which are filled with marrow on the inside. When broken or dislocated bones cannot be restored to themselves and their naturall place, the part wasts for want of nourishment; both for that the naturall site of the veines, arteries and nerves is perverted, as also because the part it selfe lyes immoveable, or scarce moveable: whereby it commeth to passe, that the spirits doe not freely flow thereto, as neyther the nutritive juice commeth thither in sufficient plentie. When the dislocated or broken member is troubled with any great inflammation, it is doubtfull whether or no a convulsion will happen, if wee attempt to restore it, or the parts thereof to their seat: therefore it is better, if it may bee done, to deferre the reducing thereof so long, untill the humor which possesses the part be dissolved, the tumor abated, and the bitternesse of paine mitigated.

The generall cure of broken and dislocated bones.

To cure a broken and dislocated bone, is to restore it to its former figure and site. For the performance whereof, the Surgeon must propose three things to himselfe: The first is, to restore the bone to its place: The second is, that he containe or stay it being so restored: The third is, that he hinder the increase of maligne symptomes and accidents; or else if they doe happen, that then he temper and correct their present malignitie. Such accidents are paine, inflammation, a feaver, abscesse, gangrene and sphacell. For the first intention, you may easily restore a broken or dislocated bone, if presently, as soon as the mischance is got, or else the same day, you endeavour to restore it: for the bitternesse of paine or inflammation, which may trouble the patient, is not as yet verie great, neyther is the contraction of the muscles upwards as yet very much or stubborne. Therefore first of all, the Patient with his whole bodie, but especially with the broken or dislocated part, as also the Surgeon, must bee in some place which hath good and sufficient light. Then let trusty and skilfull attendants be there, good ligatures, and also, if need so require, good engines. His friends which are present, let them see and hold their peace, neyther say, nor do any thing which may hinder the Worke of the Surgeon. Then putting one hand above, that is, towards the center of the body, and the other below, as neare as hee can to the part affected, let him stretch forth the member: for if you lay your hand any distance from the part affected, you wil hurt the sound part by too much compression, neyther will you much avayle your selfe by stretching it at such a distance. But if you only endeavour below with your hand or ligature, assisting to make extension thereof, it will be dangerous if there bee nothing above which may withstand or hold, lest that you draw the whole bodie to you. This being done, according as I have delivered, it is fit the Surgeon make a right or straight extension of the part affected: for when the bone is eyther broken or out of joynt, there is a contraction of the muscles towards their originall, and consequently of the bones by them, as it is observed by Galen. Wherefore it is impossible to restore the bones to their former seat, without the extension of the muscles. But the part being thus extended, the broken bones will sooner and more easily be restored to their former seate. Which being restored, you shall presently with your hand presse it downe, if there be any thing that bunches or stands out. And lastly, you shall binde it up, by applying boulsters and splints as shall bee fit. But if the bone bee dislocated or forth of joynt, then presently after the extension thereof^ it will be requisite to bend it somwhat about, and so to draw it in. The Surgeon is sometimes forced to use engines for this worke, especially if the luxation be inveterate, if the broken or luxated bones be great; and that in strong and rustick bodies, and such as have large joynts: for that then there is need of greater strength, than is in the hand of the Surgeon alone. For, by how much the muscles of the Patient are the stronger, by so much will they bee contracted more powerfully upwards towards their originals. Yet have a care that you extend them not too violently, lest by rending and breaking asunder the muscles and nerves, you cause the forementioned symptomes, paine, convulsion, a palsie and gangrene: all which sooner happen to strong and aged bodies, than to children, eunuches, women; youthes, and generally all moyst bodies, for that they are lesse hurt by violent extension and pulling, by reason of their native and much humiditie and softnesse. For thus skins of leather, moystened with any liquor, are easily retched and drawn out as one pleaseth: but such as are dry & hard, being lesse tractable, will sooner rend and teare, than stretch further out. Therefore the Surgeon shall use a meane in extending and drawing forth of members, as shall be most agreeable to the habits of the bodies. You may know the bone is set, and the setting performed as is fit, if the paine be asswaged; to wit, the fibres of the muscles, and the other parts being restored to their former site, and all compression, which the bones moved out of their places have made, being taken away; if, to your feeling there bee nothing bunching out, nor rugged, but the surface of the member remaine smooth and equall; and lastly, if the broken or dislocated member compares with its opposite in the composure of the joynts, as the knees and ancles answer justly and equally in length and thick- nesse. For which purpose it must not suffice the Surgeon to view it once, but even as often as he shall dresse it. For it may happen, that the bone which is well set, may by some chance, as by the Patients unconsiderate turning him- selfe in his bed, or as it were a convulsive twitching of the members or joynts whilest he sleepes, the muscles of their owne accord contracting themselves towards their originals, that the member may againe fall out; and it will give mani- < fest signes thereof by renewing the paine, by pressing or pricking the adjacent bodies: which paine will not cease, before it bee restored to its place: and hereof the Surgeon ought to have diligent care. For if, whilest the *Callus* is in growing, one bone ride over another, the bone it selfe will afterwards be so much the shorter, and consequently the whole member; so that if this errour shall happen in a broken legge, the Patient will halt ever after, to his great griefe, and the Surgeons shame. Wherefore the Patient shall take heed, as much as in him lyes, that he stirre not the broken member, before that the *Callus* be hardened. Such diligent care needes not bee had in dislocations. For these once set, and artificially bound up, doe not afterwards so easily fall forth as broken bones.

The second scope is, that the bones which shall be restored may bee firmely kept in their state and place. That shall be done by Bandages; as ligatures, boulsters, and other things, whereof hereafter we shall make particular mention. Hither tend proper and fit medicines, to wit, applying of oyle of Roses with the whites of Egges, and the like repelling things; and then resolving medicines, as the present necessity shall require. It will be convenient, to moysten your rowlers and boulsters in oxycrate for this purpose, or else in Rose vinegar, if the Fracture be simple, or with red wine, or the like liquor warme (in Galens opinion) if a wound bee joyned to the fracture; and it will be fit to moysten fractures oftner in Summer: For so the part is strengthened, the defluxion being repelled, whereby the inflammation and paine are hindred. You must desist from humecting and watering the part when the symptomes are past, lest you retard the generating of a *Callus;* for which you must labour by these meanes which wee shall hereafter declare. To this purpose also conduces the rest and lying of the part in its proper figure and site accustomed in health, that so it may the longer remaine in the same place unstirred. Besides also, it is expedient then only to dresse the part, when it is needfull, & with those things that are requisite, shunning, as much as may be, inflammation and paine. That figure is thought the best, which is the middle, that is, which containes the muscles in their site, which is without paine; so that the Patient may long endure it without labour or trouble. All these things being performed, the Patient must be asked, Whether the member be bound up too strait? If he answer, No, (unlesse peradventure a little upon the fracture or luxation, for there it is fit it should bee more straitly bound) then may you know that the binding is moderate. And this same first ligation is to bee kept in fractures without loosing for three or foure dayes space, unlesse peradventure paine urge you to the contrary. In dislocations the same binding may bee kept for seven or eight daies, unlesse by chance some symptome may happen, which may force us to open it before that time: for the Surgeon must with all his art have a care to prohibite the happening of evill accidents and symptomes, which, how he may bring to passe, shall bee declared in the following Chapter.

By what meanes you may performe the third intention in curing fractures and dislocations, which is, the hindring and correction of accidents and symptomes.

That we may attaine unto this third scope, it is requisite we handle as gently and without paine, as we may, the broken or dislocated member; we drive away the defluxion ready to fall downe upon the part by medicines, repelling the humour, and strengthning the part; wee, by appointing a good diet, hinder the begetting of excrements in the bodie, and divert them by purging and phlebotomie. But if these accidents be already present, we must cure them according to the kinde and nature of each of them: for they are various. Amongst which is reckoned itching, which in the beginning torments the Patient: this ariseth from a collection and suppression of subacride vapours, arising from j the blood, and other humors under the skin. Whence a light biting, which causeth a simple itch, or else a more grievous and acride one, from whence (in Galens opinion) proceeds a painefull itching. Wherefore such matter, as the cause, being evacuated, all itching ceaseth. But this cannot J easily and freely be evacuated and breathed out, because the pores of the part are shut up, and as it were oppressed with the burden of the emplaisters, boulsters, and ligatures, which are put about the part. Hereunto may be added, that the part its selfe doth not so perfecdy performe and enjoy its wonted faculties and actions: by which it commeth to passe, that the heat thereof is more languide than may suffice to discusse the fuliginous matter there collected. Wherefore it will be convenient to loose the ligatures everie third day, that, as by loosing their tyes, their sanious and fuliginous excrements, shut up under the skinne, may freely passe forth, lest in continuance they should fret and ulcerate it; as it happens to most of those who provide not for it by loosing their ligatures. Besides also, the part must bee long fomented with hot water alone, or else with a decoction of sage, chamomile, roses, and melilote made in wine and water: for long fomenting attenuates and evacuates, but shorter fils and mollifies, as it is delivered by Hippocrates. Also gentle frictions, performed with your hand, or a warme linnen cloath upwards, to the right side and left, and circularly to everie side, are good. But if the skinne be already risen into blisters, they must be cut, lest the matter contained thereunder may corrode and ulcerate the skinne: then must the skinne be annointed with some cooling and drying medicine; as, *Ung. album Camphoratum Rhasisy Desiccativum rubrum, unguentum rosatum sine aceto;* adding thereto the pouder of a rotten poste, or prepared *Tutia,* or the like. Other accidents more grievous than these, doe often happen, but we will treat of them hereafter. But if the scales of the bone underneath bee quite severed from the whole, then must they be presently taken forth, especially if they prick the muscles: But if the bone be broken into splinters, and so prominent out of the wounded flesh as that it cannot be restored into its seat, it must be cut off with your cutting mallets, or parrats beake, as occasion shall offer its selfe. In the interim, you must have a care that the part enjoy perspiration, and by change of place and rising, now and then it may be as it were ventilated: also you must see that it be not over-burdened, neyther too strait bound, otherwise it will be apt to inflammation.

OF DISLOCATIONS OR LUXATIONS

Of the kinds and manners of Dislocations.

A dislocation is the departure or falling out of the head of a bone from its proper cavitie, into an unaccustomed place beside nature, hindring voluntarie motion. There is another kinde of Luxation, which is caused by a violent distention, and as it were a certaine divancation, and dilatation, or extension into length and breadth of the ligaments, and all the nervous bodies, which containe, strengthen, and binde together the joynts. Thus those who have beene tormented and racked, have that thick ligament which is in the inner cavitie of the huckle bone too violently extended: Those who have suffered the Strappado, have the ligaments, encompassing the articulation of the Arme-bone, with the shoulder-blade, forcibly and violendy distended. Such also is their affect whose foot is strained by slipping. There is a third kinde of Luxation, when as those bones which are joyned contiguous, and one (as it were) bound to the sides ot another, gape or flye asunder: as in the Arme, when the ell parts from the wand; in the legge, when the one focile flyes from the other: yet this may be referred to the second sort of dislocations, because it happens not without dilatation, or else the breaking of the ligaments. There is also a fourth added to these, as when the *Epiphyses* and heads of bones are plucked from the bone whereon they were placed or fastened: which unproperly called kinde of Luxation, hath place chiefly in the bones of yong people, and it is knowne by the impotencie of the part, and by the noise and grating together of the crackling bones when they are handled. Now the bones of yong folks are also incident to another casualtie: for as the bones of old people are broken by violence by reason of their drinesse and hardnesse, thus the bones of children are bended or crooked in by reason of their naturall softnesse and humiditie.

Of the differences of Dislocations.

Some Dislocations are simple, others compound. We terme them simple which have no other preternaturall affect joyned with them; and such compound, as are complicated with one or more preternaturall affects; as when a dislocation is associated with a wound, fracture, great paine, inflammation, and an abscesse. For, through occasion of these we are often compelled so long to let alone the luxation, untill these bee remitted of themselves, or by our art. Some Dislocations are complete and perfect, as when the bone wholly fals out of its cavitie: othersome are imperfect, as when it is only lightly moved, and not wholly fallen out; wherfore we only call them subluxations or strains. Differences of Luxations are also drawne from the place: for sometimes the bone is wrested forwards, other- whiles backwards, upwards, downwards; somewhiles it may be wrested, according to all these differences of site, and otherwhiles onely according to some of them. Differences are also taken from the condition of the dislocated Joynt in greatnesse and littlenesse, from the superficiarie or deepe excavation of the *sinus* or hollownesse; and lasdy from the time, as if it be lately done, or of some long continuance. I have judged it fit to set downe all these, for that there are severall indications of curing, according to the varietie of each of these, as we shall teach hereafter.

Of the causes of Dislocations.

There are three general causes of Luxations, internall, externall, and hereditarie. The internall are excrementitious humors and flatulencies, which, settling into the ioynts with great torce and plentie, doe so make slippene, sorten & relaxe the ligaments which binde together the bones, that they easily fall out of their cavities; or else they so fill and distend these ligaments, and make them so short, that being contracted, they also contract the *appendices* of the bones from whence they arise, and so pluck them from the bone whereon they are placed, or else draw the heads of the bones out of their cavities, chiefly if the violence of a noxious humor doth also concurre, which possessing and filling up the cavities of the joynts, puts them from their seats, as it oft times happens to the joynt of the hip by Sciaticaes, and to the *Vertebræ* of the spine, by whose Luxation people become gibbous, or otherwise crooked. But externall causes of Dislocations are, fals from high, bruising and heavie blowes, the Rack, Strappado, slipping in going, and all such like things, which may force the heads of the bones to fly out of their seats, or cavities, which also happens somtimes to infants in their birth, when as they are too carelesly and violently drawne forth by the Midwife, so that eyther their armes or legges are put out of joynt. Hereditarie causes are such as the Parents transfuse into their off-spring: hence it is, that crooked not necessarily, but often times, are generated by crooked, and lame by lame. The truth whereof is evident by daily experience. Besides also Hippocrates himselfe averres, that infants in the very wombe may have their Joynts dislocated by a fall, blow and compression, & by the too much humidity and loosenes of the Joynts: whence also we see many crooke legg'd and footed from their nativitie; so that none need marvell or make any doubt hereof. We have read it observed by Galen *In librum de Artic.* that children may have impostumes in their mothers wombs, which may cast forth quitture,[4] the ulcers being opened of their own accord, and be cicatrized by the only benefit of nature. It also happens to many from their first conformation, that the cavities of their Joynts are lesse deprest than they should bee, and that their verges are more dilated than they ought to be; whereby it happens that the heads of the bones can the lesse enter into them. It fals out, that othersome have the ligaments, appointed by nature for fastening together the bones of the joynt, whether inserted or placed about, so weake, that from their first originall they are not of sufficient strength, or else abound with much phlegme, eyther bred together with them, or flowing from some other place; so that by their too much slipperinesse they lesse faithfully containe the knittings or articulations of the bones. In all these, as the bones are easily dislocated, so they may presendy be easily restored without the assistance of a Surgeon, as I have sometimes observed in some.

The signes of dislocations.

Some of the signes whereby we come to the knowledge of a luxated bone, are common to all dislocations; others are Proper only to severall Luxations. It is a common signe, that there is alwaies a tumor in that part whereto the bone runnes, and a hollownesse on that side from whence it is flowne. Now the proper signes shall be shewed, when as we come to treat of the particular kindes of Luxations. We know a perfect Dislocation by the lost action of the part, that is to say, the lost motion; paine also breeds a suspicion of a dislocation: for the head of the bone, which (moved out of its place) is forced into another, presses the flesh, and distends the nerves also moved out of their place. Hereto also conduces the comparing of the sound joynt with that which is hurt, in which collation, it is fit the sound part, which is compared with the hurt, be no waies, neyther by nature nor any accident, wronged, nor deformed, nor withered or decayed, nor swolne above measure, otherwise it may cozen and deceive you, if you bee lesse wane. Labour and difficultie of action in moving, is a signe of an uncomplete Luxation, or strain. Now we thus know, that the ligaments, serving to the connexion of the articulations, are extended and relaxed, if the head of the bone, pressed with your fingers, be easily driven unto the contrary part, and suddenly flye

4 i.e. a purulent discharge.

thence backe againe; if thrusting your finger into the joynt, it easily enter, nothing resisting it, as though all were empty within; if the motion be difficult, or none at all.

Of Prognosticks to be made upon luxations.

All Joynts may bee perverted or luxated, but all of them cannot in like manner be restored. For the head may be dislocated, but therupon present death ensues, by reason of the compression of the whole spinail marrow presendy at the originall thereof; such also is the dislocation of a *vertebra* of the spine, and of the Jaw-bone, which, slipped forth on both sides, hath caused inflammation, and a great tumor before that it be set. The bones of other Joynts, as they are more or lesse dislocated, and moved out of their seats, so may they bee more easily or difficuldy restored. For, by how much they are the lesse moved out of their places, by so much they are the more quickly, and by how much they are the further, by so much they are the more slowly and difficuldy set. Also an indication, taken from the figure of the luxated bone, gives a signe of the easie or hard restoring of the dislocation; as in the Arme, by how much the bones be the more easily dislocated, by so much once luxated they are the more easily restored. Bones doe not easily fall out of joynt in fleshie bodies; but when they chance to be put out, they are not easily got in againe. For in such, the articulation is straidy on everie side held in by the thicknesse of the muscles, and the plenty of the fat lying thereabouts. On the contrarie, such as are leane, especially those who formerly have beene more fat, have their joynts more laxe, whereby it comes to passe, that their bones may easily be put forth of joynt: besides also, through the default of the digestive facultie, they have their joynts replete with mucous humors; whence it is, that the heads of the bones, as standing in a slipperie place, are the lesse stable, as it is recorded by Hippocrates. But slender bodies, which are naturally dry, compact and dense, have their muscles and ligaments more strong and dry; wherefore their bones are the more difficultly displaced; and displaced, the more difficultly set. Some bones, joyned amongst themselves, doe sometimes flye asunder, as when the shoulder blade flyes from the collar-bone at the *Acromion*, and in the Arme the Ell from the Wand, and in the Legge the one focile from the other, and the Heele-bone from the Ancle. Bones thus separated will never be joyned together againe, will never recover their former comely figure, never their strength of action. For, then it most usually happens, that the ligaments are either broke asunder, or else resolved and become laxe. Those whose bones are dislocated by an externall cause, they, after they be set, may easily fall out againe, for that the ligaments, moystened and bedewed with an excrementitious humor, cannot firmely hold them: oft times the ligaments are not wholly broken, but onely in some portion thereof; and hence the action of the part either perishes, or is debilitated. Also that dislocation is uncureable, when as the ligaments, steeped and swolne up with an excrementitious humiditie, are so much shortened and contracted in their length, as they have acquired in their breadth: and thus they draw away and plucke off the *appendices* of the bones from whence they arise, and by reason the bone and the *appendix* doe enter and receive each other by manie cavities and prominencies, therefore they cannot, by how skilfull hand so-ever they be handled, be againe fitly placed and put together. Old and inveterate dislocations, wherin a tough humor possessing the cavitie is concrete in stead of the head of the bone, are not to be restored; as neither when the heads of the luxated bones have by continuall attrition made themselves a new cavitie in the neighbouring bone: neither if they be restored, is the restitution firme and of continuance; because the naturall cavitie is possessed by another matter, and the new made neare thereto cannot well and faithfully containe the received head of the bone. Those who have their shoulder dislocated, may use their hand for many actions, as well as the opposite sound hand; for the weight of the bodie is not sustained by the hands, as it is by the legs. And by how much the hand is the more exercised, by so much the arme becoms the more corpulent. Contrarily, if the thigh-bone bee dislocated, especially if it bee wrested inwards, the whole legge quickly decayes by an *atrophia,* because the part doth absolutely lose all motion: for by the opinion of Hippocrates, the performance of the proper action encreases strength, and makes the part in better plight; but idlenesse debilitates and makes it leane. If a great wound and fracture bee joyned with a luxation, there is danger, lest while wee use extension for restoring the part, we draw the nerves too violendy, and so break the nerves, veines and arteries, whence would ensue feare of inflammation, convulsion, and other maligne symptomes. Wherefore Hippocrates judges it better in such a concourse and complication of preternaturall affects, absolutely not to meddle at all with the setting of the dislocated bone: for, by attempting the restitution, certaine death; but by omitting it only lamenesse is to be feared. Everie dislocation must be restored before inflammation come; but if it be already present, you must presendy be carefull to take it away. For other things, let the Patient rest, lest if the affect be irritated, the increase and excesse of paine cause a convulsion, gangrene, and lasdy death, as I remember I have somtimes observed. Therfore when inflammation, and other maligne symptomes shall be mitigated and corrected, then may you endeavour to restore the luxation, especially if the habit of the bodie and member affected may admit it. For if the bodie be slender, delicate and tender, then the restitution will bee more speedy and facile. But on the contrarie, more difficult, if it be grosse and compact; And let thus much suffice for prognosticks in Luxations.

Of the generall cure of Dislocations.

For all that I have heretofore delivered the generall methode of curing Fractures and dislocations, yet it shall not bee unprofitable to repeat here in this place, those things which may be accommodated to this Treatise of curing Luxations. Now he that will cure Dislocations, must have regard to five intentions, which it will be fitting to performe in order. The first is, of Holding; The second, of Drawing or Extending; The third, of Forcing in; The fourth, of Placing in convenient figure and site; The fifth, of Correcting the concomitant, or following symptomes.

The first scope, which we said was of Holding, is meant eyther of the whole body, or else of some part thereof only. The whole bodie must bee holden by the strong embracement of your servant or attendant, when as the shoulder, the *vertebræ,* or the thigh-bones are dislocated. But in the dislocation of the Collar-bone, elbow, hand, knee, or foote and legge, it is sufficient onely to hold the part straidy in your hands. There is necessitie of holding eyther the bodie, or else some part thereof, lest, while the dislocated bone is extended, the whole bodie follow by continuance of parts, if there be nothing which may hinder: for if the bodie should follow him that drawes or extends, all the work- masters labour and endeavour to restore it, is to no purpose. The use of the second scope, that is, of Drawing or Extending, is, that there may be a free space and distance betweene the luxated bones, by which distance the dislocated bone may the more freely be forced into its cavitie. But the manner of drawing or extending is different in quantity and manner, according to the various strength of the muscles and ligaments, and dislocation of the bones to this or that part. Therefore this worke is almost alwaies performed by the hands; which when they cannot suffice, we must use the assistance of instruments and engins, whose figures you shall see hereafter delineated. But that you may not doe amisse, you may so farre use extension, untill the head of the bone be brought just against its cavitie. When the Surgeon hath brought it to this passe, then must he hasten to the third intention, which is, to put the head of the bone first moved and gently bended, into its cavitie. For hee must have a speciall care, that hee force it no other way than into its proper cavity: for it would be dangerous, lest he should turne it from one extreme into another, and the bone, for examples sake, of the thigh, which was dislocated into the forepart by too violent forcing, by exceeding the middle cavitie, may be driven and dislocated into the hinder part. To shun this, the bone shall be put backe the same way that it fell out, which may bee easily done in fresh and late happening dislocations. We understand that the bone is set by the noyse, or as it were a popp, or sound like that, which solid and sounding bodies, being fully and forcibly thrust into their cavities, do make; by the similitude and consent in figure, magnitude and all conformation of the affected part with the sound, and lasdy, by the mitigation of the paine. The fourth scope, which is of the convenient site of the part, must bee so fulfilled, that the bone after it is set may bee kept in its cavity, and not flye forth againe. Wherefore if the arme be dislocated, it shall be carried bound up in a scarfe: if the thigh, knee, legge, or foote be luxated, they shall be fitly layd in a bed; but in the *interim* the Surgeon, presendy after hee hath set them, shall have a care, that the affected joynt be wrapped about with stoups and clothes, or compresses steeped in rose vinegar, and spred with convenient medicines; then let it be bound with an artificiall deligation, rowling the ligatures unto the part contrary to that whereto the dislocated bone flew. For the which purpose thicker boulsters shall be there applied whence the bone came out, otherwise there will be some danger, lest it should be againe displaced: when these things are done, he shall for foure or five dayes space meddle with nothing about the Dislocation, unlesse paine, or some such like symptome happen. For then the fifth scope will call us from that cessation and rest, which is, to correct the symptomes and complicate affections, as paine, inflammation, a wound, fracture, and others, wherof wee have spoken abundantly in our Treatise of Fractures. Before wee attempt to set inveterate dislocations, wee must endevour to humect the ligaments, tendons and muscles by fomentations, cataplasmes, emplaisters, liniments, and other remedies, that so these parts may be more obedient to the Surgeons hand: then must the dislocated bones be moved, with a gentle motion up and down, to and againe, that by this meanes the excrementitious humor, which by continuance of time hath flowed downe, may waxe hot, be attenuated, resolved or made slipperie, and also the fibres of the muscles, ligaments, and nervous bodies, placed about the joynt for the defence thereof, may be loosed, that so they may presendy be more freely extended. But if a great swelling, paine and inflammation urge, we must first think of asswaging and curing them, then of the restoring the Dislocation.

Of Cataracts

By what signes ripe and curable cataracts may bee discerned from unripe and uncurable ones.

If the sound eye being shut, the pupill of the sore or suffused eye, after it shall be rubbed with your thumbe, bee presently dilated and diffused, and with the like celerity returne into the place, figure, colour and state, it is thought by some to shew a ripe and confirmed cataract. But an unripe and not to bee couched, if the pupill remaine dilated and diffused for a long while after. But it is a common signe of a ripe, as also more dense and consequently uncurable suffusion, to bee able to see nor distinguish no visible thing beside light and brightnesse; for to discerne other objects sheweth that it is not yet ripe. Therefore the sound eye being shut and pressed, the pupill of the other rubbed with your thumbe, is dilated, enlarged, swelleth and is more diffused; the visive spirits by this compression being as it were forced from the sound into the sore eye. But these following cataracts are judged uncurable, that is, such as are great, such as when the eye-lid is rubbed are nothing dilated or diffused, whose pupill becommeth no broader by this rubbing: for hence you may gather that the stopping or obstruction is in the opticke nerve, so that how cunningly and well soever the cataract bee couched, yet will the Patient continue blind; you shall do no more good in couching a cataract, which is in an eye consumed and wasted with a *Phthisis.* Also that cataract is uncurable which is occasioned by a most grievous disease, to wit, by most bitter and cruell paines of the head, or by a violent blow. Such as are of a plaister-like, green, blacke, livid, citrine and quicksilver-like colour, are usually uncurable. On the contrary, such as are of a Chesnut colour, or of a skye or sea-water colour, with some litde whitnesse, yeeld great hope of a happy and successefull cure.

Of the couching a Cataract.

After you shal know by the forementioned signes, that the Cataract is curable, it remains that you attempt the couching thereof, but so, that there be nothing which may hinder. For if the paine of the head, cough, nauseousnes or vomiting at that time trouble the patient, you shal then bestow your labour in vaine: Wherefore you must expect untill these symptomes be gone. Then make choice of a season fitting for that purpose, that is, in the decrease of the moon, when the aire is not troubled with thunder nor lightening, and when as the Sunne is not in Aries, because that signe hath dominion over the head. Then let the Sturgeon consult a Physitian whether purging or bloud-letting be convenient for the Patient, so to resist plethoricke symptomes, otherwaies ready to yeeld matter for relapse. Two dayes after you must make choice of a place furnished with indifferent or competent light, and the Patient being fasting shall be placed in a strait chaire, so that the light may not fell with the beames direcdy upon him, but sidewise. The eye which shall bee cured must bee made more steddy, by laying and binding wooll upon the other: Then the Surgeon shall seate and place himselfe directly against the Patient upon a seat somewhat higher, and bidding the Patient put his hands downe to his girdle, he shall hold the patients legges betweene his knees. One shall stand at the Patients backe who shall hold his head and keepe it from stirring; for by a litde stirring hee may lose his sight for ever. Then must you prepare and make ready your needle, and thrust it often into some strong thicke cloth, that it may bee as it were smoothe by this motion, and for the performance of the worke in hand with the lesse paine somewhat warmed. It must bee made of iron or Steele, and not of gold or silver, it must be also flatted on the sides, and sharpe pointed, that so it may the better pierce into the eye, and wholly couch the Cataract once taken hold of; and lest it should slip in the Surgeons hand, and be lesse steddy, it shall bee put into a handle, as you may see by the following figure.

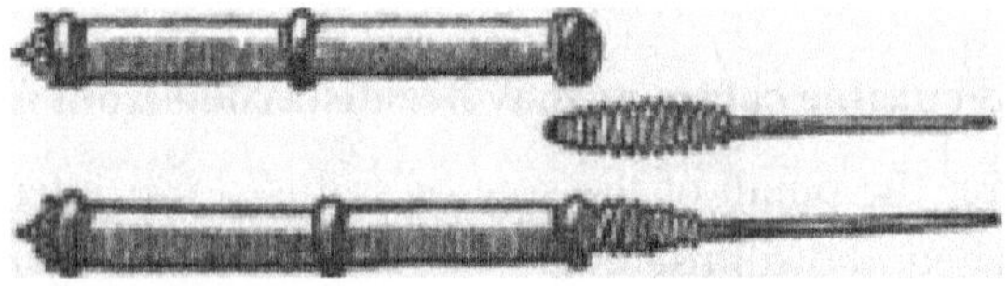

A needle inserted in a handle for the couching of Cataracts

All things being thus in a readinesse, you must bid the patient to turne the sight of his eye towards his nose, and the needle must be boldly thrust (for it is received in a place that is voyde, and onely filled with spirits) directly by the coat *Adnata,* in the middle space between the lesser corner & the horny coat, just against the midst of the Cataract, yet so, as that you hurt no vein of the *Adnata,* & then by stirring it as it were diversly untill it come to the midst of the pupill and suffusion. When it is come thither, the needle must bee inclined from above downewards to the suffusion, and there to be stirred gently untill by little and little it couch or bring downe the Cataract as whole as may be beneath the compasse of the pupill; let him still follow it though couched with his needle, and somewhat violently depresse, and keep it down for some short space, that so it may rest and stay in that lower place whether it is depressed.

The Surgeon shall try whether it firmely remaine there or no, bidding; the patient presendy to move his eye; For if it remaine constantly so, and doe not returne againe, the cure is perfect. Then must the needle be lifted up by little and little, neither must it presently be taken forth, that if the Cataract should beare up, or rise againe, that it might againe, and so often (whilst the worke is yet hot, and all things in a readinesse) be couched towards the lesser corner, untill it be fully and surely hid. Then must you draw backe the needle gently, and after the same manner as you put it in; lest if you use not moderation, you bring backe the Cataract, from whence you couched it, or grievously offend the crystalline humour, the prime instrument of sight, or the pupill with clanger of dilating thereof. Some as soone as the worke is done, give the patient something in his hand to looke upon: but *Paulus* approves not thereof, for hee feares lest his endeavouring or striving to see, may draw backe the Cataract. Wherefore it is more wisedome and better, presendy after the drawing forth of the needle, to put on a soft ragge the white of an egge beaten in rose-water with a litde choice alume, and so apply it to the eye and neighbouring parts for to binde and hinder the inflammation; then also you must together therewith bind up the sound eye, lest by stirring to see, it might together therewith draw and move the sore eye, by reason of the sympathy and consent they mutually have by the opticke nerves. After all things are thus performed, the patient shall bee laid in a soft bed, & so placed, that his head may lye somwhat high; let him be laid far from noise, let him not speake, nor eate any hard thing that may trouble his jawes, wherefore let him feed upon liquid meats, as ponado, barly cream, cullisses, gellyes, reare egs, and other meates of the like nature. At the end of eight dayes the ligature that binds up his eyes shall be loosed, and his eyes washed with rose water, and putting on spectacles, or some taffaty, the patient shall by little and litde accustome himselfe to the light, lest hee should bee offended by the sudden meeting with light. But if the suffusion, after some short while after, lift it selfe up againe, it must bee couched againe, but through a new hole, for the eye is pained and tender in the former place. It sometimes happens by the touch of the needle that the Cataract is not couched whole, but is broken into many peeces; then therefore each of them must be followed, and couched severally: if there be any very small particle which scapes the needle, it must bee let alone, for there is no doubt but that in processe of time it may be dissolved by the force of the native heat. There are also some Cataracts which at the first touch of the needle are diffused & turne into a substance like to milke or troubled water, for that they are not throughly ripe, yet these put us in good hope of recovery, and it bee but for this, that they can never afterwards concrete into one body as before. Wherefore at the length they are also discussed by the strength of the native heat, and then the eye recovers its former splendor. If that any other symptomes come unlooked for, they shall be helped by new counsels and their appropriate remedies.

THE TREATMENT OF GUNSHOT WOUNDS

... TRULY I HAVE not put my hand to the pen to write in such a manner, had it not been that some have impudently taxed and insulted me and disgraced me, more by particular hate than by any good zeal they should have to the public, concerning my manner of tying the veins and arteries, writing that which follows:

"Badly then and too arrogantly, indiscreetly, and temerariously, a certain personage has wished to condemn and blame the cauterization of the vessels after the amputation of a corrupt and rotten member, much praised and recommended by the ancients and always approved, wishing and desiring to

Ambroise Paré, "The Treatment of Gunshot Wounds," *The Life and Times of Ambroise Paré*, trans. Francis R. Packard, pp. 130-134, 160-164, 262-273.

show and teach us, without reason, judgment or experience, a new way of tying the vessels, against the opinion of all the ancient physicians, giving no caution nor advice that there frequently happen many more great perils and accidents from this new fashion of tying the vessels (which he wishes to be done by a needle piercing profoundly the healthy part) than by burning and combustion of the said vessel. Because, if with the needle one should prick some nervous part, to wit, even the nerve itself, when he wishes by this new and untried means grossly to constrain the vein in tying it, necessarily there will follow a new inflammation, from the inflammation a convulsion, from the convulsion death. For fear of which accidents Galen never dared to stitch a transverse wound (that which is always less dangerous) before uncovering the aponeuroses [membranous sheaths] of the muscles.

"Moreover, this forceps, with which, after the section he once more tears the flesh, while he thinks it possible to draw forth the vessels which are drawn back towards their origin, causes no less pain than the hot iron. And if anyone, having experienced this new fashion of cruelty, has recovered from it, he should render thanks to God forever, by the goodness of whom he has escaped such cruelty, feeling it was rather his executioner than his methodical chirurgeon [surgeon]."

Oh, what beautiful words! for an aged man, who calls himself a wise doctor. He does not remember that his white beard admonisheth him not to say anything unworthy of his years, and that he should put off and drive out from him all envy and rancor conceived against his neighbor. But, now I wish to prove to him by authority, reason, and experience that the said veins and arteries should be tied.

As to authorities I will come to that of that grand man Hippocrates,[5] who wills and commands the recovery of fistulas [ulcers] of the fundament [rectum] by ligature, as much to absorb the callosity as to avoid haemorrhage.

Galen, in his *Method*, speaking of a flow of blood made by an external cause, of whom see here the words. "It is," saith he, "most sure to tie the root of the vessel, which I understand to be that [part] which is most near to the liver or to the heart."

Avicenna commands to tie the vein and the artery, after having uncovered it towards its origin.

Gui de Chauliae, speaking of wounds of the veins and arteries, enjoins the surgeon to make the ligature on the vessel.

Monsieur Hollier, in Book III, chapter 5, of his *Matiére du Chirurgie*, speaking of the flow of blood, commands expressly to tie the vessels.

Calmetheus, in his chapter on the *Wounds of Veins and Arteries*, treats of a very sure means of arresting the flow of blood by ligature of the vessels.

Celsus, from whom the said physician hath taken the greater part of his book, recommends expressly to tie the vessels in the flow of blood following wounds as a very easy and very sure remedy.

Vesalius, in his *Surgery*, directs that the vessels be tied in a flow of blood.

Jean de Vigo, treating of haemorrhage from recent wounds, commands to tie the vein and artery.

Tagault, treating of the means of arresting a flow of blood, commands to pinch the vein or artery with a crow beak, or a parrot beak, then to tie it with a strong enough thread. …

The Journey to Turin in 1536

Moreover, I will here show to my readers the towns and places where I have been enabled to learn the art of surgery, always the better to instruct the young surgeon.

---

5 Paré cites here a number of medical authorities, beginning with Hippocrates and Galen, the classical Greek physicians, taking in Celsus and Avicenna, the most famous Roman and Arabic writers on medicine, and coming down to men of his own time, including Vesalius, on whom see above, p. 465.

And first, in the year 1536, the great King Frangois [Francis I] sent a great army to Turin to recover the cities and castles which had been taken by the Marquis de Guast, lieutenant-general of the Emperor [Charles V]; when Monsieur the Constable, then grandmaster, was lieutenant-general of the army, and Monsieur de Montejan was colonel general of the infantry, to whom I was then surgeon. A great part of the army having arrived at the Pass of Suze, we found the enemy holding the passage and having made certain forts and trenches, insomuch that to make them dislodge and quit the place it was necessary to fight. There were many killed and wounded, as many on one side as on the other, but the enemy were constrained to retire and gain the castle, which was taken in part by Captain Le Rat, who climbed with many soldiers from his company on a little hill, from whence they fired directly on the enemy. He received a shot from an arquebus in the ankle of his right foot, wherewith he suddenly fell to the ground and then said: "Now the Rat is taken." I dressed him, and God healed him.

We thronged into the city and passed over the dead bodies and some that were not yet dead, hearing them cry under the feet of our horses, which made a great pity in my heart, and truly I repented that I had gone forth from Paris to see so pitiful a spectacle. Being in the city, I entered a stable, thinking to lodge my horse and that of my man, where I found four dead soldiers and three who were propped against the wall, their faces wholly disfigured; and they neither saw, nor heard, nor spake, and their clothes yet flaming from the gunpowder which had burnt them. Beholding them with pity, there came an old soldier who asked me if there was any means of curing them. I told him no. At once he approached them and cut their throats gently and without anger. Seeing this great cruelty, I said to him that he was a bad man. He answered me that he prayed God that when he should be in such a case, he might find someone who would do the same for him, to the end that he might not languish miserably.

And, to return to our discourse, the enemy was summoned to surrender, which they did, and went forth, their lives only saved, and a white staff in their hands; but the greater part went on to gain the Chateau de Viliaine, where there were about two hundred Spaniards. Monsieur le Connestable would not leave them in his rear, in order to render the road free. The Chateau is seated upon a little mountain, which gave great assurance to those within that we could not place the artillery so as to bear upon them. They were summoned to surrender themselves or they should be cut in pieces, which they flatly refused, making answer that they were as good and faithful servants of the Emperor as Monsieur le Connestable could be of the King his master. Their answer heard, we mounted two great cannon by night with ropes drawn with the strength of arms by the Swiss and the Lansquenets [mercenary troops], when, as ill-luck would have it, the two cannon being placed, a gunner by inadvertence set fire to a sack full of gunpowder, by which he was burned together with ten or twelve soldiers; and further, the flame of the powder was the cause of discovering our artillery, which caused those in the Chateau to fire all the night many arquebus shots at the place where they had been able to discover the two cannon, which killed and wounded a number of our men.

The next day, early in the morning, we fired with the battery, which in a few hours made a breach; which being done, they demanded a parley; but it was too late, for in the meantime our French infantry, seeing them surprised, had mounted in the breach and cut them all in pieces, except a very pretty, young, lusty girl of Piedmont, whom a great seigneur wished to have to keep him company in the night for fear of the greedy wolf (loupgarou). The captain and the ensign were taken alive, but soon after hung and strangled on the battlements of the gate of the city, to the end that they might give example and fear to the imperial soldiers not to be so rash and foolish as to wish to hold such places against so great an army.

Now all the said soldiers at the Chateau, seeing our men coming with a great fury, did all they could to defend themselves, and killed and wounded a great number of our soldiers with pikes, arquebuses, and stones, wherefore the surgeons had much work cut out for them. Now I was at that time a freshwater soldier; I had not yet seen wounds made by gunshot at the first dressing. It is true that I had read in Jean de Vigo, first book, *Of wounds in General*, chapter eight, that wounds made by firearms partake of venenosity [poison] because of the powder, and for their cure he commands to cauterize them with oil of elder, scalding hot, in which should be mixed a little theriac [healing ointment]. In order not to err before using the said oil, knowing that such a thing would bring great pain to the patient, I wished to know first how the other surgeons did for the first dressing; which was to apply the said oil as hot as possible into the wound, with tents [drains] and setons [wicks]; of whom I took courage to do as they did.

At last my oil lacked and I was constrained to apply in its place a digestive [substance to promote suppuration] made of the yolks of eggs, oil of roses and turpentine. That night I could not sleep at my ease, fearing by lack of cauterization that I should find the wounded on whom I had failed to put the said oil dead or empoisoned; which made me rise very early to visit them, where, beyond my hope, I found those upon whom I had put the digestive medicament feeling little pain and their wounds without inflammation or swelling, having rested fairly well throughout the night; the others, to whom I had applied the said boiling oil, I found feverish, with great pain and swelling about their wounds. Then I resolved with myself never more to burn thus cruelly poor men wounded with gunshot.

Being at Turin, I found a surgeon who was famous above all for good treatment of gunshot wounds, into whose grace I found means to insinuate myself, to have the recipe which he called his balm, with which he treated gunshot wounds, and he made me court him for years before I could draw his recipe from him. At last by gifts and presents he gave it to me, which was to boil in oil of lilies little puppies just born, with earthworms prepared with Venetian turpentine. Then I was joyful and my heart made glad to have understood his remedy, which was like to that which I had obtained by chance.

See how I learned to treat wounds made by gunshot, not from books. …

The Journey to Flanders

Monsieur Le Due D'Ascot did not fail to send a gentleman to the King with a letter to pray him humbly that he would do him so much good and honor as to permit and command his premier surgeon to come to see Monsieur le Marquis d'Auret, his brother, who had received an arquebus shot near the knee, with fracture of the bone, about seven months ago, and that the physicians and surgeons of those parts were much troubled to cure. The King sent for me and commanded me to go to see the said Seigneur d'Auret, and to help him by all that which I could for the cure of his wound. I told him that I would use all the little knowledge which it had pleased God to give me.

I went away, accompanied by two gentlemen, to the Chateau d'Auret where the Marquis was. As soon as I arrived, I visited him and told him that the King had commanded me to come to see him and dress his wound. He said to me that he was very glad of my coming, and was greatly beholden to the King for having done him so much honor in sending me to him.

I found him with great fever, his eyes very much sunken, with a moribund and yellowish face, his tongue dry and parched, and all his body very emaciated and thin, his voice low as of a man very near to death; then I found his thigh much swollen, abscessed and ulcerated, discharging a greenish and fetid sanies [pus]. I probed it with a silver probe. By it I found a cavity near the groin, ending in the middle of the thigh, and others around the knee, sanious and caniculate [pussy and unwholesome]; also certain splinters of bone, some separated and others not. The leg was very swollen and imbued with a pituitous humor [watery mucus], cold and humid and flatulent, in such sort that the natural heat was by way of being suffocated and extinguished, and bent and drawn towards the buttocks; the buttocks ulcerated of the size of the palm of the hand. And he said he felt there extreme heat and pain and likewise in his loins, in such sort that he could not rest day or night, and had not appetite to eat, but to drink enough. It was told me that he often fell with weakness of the heart, and sometimes as in epilepsy, and often desired to vomit, with a trembling such that he could not carry his hands to his mouth.

Seeing and considering all these great complications, and his strength much abated, truly I had a very great regret to have gone to him, because it seemed to me there was little appearance that he could escape from death. Notwithstanding, to give him courage and good hope, I told him I would soon set him right, by the grace of God and the help of his physicians and surgeons.

Having seen him I went away to walk in a garden, and there I prayed God that he would do me this grace that he should recover; and that he would bless our hands and the medicaments to fight against so many complicated maladies. I discussed in my mind the means it would be necessary for me to hold to do this. They called me to dinner; I entered by the kitchen, where I saw taken out of a great pot half a sheep, a quarter of veal, three great pieces of beef, and two fowls and a very great piece of bacon, with abundance of good herbs; then I said to myself, that this broth of the pot was succulent and of good nourishment.

After dinner, all the physicians and surgeons assembled; we entered into consultation in the presence of Monsieur le Due d' Ascot and some gentlemen who accompanied him. I began by saying to the surgeons that I was greatly astonished that they had not made openings in the thigh of Monsieur le Marquis, which was all abscessed, and the pus which went forth from it very fetid and stinking, which showed it had been stagnant there a long time; and that I had found with the probe caries of the bone and splinters of bone which had already separated. They answered me that he never would consent to it and, indeed, that it was near two months that they had not been able to get leave to put clean sheets on his bed; and they scarcely dared to touch the coverlet, so great was his pain.

Then I said that to cure him it was necessary to touch other things than the coverlet of the bed. Each said what he thought of the sickness of the said seigneur, and for conclusion held it altogether hopeless. I said to them there was yet some hope because of his youth, and that God and Nature sometimes do things which seem to physicians and surgeons to be impossible.

My advice was that the cause of all these accidents came (reason of) the bullet hitting near the joint of the knee, which had broken the ligaments, tendons, and aponeuroses of the muscles, which bound the said joint together with the femoral bone, as well as the nerves, veins, and arteries; from which had followed pain, inflammation, abscess formation, and ulceration; and that we must commence the cure by that of the disease that was the cause of all the aforesaid accidents, to wit, to make openings to give issue to the sanious matter retained in the spaces between the muscles and in their substance; likewise to the bone [splinters], which caused a great corruption in the whole thigh, from which the vapors arose and were carried to the heart, which caused syncope [collapse] and fever, and from the fever a universal heat in all the body, and by consequence depravation [degeneration] of the economy.

Likewise the said vapors were communicated to the brain, which caused the epilepsy and tremors and nausea of the stomach and prevented it from performing its functions, which are chiefly to digest and concoct the viands and convert them into chyle, which if they are not well concocted, ingender crudities and obstructions, which makes that the parts are not nourished, and in consequence the body dries and becomes emaciated, and likewise because it gets no exercise.

And as to the edema [swelling caused by accumulation of serous fluid in the tissue] of his leg, that had come because of lack of aliment and of the arrest of the natural heat through all the thigh, and also because it had no power of movement, because every part which is incapable of movement remains languid and atrophied, because the heat and [vital] spirits are not sent nor drawn hither, from which ensues mortification. "And to nourish and fatten the body it is necessary to make universal frictions with warm linen cloths, above, below, on the right and on the left and round about, for the purpose of drawing the blood and [vital] spirits from within outwards; and for dispersing any fuliginous vapors retained between the skin and the flesh. Thus the parts shall thereafter be nourished and restored (as I have said before in Book Nine, treating of arquebus wounds). But it is necessary to stop when we see heat and redness in the skin, for fear of dispersing that which has been drawn out and in consequence make it more emaciated.

"Now the bedsore on his buttock has come from having been too long a time lying on it without moving himself, which has been the cause that the [vital] spirits have not been able to shine in it. From this cause there has been inflammation, from the inflammation abscess, then ulceration, even with loss of substance of the flesh subjected, with very great pain, because of the nerves which spread through this part. It is necessary, likewise, that we should put him in another bed, very soft, and give him a clean shirt and sheets.

Otherwise all the things which one could do for him would be of no service, because the excrements and vapors of the discharges, retained for so long a time in his bed, are drawn in by the systole and diastole of the arteries, which are carried through the skin, and cause the [vital] spirits to change and acquire a bad diathesia, or quality, and corruption, which is seen in those who lie in a bed whereon a smallpox patient has lain and sweat, who get the smallpox by the putrid vapors which are imbued and remain in the sheets and coverlets.

"Now the reason that he cannot sleep and is almost in a consumption is because he eats little and takes no exercise and is vexed with great pains; because there is nothing which lowers and prostrates the [body] forces more than pain. The cause of his parched, dry tongue comes from the vehemence and heat of the fever,, through the vapors which ascend from all the body to the mouth, for, as is said in a common proverb, 'When an oven is well heated, the mouth feels it/ "

Having discoursed of the causes and complications, I said that it was necessary to cure them by their contraries; and first, to ease the pains, make incisions in the thigh to evacuate the retained pus, not letting it out all at a time, for fear that a sudden great evacuation would cause a resolution of the [vital] spirits, which would greatly debilitate the patient and shorten his days. Secondly, having regard to the great swelling and coldness of the leg, fearing lest it should fall into a gangrene, and that it would be necessary to apply actual heat (the actual cautery); ... for this reason we should apply about it hot bricks, on which should be sprinkled a decoction made of nerval herbs [herbs soothing to the nerves], boiled in wine and vinegar and then wrapped in napkins; and to his feet an earthenware bottle filled with the said decoction, corked and wrapped in linen. Also it is necessary to make fomentations on the thigh and the whole of the leg of a decoction made of sage, rosemary, thyme, lavender, flowers of camomile, and melilot, red roses boiled in white wine, and a desiccant [dryer] made of oak ashes, and a little vinegar, and half a handful of salt. This decoction has the property to subtilize, attenuate, incise, resolve, wither and dry up the thick, viscous humor. The said fomentations should be kept up a long time to the end that the resolution should be greater, because being thus made for a long time, more is resolved than is attracted, because as one liquefies the humor contained in the part, the skin and the flesh of the muscles are rarefied [dried up].

Thirdly, there must be applied on the buttock a large plaster made of desiccative red ointment, and *unguentum comitissae*, equal parts mixed together for the purpose of easing his pain and drying the ulcer; also we should make him a little pillow of down to keep his buttock in the air without his being supported on it. Fourthly, to refresh the heat of his loins, we should apply over them the refrigerant ointment of Galen, freshly made, and over it fresh leaves of the water-lily, and then a napkin soaked in oxycrate, frequently sprinkled and renewed. And to support the heart, we must apply over it a refrigerant medicament, made of oil of water-lilies, ointment of roses and a little saffron, dissolved in rose-vinegar and theriac, spread on a piece of scarlet cloth.

For the syncope, which proceeded from the exhaustion of the natural forces troubling also the brain, it was necessary to use good succulent food, such as soft-boiled eggs, plums stewed in wine and sugar, also broth of the juice of the great pot, of which I have spoken before; with the white meat of capons, wings of partridges minced small, and other roasted meats easy to digest, as veal, kid, pigeons, partridges, thrushes, and the like. The sauce should be oranges, verjuice, sorrel, bitter pomegranates; and he should likewise eat them boiled with good herbs, as sorrel, lettuce, parsley, chicory, bugloss, marigolds, and the like. At night he can take barley-water, with the juice of sorrel and water-lilies, of each two ounces, with four or five grains of opium, and of the four cold seeds bruised, of each a half an ounce, which is a nourishing and medicinal remedy and will make him sleep. His bread should be that of the farm, neither too stale nor too fresh.

And for the great pain in his head, it would be necessary to cut his hair and to rub it with oxyrrhodinum, a little warm, and to leave on it a double cloth soaked in it; also, on his forehead, one with oil of roses and water-lilies and poppies, with a little opium and rose-vinegar and a little camphor, renewed at times. Moreover, he should smell flowers of henbane and water-lilies, bruised with vinegar and rose-water, with a little camphor, wrapped together in a handkerchief, which should be held for a long time against the nose, so that the odor can communicate itself to the brain; and these things should be continued only until the great inflammation and pain shall be passed, for fear of refrigerating too much the brain. Furthermore, one should make artificial rain, by making water run from some high place into a cauldron, that it may make such a noise that the patient can hear it; by these means sleep will be provoked in him.

And as to the retraction of his leg, there was hope of correcting it when one should have made evacuation of the pus and other humors contained in the thigh, which by their extension, made by repletion, have drawn back the leg. It would remedy itself after first rubbing all the knee joint with ointment of althea and oil of lilies and a little brandy, and putting above it black wool with the grease in it, likewise by putting under the knee a feather pillow, folded double; and little by little we shall extend his leg.

This my discourse was well approved by the physicians and surgeons.

The consultation ended, we went to the patient, and I made three openings in his thigh, from which went forth a great quantity of pus and sanies, and at the same time I took from him some little splinters of bone, but did not wish to let go forth too great a quantity of the said sanies for fear of too much exhaustion of his forces. Two or three hours afterwards, I had a bed made for him near his own, on which were clean white sheets; then a strong man placed him in it, and he was glad to be taken out of his dirty, stinking bed. Soon after, he asked to sleep, which he did for near four hours; whereat everybody in the house commenced to rejoice, and especially Monsieur le Due d'Ascot, his brother.

The following days I made injections into the depth and cavities of the ulcers, composed of aegyptiacum dissolved sometimes in brandy, other times in wine. I applied compresses to the bottom of the sinuses, to cleanse and dry the spongy soft flesh, with tents [drains] of lead cannulas [tubes] for the purpose of always giving issue to the sanies; and over them a large plaster of diacalcitheos, dissolved in wine. Likewise I bandaged him so dexterously that he had no pain, which ceasing, the fever began to diminish very much. Then I made him drink wine moderately tempered with water, knowing that it restores and quickens the forces. And all the things that we had ordered in the consultation were accomplished according to their time and order; his pains and the fever ceased and he began always to grow better. He discharged two of his surgeons and one of his physicians so that we were but three with him.

… In one month we had so wrought that he could sit up in a chair; and he had himself carried to and fro in his garden and to the gate of his chateau to see the people pass. … And the citizens of Mons in Hainault and other gentlemen, his neighbors, came to see him in wonder, as a man coming forth from the grave; and from then that he was so well, he was never without company; and as one went forth, another would enter to visit him. …

Explanation of the fashion and use of three and fifty Inftruments of Chirurgery.

Gathered out of *Ambrofius Pareus*, the famous French Chirurgian, and done into Englifli, for the behoofe of yone Practitioners in Chiru'rgery, by H. C.

The Practise of Chirurgery

Chap. I.

For the opening of Tumors.

When a Tumor is ripe, that is, when there is in it *Pus confectums,* at which time all symptomes of heate, paine, and the like, are mitigated, and the head of it is growne mucronated and soft, then it is time to open it, and not before. Neither ought the Chirurgian afterward to linger, for feared the humour shut up in the flesh,should contrast a venomous, or at least a malignant disposition, and by his contagion, infects the neighbouring parts. And this is especially to be feared, where the adjacent parts are of more exquisite sense, or of greater dignity: as also where they are more subject to the confluence of excrements, or in a more prone portion; for the weight of humours will naturally decline.

This apertion is made sometimes by a phlegme or lancet, sometimes by a penknife, as we call it, sometimes by Cauteries.

The phlegme or lancet, is that Instrument wherewith they use to open a Veine, and may be of use in tender and soft parts, and where the Apostemation is outward: The figure of it you have here under fet.

The forme of a Phlegme.

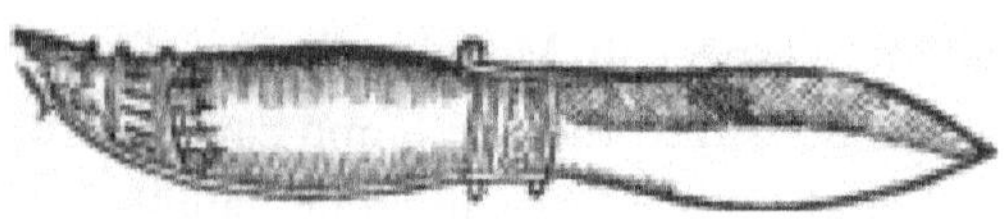

But if the Apostemation lie deeper, or if the Tumor be harder, or the skin thicker, then the Penknife is fitter, for with it the hand may be carried more steadily; you may strike deeper (if need be) and without danger that your Instrument should faile you. Heere you have the figure joyned to the handle, but turned our, to shew the crooked blade marked with [C] for that is most fit for almost all manner of incisions. Where there is any different forme to be used, you shall have it expressed.

Ambroise Paré, from *Three and Fifty Instruments of Chirurgery*, no. 141. The English Experience: Its Record in Early Printed Books Published in Facsimile, trans. H.C, pp. 3, 9, 12, 14, 49.

The forme of the Penknife standing out of his handle

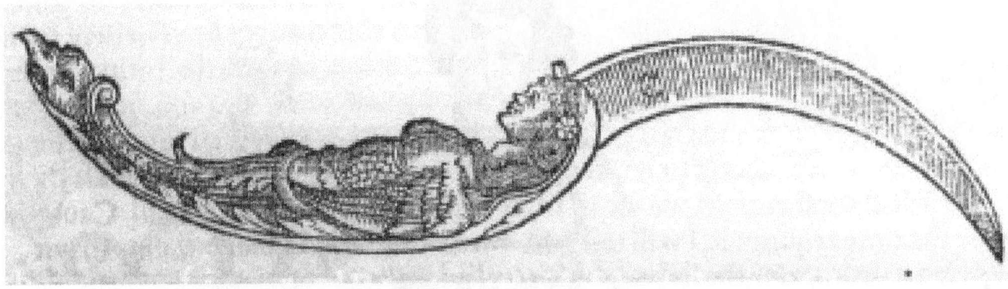

But because some faint-hearted Patients are afraid of this Instrument, Chirurgtans have decided to fasten the point of a Lancet or Knife in the midst of a piece of Coune, to stand out as far as they would have the wound to be deep. That coyne they couer with some thin Cearecloath, to hide the edge or point, pretending that Cearecloath to be the Medicine which shall make way for the matter to issue; but when they have cunningly conveyed the Coyne upon the Apostemation, suddenly they presse it as hard as they meane to make the Incision deepe.

Of Ruptures.

There be many sorts of Ruptures, or Relaxations, whose names are taken from that which falleth downe: for it is the *Peritoneum* or Rimme of the belly onely which is broken or relaxed in them all. Sometimes the gut, sometimes the kell, sometimes both fall together; and the Relaxation is at the productions of the *Peritoneum.* Unlesse it be that we call *Exomphalos,* when the *Peritoneum,* at the Nauell is relaxed or broken, and the guts or kell, or wind, or flesh, or humor, make a Tumor in that place, which I have seene as big as a mans head. I will not particularise heere of all the kindes, onely let me tell you, that in children a cure may be made according to the first intention as we say, but after childhood not so, or at least very rarely, and by accident, as it happened to the Priest *Pareus* makes mention of; then the Trusse is most in use. Sometimes also the golden ligature.

For the Trusse, it is made diuers wayes by diuers men, some of Holland, some of Suftian, of Taffata, & etc. Some stuffed with Bumbast, some are made of Steele which in my opinion are the best and the easiest, if they be made light and fit. All the skill is in fitting them to the Patients body, but first the Tumor must be gently returned up. I know there is a tricke lately brought out of *France* to trusse a man up with I know how many Ells; of Holland, and I believe there may be some skill in the manner of the tying of the Fascia, but I have experience that it hath done more harme in heating the backe and sides then good, by the fastnesse of the Ligature. Neither doe I thinke it possible to make any Ligature of that kinde so firme as the ordinary Trusses are, especially if we would use the backe and shoulder band to our Trusses, which I see few do. Wherefore my Counsell is, that men thus affected, resort to such Chirurgians as make their trusses themselves, and can fit them precisely. I have exhibited two figures of them hereunder.

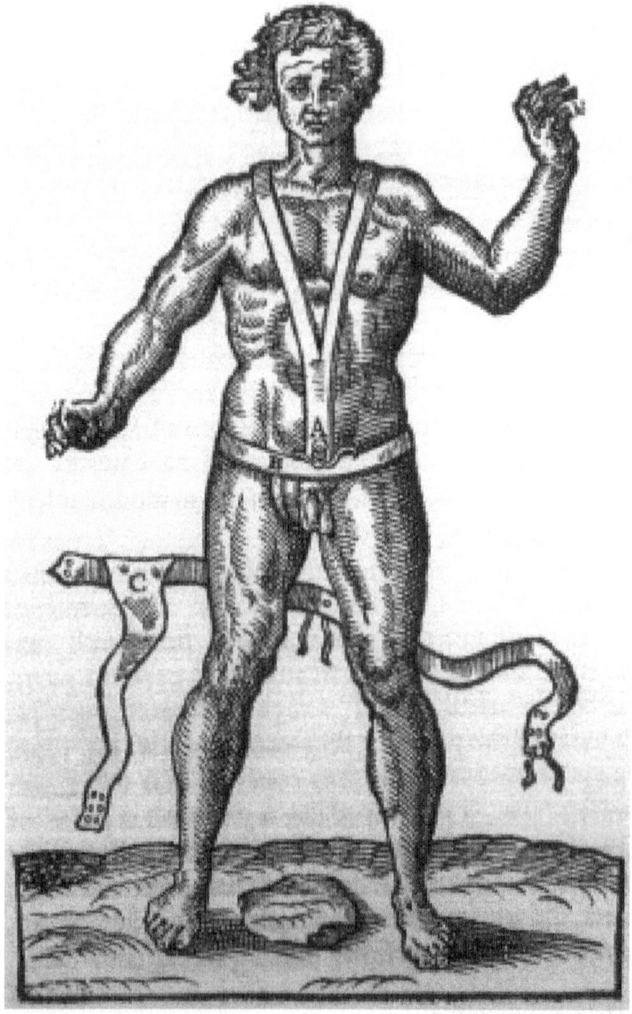

The figure of a man broken en one fide, together with his Truffe, whofe boulfter bath three fwelling inequalities, two in the up per part, and one in the neather, and betwixt them fomewat bollowed, that it may not ly too hard vpon the fhare bone. This will ferue when the gut or the kell falls in-to the groyne.

A, A *Fascia* or band that goes over the shoulder, and is fastened behind and before to the girdle of the Trusse to keepe it in due place.

B, The girdle or Trusse.

C, The cavity of the Boulder in the middest of the swelling inequalities where it is better stuffed.

But if a man be bursten on both sides of the Groyne, which is a thing not very unusual, then the Girdle is made like the former, but there must be two Boulsters, or at least a Boulster fitted for both sides, having a hole through it, whereat the Yard may issue; the fashion of it is such.

Next, that the future be immediately made after the wound is given, or as soon as may be; and again, that the deeper the wound is into the flesh, the more flesh be also taken up with the needle, otherwise if the surface onely be sewed, the flesh underneath the suture which is wounded, will turn into quitture, and apostemate into a cave or hollow Ulcer.

There are five kinds of sutures.

The first used in fleshy parts, not fit to be swathed, is after this manner.

The needle must be long and slender, and toward the point three-square, like a Glouers needle, for so it will pierce better; the eye somewhat hollowed that the thread may be hidden, as it were, in the gutter of it, and so it will more easily follow the needle. You must also prepare a silver quill, with a window cut out toward the end, whose whole side you shall place against the lip of the wound which you meane to pierce with the needle, as well to keepe it steady and firme against the force of the needle, as also that by that window, you may perceive when the needle hath pierced so much of the skinne and flesh as you desire, and through it may also draw the needle and his thred without shaking or moving the sides or lips of the wound. When the wound is stitched up, tye a knot upon the thred, as neere the skin as you can, and cut off the rest that it sticke not to your Emplaisters.

But in the stitching you must observe, that if the wound be any thing large, you must take the first stitch about the middest of the wound, and the second in the midway between the first stitch and the end of the wound, and the third answerable to the second, for betwixt every stitch there should be aboue halfe an inch distance. Neither must you draw the lips of the wound close together with your stitches, but leaue a distance betwixt, that out of that distance the quitture may vent it selfe as it groweth, for otherwise it will not onely cause paine and inflammation, but so tumisie, that either the stitch or the thread, or both, will breake. Observe also that in taking up the skin with the needle, you take not up too muck flesh with it, for that will increase the paine and inflammation, and make the Cicatrice or scarre more deformed. But have due regard to the depth of the wound, and the shallower it is take up lesse flesh, the deeper more. Yea, sometimes the wound in fleshy and brawny parts will be so deepe, that it will be necessary to provide a crooked needle, and a crooked quill or Canule, to performe the worke, and therefore you have hereunder described of both sorts as well straight as crooked, for several uses.

A type of the Quils and Needles required for the making of a Seameer Suture.

Observe by the way that the silke thread waxed, is to be preferred before the thread of Line; and *Blondus* gives a good reason for it, for it will not so soone rot as the other.

The second kinde of Seame or Suture, is like that of Glouers, or that of the Skinners in sewing their Skinnes together. And it is used when the entrals are wounded, left the excrement should issue out. I do not beny but that it is possible such a cure may be wrought, but how hard it is to come to them, to do the worke, and how dangerous after it is done no man doubteth; yet any thing almost maybe attempted to save life; if it may be, and Nature sometimes doth incourage us to that which Art would thinke and leave as desperate.

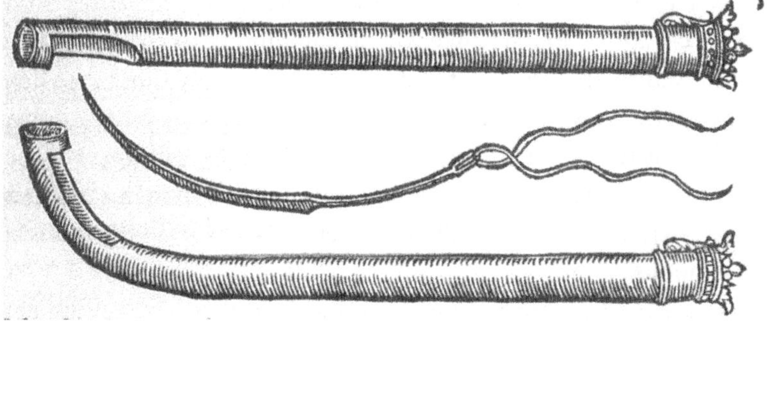

The third kinde of Seame,is that which Chirurgians use in the Cure of the Flax-lip, that is, when the upper lip in the middest, is separated the one halfe from the other, and that from the birth, as it hapneth many times. They use the same Suture also when the lip is so wounded by accidents, as also in maine deep wounds of the flesh, whose lips are farre distant. The needles (for they must be diuers, sometimes many) must be triangular or foure-square, almost throughout the length, and the thread well waxed that it breake not. That needle (if one stitch will serve) must be thrust through both sides of the wound or breach, and take up all the flesh of both lips and there …

Chap. VIII. Of some offences of the Eyes.

We spake last of the wounds of the face in the end of the last Chapter, wherefore here I will also prosecute some accidents which happen about the face also, and absolve what I have to say concerning it, yet so that I will meddle onely with such accidents as require the use of the Instruments I have to describe, to which in this small additament I tye my selfe.

First therefore many small motes fall into the Eye which are sometimes hard to get out, and being sharpe, or otherwise of euill qualitie, breed an extreame and insufferable offence. If by turning the eyelid over the end of a *patula*, you cannot finde that which offends, then you many use the Instrument hereunder described. You must insinuate it under the eye-lids next to the white of the eye-lids next to the white of the eye, and so separate the you cannot finde that which offends, then you may use the Instrument hereunder described. You must insinuate it under the eye-lids next to the white of the eye, and so separate the liddes as farre asunder as you can without too much violence, and withal, hold the eye steady, that with a paire of small Pincers you may pull out that which offends, which sometimes will be fast fixed, or adheere close to the membranes. This Instrument must be so artificially made that according to the bignesse or smallnesse of the eye, or as you would have it extended or drawne in, it may be made wider or narrower, at your pleasure. This is the forme of it.

Againe, the Eyes are often vexed with sharp and most importanate Defluxions, so that sometimes the Horny coat of the Eye is broken therewith.

Beside, you have here expressed the figure of a man wounded with all kinde of Weapons and inetiery part of the body.

Againe, there is great difference in respect of the wounded part, whether to be fleshie, bony, nervous, in a joynt, or neere a joynt, or farther off, it a noble partes the Braine, the Longues, the Heart, the Stomacke, the Liver, the Guts, or such like; or in a part more ignoble man inward or an outward part, and according to these differences, such wounds are more or lesse mortall. In all mortall wounds it shall be for the honour of the Chirurgian and his Art, to foretell the danger. Yet not to leave any thing unattempted which may give hope of recovery, because as in diseases as in wounds, it falleth often out, that what the Physitian or Chirurgian gives over as desperate, that either some good old Wife, or which is worse, some cheating Mountebanke will take upon him to cure, and if he, while time, with a little herbe *Robert,* till Nature prevaile over the disease (which many times thee doth above and against our expectation) then is he famed for a second *Aesculapius.* How soever it is a great disparagement to a Chirurgian, if he be called while the Patient lives to let him die with the weapon in his body, yea as much honour may be gotten by the Artificial getting out of the weapon in a desperate case, as by curing him that is not desperately wounded. It shall not therefore be amiss a little to insist upon the Artificial extraction of such weapons.

And in the first place,the Chirurgian must be forewarned that he take care he does not his worke butcherly, with too much cutting or tearing the flesh, but especially veines, artries, nerves or tendons, least it be said of him that his hand hath done more harme then the weapon,which would be an extreme dishonour to him and to his Art.

But to the matter. There be two wayes to get out a weapon: one by the way, it went in, and that we call extraction,the other by the part which is adverse, and that we called expulsion.

After the very first dressing, these workes must be done, and with more ease and felicity performed if you place your Patient in the same posture he was in when he received the wound, as hath beene before signified. Againe,you shall have at hand all your Instruments, as for example. A paire of Pliers whose handles when you presse together the shankes will be divided; those are fit to take out an Arrowhead, or the head of any weapon which is hollow, for the shankes being divided in that hollownesse, will hold the Arrow head firme and fast, and so draw it out. The next is a hollow instrument of Steele like a Cane clouen in the lengthen which runnes a slender and sharpe probe, and at the handle a large screw answerable to the hollownesse of the Cane of Steele: this screw doth not only serve to divide the clouen cane, which by that meanes fills the hollownes of the head of the Iauelin or such like, and so drawes it out as the former Instrument did, but also if a piece of the wood remained in the head, it presses the sharpe probe into that wood, and so drawes it out.

The next is a paire of small plyers, a little compassed at the end, and toothed within; that if the wound be oblique it may attaine to the bottome of it and meet with any small pieces of its may be or the like, which lie there, and bring them away. The next is a paire of plyers, with a screw running crosse the shanks of the handle, but the end of the pliers is like the Crowes Bill, or a little flatter. This screw in the handle doth open and close.

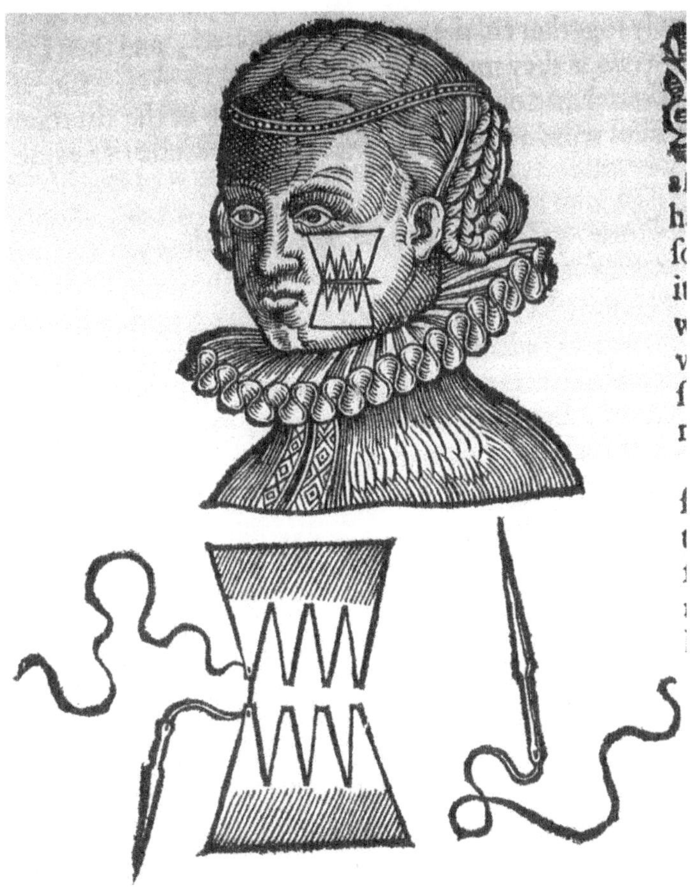

One of the suturing techniques utilized by Ambroise Pare on the face.

Chapter 10

Miguel Serveto: *Christianismi Restitutio* (1553)

HISTORICAL HIGHLIGHTS

- Miguel Serveto (1509–1553). Also known as Michael Servetus
- Born at Villanueva de Sigiena, Aragón, Spain
- Entered service of Franciscan friar Juan de Quintana (1524)
- Studied at Collége de Calvi, Paris (1533)
- Also studied medicine in Paris (1536)
- Obtained Doctor of Medicine from Montpellier (1539)
- Was a theologian, cartographer and humanist as well
- Correspondence with Calvin offended Calvin's religious views
- Became first European to describe the function of the pulmonary circulation
- Published his notable book, *Christanismi Restitutio* (1553)
- Burned at the stake in Geneva, Switzerland at the insistence of Calvin because of heretical views on non-Trinitarianism and anti-infant baptism

THE WRITINGS OF MIGUEL SERVETO

... body (see Ch. IV). He is less well known for his anatomical studies of heart muscle in which he demonstrated that individual contractile fibers of the cardiac ventricle are disposed in a "figure-of-eight" fashion such that when they contract, the fibers tend to obliterate the ventricular cavity completely on both sides of the heart. He was also aware that this occlusion of the two ventricular cavities occurs virtually simultaneously during ventricular systole.

Lower's studies are noteworthy for his clear vision into the functional significance of the facts of anatomical structure. Like Charles Sherrington, another Oxford physiologist of over two centuries and a half later, Lower "turned anatomical facts into physiological language." Professor Kenneth Franklin has pointed out that he gave definite proof of the myogenic nature of the heart beat, and an estimation of the heart's output and of the rapidity of blood flow, that he missed by a narrow margin anticipating

Michael Servetus, "Christianismi Restitutio," *Memoirs of the American Philosophical Society*, vol. 34, ed. Charles D. O'Malley, pp. 202–208. Readings selected and historical highlights written by Luis Horacio Toledo-Pereyra.

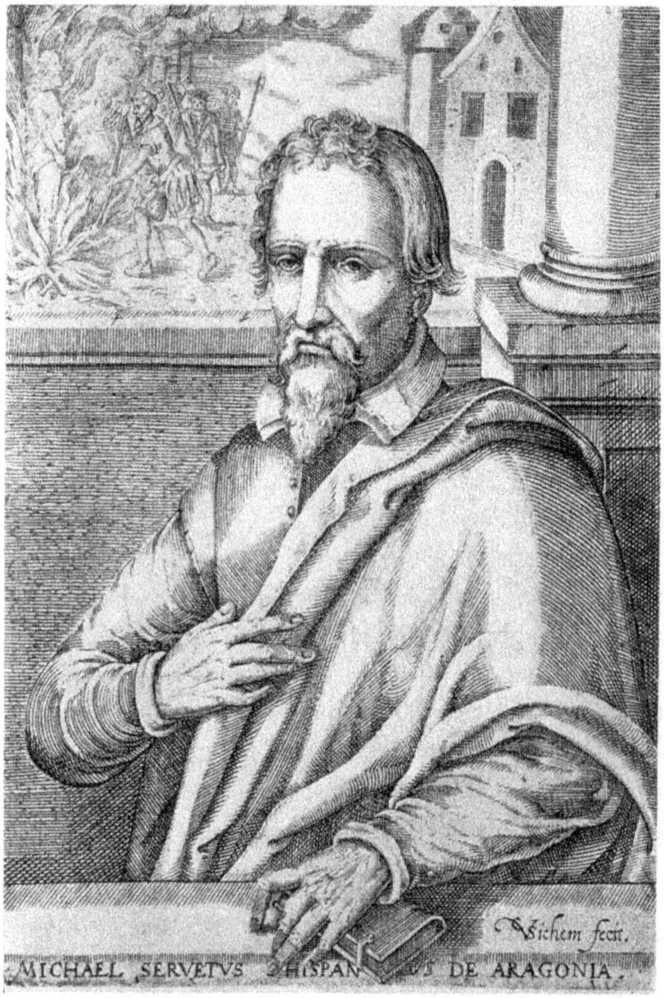

MICHAEL SERVETUS Copper-plate engraving by Christoffel van Sichem (1607)

the Webers' discovery of vagal inhibition, and that he was the real inventor of transfusion, having first demonstrated the technique in February of 1665.

Structure of the Heart

[P. 30 of original Latin ed.] But in this ventricle also the whole of the fibres do not reach from the base to the apex, and, only after a number have been removed, can the others be separated that far; for several are deflected from the general course and path in the middle of their passage across the Heart, and disappear under the next preceding fibres to ascend obliquely to the tendon of the opposite side, and so describe by their passage a shorter circle. As was seen above in Fig. 5 [Fig. 2].

The inner fibres, on the other hand, all ascend obliquely upwards and to the left, in exactly the opposite direction to the outer fibres, to reach the base of the heart. They are inserted into the tendon at the base and form the inner wall of the ventricle.

The longer fibres of the opposite set run together to the apex of the Heart, and pass round it to form a whorl, in such a way, however, that the space which is left in the centre becomes the thinnest part of the Heart. The fashion of this whorl, and the meeting in it, at the apex of the Heart, of the fibres of the outer wall of the left ventricle with those [p. 31] of the inner wall, are quite well shown in Fig. 7 [Fig. 3]. In this figure

a is the tendon of the right side.

b is the tendon of the left side.

c are some fibres of the outer wall.

d are fibres of the inner wail, together with the whorl formed by fibres of both sets near the apex.

Not[1] only because of such gifts, but by reason of that one alone who breathes the divine spirit into us, God is said to give us his spirit, Gen. 2 and 6. Our soul is a kind of lantern of God, Prov. 20. It is like a spark of the spirit of God, a reflection of the wisdom of God, created yet very similar to that spiritual wisdom, incorporated in it, retaining the innate light of divinity, the spark of that prime wisdom and the very spirit of divinity. God himself testifies, in chapter 6 above, that the spirit of divinity was innate in man even after Adam's sin. The dispensation of our life is given and is sustained through grace from his breath, as Job says, chap. 10 and 32 and following. God breathed the divine spirit into Adam's nostrils together with a breath of air, and thence it remains, Isaiah 2 and Psa. 103. God himself maintains the breath of life for us by his spirit, giving breath to the people who are upon the earth and spirit to those treading it, so that we live, move and exist in him, Isaiah 42 and Acts 17. Wind from the four winds and breath from the four breaths gathered by God revive corpses, Ezek. 37. From a breath of air God there introduces the divine spirit into men in whom the life of the inspired air was innate. Hence in Hebrew "spirit" is represented in the same way as "breath." From the air God introduces the divine spirit, introducing the air with the spirit itself and the spark of the very deity which fills the air. The saying of Orpheus is true, that the divine spirit is carried by the winds and enters through full inspiration, as Aristotle cites in the books, *De anima*. Ezekiel teaches that the divine spirit contains a kind of elemental substance and, as God himself teaches, something in the substance of the blood. I shall explain this matter at greater length here so that you may thence understand that the substance of the created spirit of Christ is essentially joined to the very substance of the holy spirit. I shall call the air spirit because in the sacred language there is no special name for air. Indeed, that fact indicates that the divine breath is in the air which the spirit of the Lord fills.

So that you, the reader, may have the whole doctrine of the divine spirit and the spirit, I shall add here the divine philosophy which you will easily understand if you have been trained in anatomy. It is said that in us there is a triple spirit from the substance of three higher elements, natural, vital and animal. Aphrodisaeus calls them three spirits. But they are not three but once again of the single spirit (*spiritus*). The vital spirit is that which is communicated through anastomoses from the arteries to the veins in which it is called the natural [spirit]. Therefore the first [i.e., natural spirit] is of the blood, and its seat is in the liver and in the veins of the body. The second is the vital spirit of which the seat is in the heart and in the arteries of the body. The third is the animal spirit, a ray of light, as it were, of which the seat is in the brain and the nerves of the body. In all these there resides the energy of the one spirit and of the light of God. The formation of man from the uterus teaches that the vital spirit is communicated from the heart to the liver. For an artery joined to a vein is transmitted through the umbilicus of the foetus, and in like manner afterward the artery and vein are always joined in us. The divine spirit of Adam was inspired

1 This translation was made from Photostats of the page-for-page reprint (Nürnberg, 1790), made available through the kindness of Professor John F. Fulton.

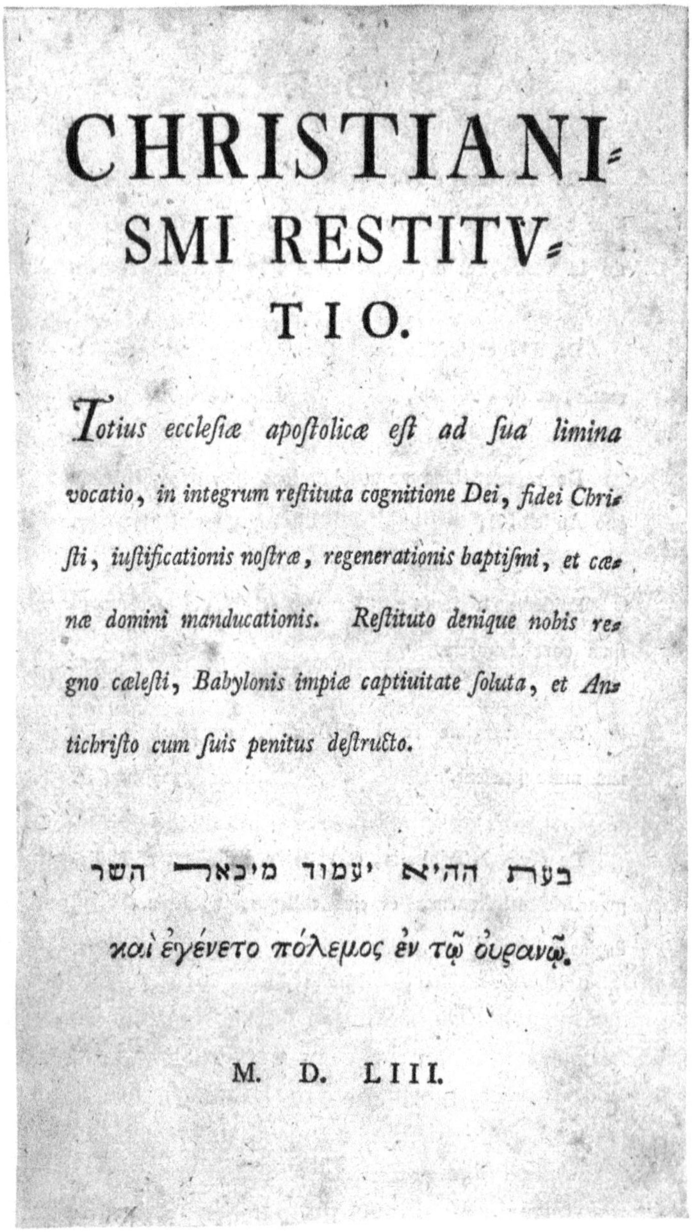

CHRISTIANI-
SMI RESTITV-
TIO.

Totius ecclesiæ apostolicæ est ad sua limina vocatio, in integrum restituta cognitione Dei, fidei Christi, iustificationis nostræ, regenerationis baptismi, et cœnæ domini manducationis. Restituto denique nobis regno cælesti, Babylonis impiæ captiuitate soluta, et Antichristo cum suis penitus destructo.

בעת ההיא יעמוד מיכאל השר

καὶ ἐγένετο πόλεμος ἐν τῷ οὐρανῷ.

M. D. LIII.

Plate 5. Title-page of the Murr reprint (1790) of the *Christianismi restitutio* of Servetus, 1553. The reprint is now almost as scarce as the original.

from God into the heart before [it was communicated into] the liver, and from there was communicated to the liver. The divine spirit was truly drawn into the mouth and nostrils, but the inspiration extended to the heart. The heart is the first living thing, the source of heat in the middle of the body. From the liver it takes the liquid of life, a kind of material, and in return vivifies it, just as the liquid of water furnishes material for higher substances and by them, with the addition of light, is vivified so that [in turn] it may invigorate. The material of the divine spirit is from the blood of the liver by way of a remarkable elaboration of which you will now hear. Hence it is said that the divine spirit is in the blood, and the divine spirit is itself the blood, or the sanguineous spirit. It is not said that the divine spirit is principally in the walls of the heart, or in the body of the brain or of the liver, but in the blood, as is taught by God himself in Gen. 9, Levit. 7 and Deut. 12.

In this matter there must first be understood the substantial generation of the vital spirit which is composed of a very subtle blood nourished by the inspired air. The vital spirit has its origin in the left ventricle of the heart, and the lungs assist greatly in its generation. It is a rarefied spirit, elaborated by the force of heat, reddish-yellow *(flavo)* and of fiery potency, so that it is a kind of clear vapor from very pure blood, containing in itself the substance of water, air and fire. It is generated in the lungs from a mixture of inspired air with elaborated, subtle blood which the right ventricle of the heart communicates to the left. However, this communication is made not through the middle wall of the heart, as is commonly believed, but by a very ingenious arrangement the subtle blood is urged forward by a long course through the lungs; it is elaborated by the lungs, becomes reddish-yellow and is poured from the pulmonary artery into the pulmonary vein. Then in the pulmonary vein it is mixed with inspired air and through expiration it is cleansed of its sooty vapors. Thus finally the whole mixture, suitably prepared for the production of the vital spirit, is drawn onward from the left ventricle of the heart by diastole.

That the communication and elaboration are accomplished in this way through the lungs we are taught by the different conjunctions and the communication of the pulmonary artery with the pulmonary vein in the lungs. The notable size of the pulmonary artery confirms this; that is, it was not made of such sort or of such size, nor does it emit so great a force of pure blood from the heart itself into the lungs merely for their nourishment; nor would the heart be of such service to the lungs, since at an earlier stage, in the embryo, the lungs, as Galen teaches, are nourished from elsewhere because those little membranes or valvules of the heart are not opened until the time of birth. Therefore that the blood is poured from the heart into the lungs at the very time of birth, and so copiously, is for another purpose. Likewise, not merely air, but air mixed with blood, is sent from the lungs to the heart through the pulmonary vein; therefore the mixture occurs in the lungs. That reddish-yellow color is given to the spirituous blood by the lungs; it is not from the heart.

In the left ventricle of the heart there is no place large enough for so great and copious a mixture, nor for that elaboration imbuing the reddish-yellow color. Finally, that middle wall, since it is lacking in vessels and mechanisms, is not suitable for that communication and elaboration, although something may possibly sweat through. By the same arrangement by which a transfusion of the blood from the portal vein to the vena cava occurs in the liver, so a transfusion of the spirit from the pulmonary artery to the pulmonary vein occurs in the lung. If anyone compares these things with those which Galen wrote in books VI and VII, *De usu partium*, he will thoroughly understand a truth which was unknown to Galen.

And so that vital spirit is then transfused from the left ventricle of the heart into the arteries of the whole body so that that which is more rarefied seeks the higher regions where it is further elaborated, especially in the retiform plexus situated under the base of the brain, and, approaching the special seat of the rational soul, the animal spirit begins to be formed from the vital. Again it is more greatly rarefied by the fiery force of the mind, elaborated and completed in the very slender vessels or hair-like (*capillaribus)* arteries which are situated in the choroid plexuses and contain the mind itself. These plexuses penetrate all the inmost parts of the brain, internally girdling the ventricles of the brain, and those vessels, enfolded and woven together as far as the origins of the nerves, serve to introduce in these last the faculties of sensation and of motion. Those vessels in a very remarkable way are woven together very finely, and even if they are called arteries, nevertheless they are the termination of arteries extending through the assistance of the meninges to the origin of the nerves. It is a new kind of vessels. For just as in the transfusion from the veins into the arteries there is a new kind of vessels in the lung, from vein and artery, so in the transfusion from the arteries into the nerves there is a new kind of vessels from the tunic of the artery in the meninx, since especially do the meninges preserve their tunics in the nerves. The sensibility of the nerves is not in their soft material, as in the brain. All nerves end in membranous filaments which have the most exquisite sensibility and to which for this reason the spirit is always sent. And from those little vessels of the meninges, or choroid plexuses, as from a source, the clear animal spirit is poured forth like a ray through the nerves into the eyes and other sense organs. By the same route, but in reverse, light images of things causing sensation, coming from without, are sent to the same source, penetrating inwardly, as it were, through the clear medium [i.e., spirit].

From these things it is sufficiently clear that that soft mass of the brain is not properly the seat of the rational soul, since it is cold and lacking in sensation. But it is like a bolster for the aforesaid vessels lest they be broken, and like a custodian of the animal spirit lest it blow away when it must be communicated to the nerves; and it is cold that it may temper that fiery heat contained within the vessels. Hence also it happens that the nerves serve the tunic of the membrane in the internal cavity, which is common to the aforesaid vessels as a faithful guardian of the spirit, and they hold this [away] from the thin meninx just as they hold another from the thick. Also those empty spaces of the ventricles of the brain which puzzle philosophers and physicians contain nothing else but the spirit. But those ventricles were made in the first place like a cloaca for the reception of the purgings from the brain so that they may test the excrementa received there, from which morbid defluxions arise, and provide a passage to the palate and nostrils. And when the ventricles are so filled with pituita that the arteries themselves or the choroid plexuses are immersed in it, then suddenly apoplexy is aroused. If a very noxious humor obstructs a part, and its vapor infects the mind, epilepsy occurs, or another disease, according to the part into which it settles when it has been expelled. Therefore let us say that it is the mind which we clearly perceive to be afflicted. From the immoderate heat of those vessels, or from the inflammation of the meninges, obvious delirium and frenzy occur. Whence from the diseases occurring by reason of site and substance, by force of heat and because of the ingenious construction of the vessels containing it, and from the actions of the mind apparent there, we always conclude that those little vessels must be given first consideration because all the rest serve them and because the nerves of sensation are tied to them so that they may receive their force from them. Finally, because we perceive the intellect exerting itself there when, as a result of concentrated thought, those arteries are pulsating as far as the temples. He who has not seen this thing will scarcely understand. Those ventricles were made for a second reason, that a portion of the inspired air penetrating through the ethmoid bones to their empty spaces, attracted by diastole from the vessels of the spirit, may refresh and ventilate the animal spirit contained within and the soul. In those vessels are mind, soul and fiery spirit requiring constant fanning; otherwise, like an external fire which has been covered up, there would be suffocation. As in the case of an ordinary fire, there is required not only fanning and blowing upon so that it may take fuel from the air, but also that it may discharge its sooty vapors into the air. And just as this common external fire is bound to a thick earthy body, because of a common dryness and because of a common form of light, so that which has the liquid of the body as its food is blown upon, supported and nourished by the air; thus that fiery spirit and our soul are similarly bound to the body, making one with it and having its blood as food; it is blown upon, supported and nourished by the airy spirit through inspiration and expiration, so that there is a double nourishment for it, spiritual and corporeal.

Chapter 11

Girolamo Hieronymus Fabricius: *De Venarum Ostiolis* (1603)

HISTORICAL HIGHLIGHTS

- Girolamo Hieronymus Fabricius (1537-1619)
- Born at Acquapendente, Italy
- Attended University of Padua
- Obtained Doctor of Medicine at Padua in 1559
- His medical school advisor, Gabriel Falloppio, was a professor of anatomy and surgery
- William Harvey studied under Fabricius
- Succeeded Fallopio as professor of anatomy and surgery at Padua (1565–1604)
- Considered "Father of Embriology"
- Published book, *De Venarum, Ostiolis* (1603), where it was demonstrated that valves were present in veins to move blood flow ahead
- Harvey used Fabricius' findings to advance his concepts on the theory of the circulation

THE WRITINGS OF GIROLAMO FABRICIUS

DOORLETS OF VEINS [hereafter translated as *valves*] is the name I give to some extremely delicate little membranes in the lumen [cavities] of veins. They occur at intervals, singly or in pairs, especially in the limb veins. They open upwards in the direction of the main venous trunk, and are closed below, while, viewed from the outside, they resemble the swellings in the stem and small branches of plants.

My theory is that Nature has formed them to delay the blood to some extent, and to prevent the whole mass of it flooding into the feet or hands and fingers, and collecting there. Two evils are thus avoided, namely, undernutrition of the upper parts of the limbs, and a permanently swollen condition of the hands and feet. Valves were made, therefore, to ensure a really fair all-round distribution of the blood for the nutrition of the various parts.

A discussion of these valves must be preceded by a feeling of wonder at the way in which they have hitherto escaped the notice of anatomists, both of our own and earlier generations; so much so that

Girolamo Hieronymus Fabricius, "Doorlets in the Veins," *Readings in the History of Physiology*, ed. John F. Fulton, trans. K.J. Franklin. Readings selected and historical highlights written by Luis Horacio Toledo-Pereyra.

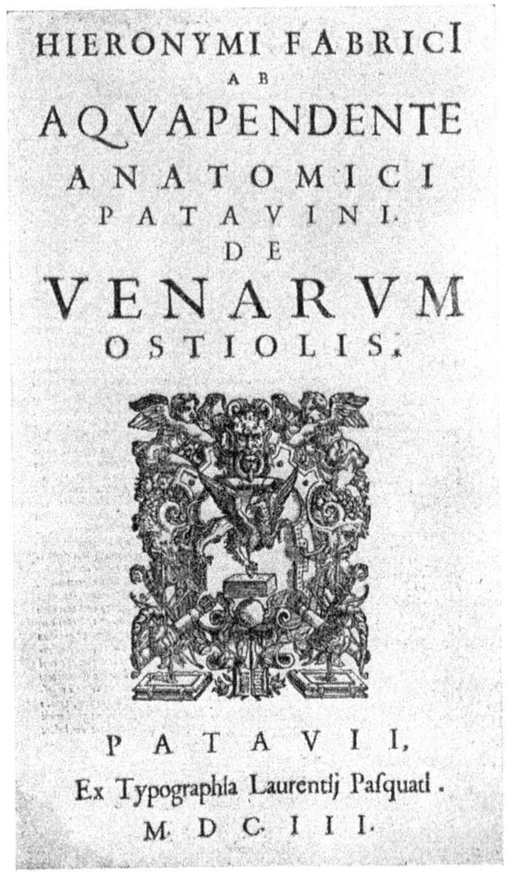
HIERONYMI FABRICI
AB
AQVAPENDENTE
ANATOMICI
PATAVINI.
DE
VENARVM
OSTIOLIS.

PATAVII,
Ex Typographia Laurentij Paſquati.
M. D C. I I I.

The title-page of Fabricius's tract on the valves of the veins, 1603

Girolamo Hieronymus Fabricius, from Fabricius's *Tract of the Valves of the Veins*, 1603.

not only have they never been mentioned, but no one even set eye on them till 1574, when to my great delight I saw them in the course of my dissection. And this despite the fact that anatomy has claimed many distinguished men among its followers, men, moreover, whose research was conducted with great care and minuteness. But a certain amount of justification does exist for them in this case, for who would ever have thought that membranous valves could be found in the lumen of veins, especially as this lumen, designed for the passage of blood to the whole body, should be free for the free flow of the blood, just as in the case of the arteries, which are valveless, yet, inasmuch as they are channels for blood, are on the same footing as veins?

But a further justification can be advanced for the anatomists. All veins are not provided with valves. The *vena cava*, where it traverses the trunk of the body, the internal jugulars, and countless superficial veins in like manner are destitute of them. On the other hand, a reasonable charge may be made against the earlier workers. Either they neglected to investigate the function of the valves, a matter, one would think, of primary importance, or else they failed to see them in their actual demonstration of veins. Nay more, when assistants pass a ligature round the limbs preparatory to blood-letting, valves are quite obviously noticeable in the arms and legs of the living subject. And, indeed, at intervals along the course of the veins certain knotty swellings are visible from the outside; these are caused by the valves. In some people, in fact, such as porters and peasants, they appear to swell up like varices [varicose veins].

But here I must correct myself. It must be clearly stated that actual varices are due entirely to the dilatation of valves and veins by too long retention and thickening of the blood at the valves; since, in the absence of valves, the veins would be expected to swell up and dilate uniformly throughout their length, differing thus from varices. From which begins to be visible one function of valves, namely, a strengthening action on the veins *per se.* For as in cases of varix, with valvular incompetence or rupture as an expected finding, one always sees a greater or lesser degree of venous dilatation, one can doubtless say with safety that the Supreme Artificer made valves to prevent venous distention. Venous distention and dilatation would, moreover, have occurred readily had the veins been of a membranous texture, and that uniformly thin. And if they were to dilate, not only would the excessive accumulation of blood in them cause damage to themselves and the surrounding parts, and a swelling be caused, as has been known to occur in cases of limb varix. There would also be a more or less defective nutrition of the parts above, with the blood rushing in force, say, to a site of venous dilatation, and collected, as it were, in a pool. Arteries, on the other hand, had no need of valves, either to prevent distention—the thickness and strength of their coat suffices—or to delay the blood—an ebb and flow of blood goes on continuously within them.

But let us, if you will, consider the number, form, structure, site, distance, et cetera, of valves. It was certainly necessary to make valves in the limb veins either of large or medium calibre—not the small ones—in order, no doubt, to slow the blood flow everywhere to an extent compatible with sufficient time being given for each small part to make use of the nourishment provided. Otherwise the whole mass of blood, owing to the slope of the limbs, would flood into their extremities, and collect there, causing a swelling of these lower parts, and wasting of the parts above.

That the blood flow is slowed by the valves, evident even without this from their actual construction, can be tested by anyone either in the exposed veins of the cadaver, or in the living subject, if he passes a ligature round the limbs as in blood-letting. For if one tries to exert pressure on the blood, or to push it along by rubbing from above downwards, one will clearly see it held up and delayed by the valves. This indeed was the way in which I was led to an observation of such nature.

Chapter 12

Conclusion: Contributions of the Founders of Medicine

By Luis Horacio Toledo-Pereyra

Just as in Volume 1 of this series of books on the Founders of Medicine, our intention in Volume 2 is to give readers exposure to some of the clear writing and actual thinking of the founders who built our medical profession.

We are captivated by the writings of our medical forefathers who focused intensely on offering us their contributions to the field, which were advanced at the time in which they were conceived.

The History of Medicine, As Written by Its Founders, Volume 2: From Roger's Chirurgia (1170) to Venarum Ostiolis (1603) presents the writings and drawings of physicians and artists who were concerned both about the state of medicine in their time and the way in which patients could be aided to improve their healthcare.

The readings in Volume 2—as in Volume 1—help us discover how the contributions of the Founders of Medicine "influence the way we think today;" it is for that reason that we study them here.[1] In essence, the Founders of Medicine in Volume 2—Roger de Frugard, Mondino De' Luzzi, Henri de Mondeville, Guy de Chauliac, Leonardo da Vinci, Andreas Vesalius, Ambroise Paré, Miguel Serveto, and Girolamo Hieronymus Fabricius—are among the best examples we have for demonstrating the practice of medicine during their time and the evolution of medicine from then to now. We hope that their works permit us to apply what we have learned from the medicine of the past in order to progress the medicine of the future.

Finally, if our audience continues to be interested in this historical journey, sustained now through two volumes, a third volume will be compiled that continues telling the story of the unique members of our profession who so deservingly should be called the Founders of Medicine.

References

1. Toledo-Pereyra, L.H. *The History of Medicine, As Written by Its Founders, Volume 1: From the Hammurabi Code to the Canon of Medicine.* University Readers, Inc., Cognella 2012, San Diego, CA.

CPSIA information can be obtained at www.ICGtesting.com
Printed in the USA
LVOW03s2122081213

364268LV00016B/129/P